MRI Atlas of Pediatric Brain Maturation and Anatomy

MRI Atlas of Pediatric Brain Maturation and Anatomy

Julie A. Matsumoto, MD, FACR
Associate Professor
Department of Radiology and Medical Imaging
University of Virginia Health System
Charlottesville, Virginia

Cree M. Gaskin, MD
Associate Professor and Vice Chair, Informatics
Department of Radiology and Medical Imaging
University of Virginia Health System
Charlottesville, Virginia

K. Derek Kreitel, MD
Clinical Instructor
Department of Radiology and Medical Imaging
University of Virginia Health System
Charlottesville, Virginia

S. Lowell Kahn, MD, MBA
Assistant Professor
Department of Radiology
Tufts University School of Medicine
Baystate Vascular Services
Baystate Medical Center
Springfield, Massachusetts

OXFORD
UNIVERSITY PRESS

OXFORD
UNIVERSITY PRESS

Oxford University Press, Inc., publishes works that further
Oxford University's objective of excellence
in research, scholarship, and education.

Oxford   New York
Auckland   Cape Town   Dar es Salaam   Hong Kong   Karachi
Kuala Lumpur   Madrid   Melbourne   Mexico City   Nairobi
New Delhi   Shanghai   Taipei   Toronto

With offices in
Argentina   Austria   Brazil   Chile   Czech Republic   France   Greece
Guatemala   Hungary   Italy   Japan   Poland   Portugal   Singapore
South Korea   Switzerland   Thailand   Turkey   Ukraine   Vietnam

© Oxford University Press 2015

Published by Oxford University Press, Inc.
198 Madison Avenue, New York, New York 10016
www.oup.com

Library of Congress Cataloging-in-Publication Data
Matsumoto, Julie A., author.
MRI atlas of pediatric brain maturation and anatomy / Julie A. Matsumoto, Cree M. Gaskin,
K. Derek Kreitel, S. Lowell Kahn ; with programming by Bing Li.
p. ; cm.
Includes bibliographical references and index.
ISBN 978–0–19–979642–7 (alk. paper)
I. Gaskin, Cree M., author.   II. Kreitel, K. Derek, author.   III. Kahn, S. Lowell, author.   IV. Title.
[DNLM: 1. Brain—anatomy & histology—Atlases.   2. Brain—growth & development—Atlases.
3. Child.   4. Infant.   5. Magnetic Resonance Imaging—methods—Atlases.   WL 17]
QP376
612.8′2—dc23
2015010015

9 8 7 6 5 4 3 2
Printed in the United States of America
on acid-free paper

With love and gratitude, this work is dedicated to Alan, Mallory, and Monica, and to the memory of sweet Lily.

—J. A. M.

To Kathy, my wife and best friend, and to our children Anna Kate, Warner, Audrey, and Arwen.

— C. M. G.

For my wife, Carrie, and my three belles, Chloe, Ella, and Kelsey.

— S. L. K.

To my parents, for your unconditional love and support.

— B. L.

DVD Atlas Design

The DVD that accompanies the print edition of this atlas provides two primary functions: one for the assessment of brain maturation and myelination, and one for use as an anatomic reference. These functions are introduced briefly here; further details about the software tools can be found in the users' manual included in the software.

The *Brain Maturation* section contains 45 complete sets of scrollable pediatric brain MRIs obtained at 24 different time points between the ages of preterm (starting at 32 weeks for 3T and at 38 weeks for 1.5T) to 3 years. The user can select a single age and view up to six sequences simultaneously, or can choose to view one sequence on up to six different ages at once in order to appreciate temporal changes in brain maturation. Annotated images are provided for most sequences, depending on the age and plane of section. The annotations, which may be toggled on or off, point out relevant aspects of myelination and brain maturation for each age and draw attention to normal appearances of structures as they mature. Six sequences (axial 2DT1, 3DT1, T2, DWI and ADC; sagittal 3DT1) may be viewed with annotations on subjects up to 1 year of age, spanning the time period when the most rapid changes in the brain are observable on MRI. Coronal images (TSE T2 and 3DT1) without annotations are also provided. By 12–15 months of age, myelination has nearly reached an adult pattern on T1W images and gray-white matter contrast has a mature appearance on DWI and ADC images. At the same time, subtler refinements in myelination become visible on T2W and FLAIR images in the older infant and young child. Thus, for subjects over the age of 1 year, annotations are available for the axial T2, axial FLAIR, and sagittal 3DT1 sequences. The remaining sequences for children over 1 year of age (axial 3DT1, DWI and ADC; coronal 3DT1 and TSE T2) are available without annotations. Annotations are displayed in different colors to enhance readability; they are not "color coded" for certain types of tracts or structures.

The *Anatomy* section contains detailed, anatomically labeled MR images of the brain of a 3-year-old (axial, sagittal, and coronal 3DT1) and a newborn (axial and coronal TSE T2). Annotated color fractional anisotropy (FA) maps in three planes of a 3-year-old brain are also provided. As in the *Brain Maturation* section, the image sets in the *Anatomy* section are all scrollable, and annotations can be toggled on or off.

Contents

Preface

This reference was created to address a widespread clinical need for a comprehensive collection of readily accessible, digital pediatric brain MR images for use as normal comparisons. During more than 25 years of practice in pediatric and adult neuroradiology, primarily at a university academic medical center where referral cases are common, I have observed that distinguishing the normal infant brain from the abnormal on MRI is challenging for nearly all practitioners, including a significant chunk of accomplished neuroradiologists. The reality is that few radiologists see the volume of infant brain MRIs and with enough frequency to become confident in their evaluation; the result may be interpretive errors that cause delays in proper diagnosis and treatment. Suggesting a disease process where none exists often stems from a lack of familiarity with the developing brain on MRI. A more common mistake, however, is a failure to recognize an abnormality of myelination or cortical formation, or the symmetric lesions that can occur in hypoxic-ischemic insults, metabolic diseases, and genetic disorders. Finally, I have observed, in more than a few instances, an incorrect radiology report (usually when the MRI has been misinterpreted as "negative") becoming a serious and very expensive point of contention in medicolegal cases alleging hypoxic-ischemic injury.

Answering the most basic question of "is this baby's MRI abnormal?" is made significantly easier when one can compare the images with normal examples and knows where in the brain to look. Authoritative textbooks describing stages of myelination are valuable resources, but these print materials are, by nature, severely limited in the size and number of images and the number of ages that can be illustrated, and can be cumbersome to use at the workstation. An alternative, but inefficient, strategy employed at my institution is to launch a hasty on-the-spot search of the PACS for an age-matched patient that has, hopefully, a normal brain MRI with which to compare. Given this frustratingly common experience, we surmised that similar scenarios must regularly play out in reading rooms around the world.

In response, countless images from our PACS were reviewed, selected, edited, and annotated over a multi-year period in order to assemble the highest possible quality sets of pediatric brain MRIs. All images were rigorously compared to reference standard MRIs of the same age to verify normal brain maturation. Electronic medical records were reviewed in each case to ensure the absence of neurological or developmental abnormalities. The resulting atlas in DVD format, when installed at the radiology workstation, puts over 13,000 non-annotated and 7,500 annotated high resolution reference images literally at one's fingertips, viewable with minimal disruption to the workflow.

The reference as a whole is targeted for use by clinicians in any type of practice and at all levels of training, from residents to experienced radiology subspecialists, who wish to both improve their skills in pediatric neuroimaging and simplify the process of interpretation. It is anticipated that pediatric neurologists, neonatologists, developmental pediatricians, and geneticists will find the use of this reference increases the understanding of their patients' MR abnormalities. The DVD format, in particular, easily doubles as an educational tool for those in an academic setting.

The DVD accompanying the print edition of this atlas contains two main sections: *Brain Maturation* and *Anatomy Images.* The *Brain Maturation* section, created to aid the user in the determination of normal from abnormal, contains 45 complete and scrollable brain MRIs, with examples at both 1.5T and 3T, acquired at 24 different ages from preterm (beginning at 32 weeks) to 3 years. Most images can be viewed with or without detailed color annotation overlays that provide concise descriptions of age appropriate myelination and highlight the changing appearance of the maturing brain. The *Anatomy* section consists of annotated multiplanar conventional MR images of a newborn and toddler, as well as annotated diffusion tensor imaging (DTI) color fractional anisotropy (FA) maps in three planes. The print edition of the atlas is on a smaller scale and is largely composed of abridged sets of images for use by those favoring this format. A new myelination timetable for quick reference can be found in the DVD and print editions, along with two previously published timetables viewable on the DVD. Both formats contain a written discussion of MR techniques, myelin and myelination, assessing myelination using MRI, and summaries of normal brain maturation and myelination grouped into ages.

The DVD is designed for use on the imaging workstation at the time of interpretation, rapidly calling up age-matched comparisons to answer questions as they arise. The annotated mode of the *Brain Maturation* section points the user to pertinent normal appearances at each age. The *Anatomy* section can be used to more precisely determine lesion location or areas involved by congenital malformations in patients of any age. Finally, it is hoped that use of the DVD atlas will improve clinical consultations in both formal conference settings and in the reading room: neuroimaging abnormalities are more easily understood by most health care providers when displayed alongside normal examples.

With this reference at hand, I hope you will find interpreting pediatric brain MRIs to be a more rewarding, enjoyable, and less daunting experience, ultimately to the benefit of your youngest patients and their families.

Julie A. Matsumoto, MD, FACR

Acknowledgments

This atlas and book, the product of years of sporadically intensive effort, rests upon the contributions of many people along the way. A special thank you goes to our former neuroradiology fellow, Ricardo Burgos, MD, for sparking the idea with his observation that an atlas of pediatric brain images was greatly needed. Dr. Paul Bunch deserves our thanks for getting things rolling as a medical student with his early investigations into potential pediatric subjects for the atlas.

We especially would like to acknowledge the long-term support and encouragement from our radiology colleagues who contributed to the collegial working environment in which we tackled this project, especially Drs. Mark Anderson, Alan Matsumoto, and Max Wintermark. A kind thank you is also offered to our compassionate and hard-working pediatric neurologists at the University of Virginia, Drs. Howard Goodkin, Russell Bailey, Kristen Heinan, Laura Jansen, Denia Ramirez-Montealegre, and Robert Rust, for their unfailing willingness to share their knowledge and keep us on our toes.

We are grateful for the dedication of the MR technologists and nurses of the University of Virginia Health System, who work tirelessly to obtain the best possible studies on our pediatric patients. This project would not have been possible without them.

Finally, we wish to express our sincere appreciation to Andrea Knobloch at Oxford University Press for her belief in our idea from the very beginning, and for her kind-hearted patience as we labored to complete this project.

MRI of Normal Brain Maturation: Preterm to Age 3 Years

Introduction

Interpretation of a brain MRI of an infant or young child poses unique challenges. Not only does the brain differ dramatically in appearance on MRI from that of adults, but it is constantly changing in the first 2–3 years of life, presenting a variety of appearances depending on the age and pulse sequence. Congenital malformations and disease processes that can affect the young brain symmetrically are easy to overlook unless one has a solid understanding of age-appropriate norms. Alternatively, the normal MR signal or morphology of an immature brain may be mistaken for abnormality, resulting in erroneous diagnoses. While visual assessment of brain maturation using anatomic images (T1-weighted [T1W] and T2-weighted [T2W] sequences) remains the standard in clinical practice, few radiologists feel confident reading these studies without referring to published myelination guidelines or searching out normal examples with which to compare. Indeed, as in most of the practice of medicine, a firm grasp of what constitutes normal is required before one can diagnose the abnormal. Such diagnostic skills are generally gained by extensive firsthand experience with imaging examinations of healthy patients, something that is in short supply for most radiologists interpreting pediatric brain MRIs. This atlas is intended to fill the gap by providing immediate access to normal comparisons with optional annotations relevant to each age.

The progression of myelination as visualized on MRI is an important indicator of normal brain function and maturation and accordingly is an emphasis of this atlas. Myelination, however, is not the only measure of brain development. In the preterm infant brain (i.e., < 37 weeks gestation), normal growth is chiefly characterized on MRI by cortical folding and sulcation, germinal matrix regression, and changes in the developing white matter that precede the actual appearance of myelin. In addition, ventricular size and shape as well as the size of the extracerebral subarachnoid spaces differ from what is found in term infants (37–42 weeks gestation) and must be evaluated based on the gestational age (GA) of the patient.

This book begins with a brief explanation of the process used for subject and image selection for the atlas and short reviews of MR techniques and normal myelin and myelination. This is followed by observations and tips on the practical assessment of myelination on MRI. Summaries of normal brain maturational changes found on MRI are provided for reference, grouped into three age ranges: preterm infant, term infant to 4 months of age, and 4 months to 3 years of age. A glossary of terms pertinent to normal and abnormal white matter, aimed at assisting clinical reporting of pediatric MR studies, concludes the book.

Subject Selection

The subjects selected for this atlas range from preterm neonates to children 3 years of age who underwent brain MRI at our institution for a variety of reasons, including benign scalp or facial skin lesions, headache, idiopathic febrile seizure, vomiting, possible apnea or minor apneic spell, suspected mild head trauma, and spell investigated for possible seizure with a subsequently normal electroencephalogram (EEG), normal neurological exam, and no recurrence at clinical follow-up. Additional indications for MRI in our subjects included developmental cyst, idiopathic nystagmus, and congenital spinal lesion not known to be associated with brain anomalies. Electronic medical records were reviewed in each case to determine estimated GA, age at MRI, absence of significant pregnancy- or delivery-related complications, absence of neurological or serious systemic disease, and documentation of subsequent normal growth and development. In some older children, birth age recorded in the medical record was simply "full term"; these cases were presumed to have a GA of 40 weeks for the purposes of this atlas. Length of clinical follow-up for the term-born children ranged from 1 to 9 years. All images selected for inclusion were strictly compared with accepted reference standards of normal age-matched MRIs and to published myelination timetables in order to confirm normal brain maturation (1–6).

The preterm neonate subjects in the atlas were imaged within 3 weeks of birth, resulting in an equivalent GA at the time of MRI of 32, 34, and 35 weeks. These subjects had lengths of clinical follow-up from 6 months to 6 years. Despite a morphologically normal brain at early MRI and normal early clinical development in these patients, we recognize that the potential for long-term neurodevelopmental sequelae exists due to their prematurity alone (7). Excluded from this atlas are any preterm infants imaged at term-equivalent age or older because brain growth and cortical development have been shown to be subsequently altered following preterm delivery, even without an obvious area of injury on MRI (8, 9). Thus, no cases used at time points of 37 gestational weeks or greater have a history of prematurity.

Although hundreds of clinical MR studies and medical records were meticulously screened to find our best normal examples at each age point, the examples in this atlas are not intended to represent age-precise normative standards for brain maturation on MRI, but rather to provide reliably normal examples at each age. Note that at some age points, sequences from more than one subject were used due to missing images or motion artifacts on the primary study. The atlas images should be considered with the complementary use of published myelination timetables and other accepted guidelines, included in this and other references, when evaluating an individual patient.

MR Techniques

The commonly used pulse sequences for assessing pediatric brain maturation include T1W, T2W, diffusion weighted imaging (DWI), apparent diffusion coefficient

(ADC) map, and a sequence sensitive to hemorrhage and calcification, such as a gradient-echo or susceptibility-weighted sequence. T2 fluid-attenuated inversion recovery (FLAIR) images are not generally considered as useful for assessing the progress of myelination in the first year (10–12), although T2 FLAIR (often referred to as simply "FLAIR") is regularly employed for older children and adults. Diffusion tensor imaging (DTI), magnetization transfer imaging, and MR spectroscopy are other MR techniques that may be used. Methods to study myelination with MRI that are not in widespread clinical use include multicomponent relaxation (MCR), automated tissue segmentation and parcellation, and T2 relaxation separation (13–15). The mainstays of routine clinical practice, however, remain conventional imaging with T1W and T2W sequences, which are well established, widely available, and easily performed.

T1W images can be obtained with conventional spin-echo (SE), fast spin-echo (FSE) (also known as turbo spin-echo [TSE]), inversion recovery, or spoiled gradient-echo techniques. Volumetric gradient-echo T1W (3DT1) techniques are useful to acquire high-resolution, contiguous images that can be reformatted in axial, sagittal, and coronal planes; however, these sequences are more vulnerable to field inhomogeneities and susceptibility and motion artifacts. The T1 shortening effect of myelin may be visible slightly earlier on heavily T1-weighted sequences than on routine 2D spin-echo T1W images, particularly on 3T systems (16), a fact that should be kept in mind when evaluating myelination stage.

T2W images are typically acquired with SE or FSE techniques. The T2 hypointense signal attributed to myelin will be somewhat more conspicuous on FSE T2 images at an earlier age, as a rule, than on conventional SE T2W images (11), although the influence of this on the estimation of myelin progress is unlikely to be significant in clinical practice (10, 17). Heavily T2-weighted images are recommended for infants under 1 year of age due to the much higher water content of the brain during this period.

The choice of imaging parameters for routine T1W and T2W sequences can alter the conspicuity of the MR signal attributed to myelin, although typically to only a small degree. In addition, the variety of MR systems and field strengths in clinical use may yield subtly different appearances to routine images of the brain. It is therefore important that radiologists and other physicians become familiar with the range of normal appearances produced on their own machines, using their specific imaging protocols. Details about optimizing sequences for imaging the pediatric brain can be found in several excellent references (12, 18, 19).

DWI sequences and ADC maps in this atlas were obtained by applying diffusion gradients in three directions with a b-value of 1000 s/mm² using spin-echo single-shot echoplanar imaging (SS-EPI); this is a standard technique also used for adult brain imaging (7). It is of interest to know that given the relatively higher ADCs of the neonatal brain, recommendations regarding the ideal b-value to use in infants vary from 600 to 3000 s/mm² (12, 20–23). Note that if a b-value greater or lesser than 1000 s/mm² is used, it may result in different degrees of tissue contrast between unmyelinated white matter, myelinated white matter, and gray matter. Should a b-value other than 1000 s/mm² be used for generating clinical images, the resultant tissue contrast differences must be taken into account when comparing patient images to those in this atlas.

FLAIR pulse sequences are obtained with an FSE technique in order to achieve a reasonably short scan time, and may be acquired as 2D or 3D image sets. The resulting images are heavily T2-weighted with signal from the cerebrospinal fluid suppressed. T1 relaxation times also influence the tissue signal in FLAIR sequences and are thought to be responsible for the complex triphasic signal change that takes place in the neonatal and infant deep cerebral white matter (5, 24). The later stages of myelination can be assessed on FLAIR in toddlers (5, 12), and at this stage it becomes a valuable tool for assessing white matter pathology. However, because FLAIR has decreased sensitivity for the detection of lesions in the posterior fossa and spinal cord compared to conventional SE or FSE T2W techniques (25, 26), it should be obtained in addition to, and not in place of, SE or FSE T2W sequences for routine brain examinations.

The images in this reference were acquired on 1.5T and 3T MR scanners (Siemens, Erlangen, Germany) at the University of Virginia Health System, spanning an 8-year period. Pulse sequences for all age points include 3DT1 ultrafast gradient-echo reformatted in three planes, axial FSE or SE T2W, coronal FSE T2W, axial DWI, and axial ADC maps. Axial T2 FLAIR images are available for subjects 1 year of age and older. For subjects younger than 1 year, T1W images are valuable for the assessment of both myelination and brain injury, so axial 2D T1W images (spoiled gradient-echo, FSE, or SE) are included, in addition to the volumetric gradient-echo T1W images. Due to the challenges of obtaining excellent field homogeneity and adequate T1W tissue contrast at 3T, more deliberate windowing of some image sets was performed and may be further adjusted by the end-user of the atlas software. The specific sequence parameters employed for cases included in this atlas varied slightly over the years due to changes in practice and equipment and will not be detailed here.

Myelin and Myelination

Myelin is the essential component of white matter in the central nervous system (CNS). It serves as a nonconductive electrical insulator of axons, markedly increasing the speed of neuronal signal transmission, and is vital in the maintenance of axonal integrity and function (27). In short, normal human cognitive, sensory, motor, and behavioral processes rely on healthy, intact myelin.

Oligodendrocytes are the glial cells that produce and maintain myelin in the CNS, with each cell providing myelin to dozens of different neuronal axons. Astrocytes also play an important role in myelin deposition and are essential to oligodendrocyte function and survival (27). Mature myelin is predominantly composed of lipids (e.g., cholesterol, phospholipids, and glycolipids) and CNS myelin proteins (e.g., myelin basic protein, proteolipid protein, and hundreds of others) with a high lipid-to-protein ratio of approximately 2.3:1 (6, 27). Myelination consists of the formation of a myelin sheath, which begins as a plasma membrane extension of the oligodendrocyte and forms as a specific lipid and protein multilayered structure. Myelin is relatively poorly hydrated, containing only 40% water compared to 80% for gray matter (27).

The process of CNS myelination begins *in utero* during the second trimester and continues through much of adulthood (28). The timing of myelination in the fetus is very precise, even though the details of the actual process and factors regulating it remain largely unknown. Myelination begins in different sites in the brain at different times and progresses to mature myelin at different rates (28). After birth, myelination continues in a systematic, predictable manner, and thus the existence of MR signal attributable to myelin in specific locations can be used as a marker of normal brain maturation. It is notable that histological studies demonstrate the onset of myelination in different parts of the brain several weeks before it can be observed on MRI, with varying estimates of the time difference depending on the histological stain used and the specifics of the MR technique.

The presence of mature myelin is associated with hyperintense signal on T1W images and hypointense signal on T2W images relative to unmyelinated white matter. These signal changes are not specific to myelin content, however, but more broadly reflect multiple biochemical and biophysical processes taking place during brain maturation (13). For practical purposes, the changes in T1W and T2W images can be thought of as reflecting an increase in lipid content and a decrease in the quantity of free water. A newborn's brain is relatively unmyelinated and consequently contains a higher proportion of water compared to an adult. After birth, the water content of the brain decreases, predominantly in the white matter, and the lipid and protein content increases as myelination progresses. The evolution of signal changes on T1W and T2W images, however, is not straightforward: the signal ascribed to myelin is usually identified earliest on T1W images and will not be visible at all, or to the same degree, on T2W images for several more weeks or months. To understand why myelination seemingly occurs at different times and proceeds at different rates on T1W versus T2W images, it is useful to keep in mind that myelin does not appear suddenly as a finished product, but rather, different components of the myelin sheath are synthesized and modified in complex ways over time. Molecular interactions of bound and free water with the developing myelin membrane lipids and proteins change during maturation and may affect T1 and T2 relaxation times differently (29). Multiple spiral wrappings, and then compaction, of the myelin sheaths around axons take place as myelin matures, a process that is associated with shortening of T2 relaxation times (29).

Although less widely appreciated, gray matter structures in the immature brain also undergo alterations in MR signal. In various parts of the basal ganglia and thalami, myelination of projectional axons probably plays a significant role in this changing appearance. However, in regions of the cerebral cortex, such as the perirolandic area, the pattern of signal change on T1W and T2W images is inconsistent with the small amount of myelination that the tissue contains. Other factors, including the degree of cortical cellularity, synaptic density, dendrite formation, capillary proliferation, and protein layering are likely responsible (11).

Assessing Myelination on MRI

Because T1W images are generally more sensitive to the presence of small amounts of myelin (10), hyperintense T1 signal is seen earlier and more prominently than the corresponding hypointense signal on T2W images, as discussed earlier. Later in infancy and early childhood, T2W images are superior for showing further, subtle refinements in myelination (10), a finding felt to reflect ongoing modifications in the lipid composition of white matter, in addition to numerous complex biochemical and physical changes taking place in the maturing myelin sheaths (5, 29). The result is that

T1W images are more useful to evaluate myelination in the first 6–8 months of life, and T2W images are more reliable after 6 months of age (1, 2). A modification of this rule applies to the preterm infant, where myelination, particularly in the brainstem and thalamic nuclei, is more easily seen on T2W sequences, and especially so with FSE techniques (3, 30). In the term infant, brainstem myelination is also better assessed with T2W images. Both the T1W and T2W sequences, nevertheless, should be scrutinized for age-appropriate myelin signal in all pediatric patients undergoing MRI of the brain. FLAIR can be used to evaluate the later stages of myelination and is mostly useful after 2 years of age, when myelination appears nearly complete on T2W images.

Understanding the normal progression of myelination on MRI is helped by familiarity with some general anatomic principles. As a rule, tracts become myelinated when they become functional. Sensory pathways myelinate prior to motor pathways and myelination occurs earlier in areas of primary function than in associative pathways (1, 28). The general topographic progression of myelination is from caudal to rostral and from central to peripheral, with some exceptions (28). Therefore, the brainstem myelinates before the cerebellum and basal ganglia, which myelinate before the cerebrum. Myelination also tends to proceed from dorsal to ventral within a region, so that dorsal brainstem structures myelinate prior to the ventrally located corticospinal tracts, and the parietal and occipital lobes myelinate before the frontal and temporal poles. Once begun, myelination progresses at a faster rate in some areas, such as the internal capsules and optic radiations, than in others, such as the frontal and temporal poles (28).

Making a side-by-side comparison of a patient's MRI with those from age-matched, healthy subjects is an easy way to evaluate the progress of myelination. Annotations on the reference images in this atlas call attention to pertinent areas of myelin maturation at each age, while also pointing out normal developmental findings. The DVD atlas contains 1.5T and 3T examples, and, in younger patients, both 3DT1 and 2D T1W images, in an effort to present a range of images for comparison. Contrasting slightly younger and older normal subjects with the clinical case in question will help to pinpoint the best match and will bring into focus abnormalities of either the white matter or gray matter that may be symmetric or diffuse. Suspected deviations from normal brain morphology, such as malformations of cortical development, may also be more confidently identified or excluded through comparison with normal subjects.

It can be useful to consult published data on normal MR milestones for myelination when interpreting pediatric brain studies in order to maintain a reference of appropriate maturation. However, a word of caution is warranted in order to avoid interpretive errors. If a particular reference is used, the radiologist should understand the method applied by the author to establish the specific milestones. While the temporal *sequence* in which myelin signal appears in different structures is generally consistent across studies, there are variations between authors regarding the *actual age* at which the signal changes are said to occur (1–3, 5, 11). These variations, though mostly small, seem to be due to two main factors: technical differences in how the MR images were produced and differences in the grading systems. The majority of studies published to date on the qualitative evaluation of brain maturation are based on nonvolumetric, conventional SE T1W images and either SE or FSE T2W images, obtained at field strengths of 1.5T or lower (3, 11, 31–34). Differences between magnet systems, pulse sequences, and image resolution may modestly affect the visibility of

T1 or T2 shortening in the brain. It is quite possible that current (and future) technology will result in the identification of signal attributed to myelin a little earlier than has been documented.

In addition to technical differences, grading systems vary between published myelination milestones. Some authors assigned the milestone age according to the age of "first appearance" of myelin signal; others used the age when a structure "should appear myelinated"; and still others listed the milestone age as the point when "myelination is complete" (1– 3, 5). It is not known which, if any, of these methods is superior, but it is clear that the first system, for example, will result in younger milestone ages than the other two. Whichever milestones or guidelines are used in practice, the radiologist should be aware of how they were created so they may be properly applied.

In early infancy, brain growth and the progression of myelination are more rapid and consistent across subjects (14) in contrast to older infants and toddlers, when myelination rate slows and the changes over time become less obvious on MRI. There is also a normal biologic range in the level of brain development and myelination with respect to the gestational and chronological age, and there are inaccuracies in estimating the dates of a pregnancy. Consequently, exactly how much temporal variation is acceptable in the progression of myelination on MRI remains unknown, and this is reflected in the ranges given in myelination tables. As a rule, the time intervals become broader and less precise in the later stages of myelination.

In summary, multiple factors need to be taken into consideration when evaluating an immature brain with MRI. The images in this atlas can be used as a guide, but whenever a significant departure from normal myelination or brain maturation is found, the pattern of abnormality should be documented and other sources consulted to formulate a differential diagnosis. If only a mild deviation from the expected stage of myelination is present, a practical approach is to report the age range with which the patient's myelination pattern most closely fits, rather than diagnosing a definite abnormality.

MRI of Brain Maturation: Preterm to Age 3 Years

The normal sequence and progression of myelination on MRI has been described previously by various authors (1–5, 10, 11). Clinically relevant, focused summaries of this topic are presented in the following sections. A detailed list of the timing of myelination signal in numerous structures throughout the brain on T1W and T2W images is provided in Table 1.

Preterm Infant

Evaluating a preterm brain MRI calls for a somewhat different focus from what is needed for term-born infants. In the preterm neonatal brain, immature cortical folding and sulcation are present and must be assessed; the ventricles and CSF spaces occupy a different proportion of the intracranial contents than in a term neonate; and zones of migrating glial cells and involuting germinal matrix should not be misinterpreted as pathology (30, 35). Knowledge of both the GA and the corrected age at imaging (i.e., the infant's chronological age minus the number of weeks born prematurely) is essential for accurate interpretation. As mentioned earlier, the MR appearance of a

Table 1:
Ages at Which Myelination Signal Is Present on MRI* (1, 3 – 5, 10, 11)

Age	T1 Hyperintensity (Relative to Unmyelinated WM)**	T2 Hypointensity (Relative to Unmyelinated WM)**
32 weeks, preterm	**Brainstem and Cerebellum**	
	Multiple dorsal brainstem GM nuclei and WM tracts	Multiple dorsal brainstem GM nuclei and WM tracts
	Midbrain tegmentum	Inferior colliculi
	Inferior cerebellar peduncles	Inferior cerebellar peduncles
	Superior cerebellar peduncles and decussation	Superior cerebellar peduncles and decussation
	Dentate nuclei (rim)	Dentate nuclei (rim)
	Vermis	Vermis
	Cerebral hemispheres	
	Subthalamic nuclei	Subthalamic nuclei
	Globi pallidi	Globi pallidi
	Ventrolateral thalamic nuclei	Ventrolateral thalamic nuclei
	Posterolateral putamina	Posterolateral putamina
	Corpus callosum (mildly hyperintense posteriorly; may be due to fiber packing and not myelination)	Corpus callosum (mildly hypointense; may be due to fiber packing and not myelination)
36 weeks, preterm	**Brainstem and Cerebellum**	
All of above, plus:	Inferior colliculi	
	Cerebral hemispheres	
	Posterior third of PLIC (by 36–37 wks GA)	
	WM tracts of pre- and postcentral gyri in corona radiata	
Term (37–42 weeks)	**Brainstem and Cerebellum**	
All of above, plus:	Most of medulla and midbrain	Most of medulla
	Middle cerebellar peduncles (beg.)	
	Cerebellar deep WM (beg.)	
	Cerebral hemispheres	
	Posterior third of PLIC (by 36–37 wks GA)	Posterior third of PLIC (smaller than on T1W images)
	Optic nerves, chiasm, tracts	Optic nerves, chiasm, tracts
	Optic radiations (beg.)	Optic radiations (beg.)
	WM tracts of pre- and postcentral gyri in centrum semiovale	WM tracts of pre- and postcentral gyri in corona radiata, centrum semiovale
	Perirolandic cortex	Perirolandic cortex

(continued)

Table 1:
Continued

Age	T1 Hyperintensity (Relative to Unmyelinated WM)**	T2 Hypointensity (Relative to Unmyelinated WM)**
1 month	**Brainstem and Cerebellum**	Middle cerebellar peduncles (beg.)
	Cerebral hemispheres	
	(Globi pallidi and subthalamic nuclei hyperintensity is fading)	
	Posterior portion of PLIC extending toward genu	
2 months	**Brainstem and Cerebellum**	
	Middle cerebellar peduncles	
	Cerebellar deep WM	Cerebellar deep WM (beg.)
	Cerebral hemispheres	
	Basal ganglia mostly homogeneous; hyperintensity of globi pallidi has faded	Basal ganglia mostly homogeneous; globi pallidi may be slightly hyperintense up to 1 year
	PLIC, entire	
	ALIC (beg.)	
	Parahippocampal WM (beg.)	
3 months	**Brainstem and Cerebellum**	
	Ventral brainstem approximately isointense w/dorsal brainstem	Ventral brainstem approximately isointense w/dorsal brainstem
		Middle cerebellar peduncles
	Cerebral hemispheres	
	ALIC, entire	Posterior portion of PLIC extending toward genu
	Calcarine fissure WM (beg.)	Optic radiations
	Splenium and posterior body of corpus callosum (beg.)	
	Corona radiata and centrum semiovale extending anteriorly	Corona radiata and centrum semiovale extending anteriorly
	Perirolandic subcortical WM	
4 months	**Brainstem and Cerebellum**	
	Cerebellar subcortical WM	Cerebellar deep WM
	Cerebral hemispheres	
	Splenium of corpus callosum	Calcarine fissure WM (beg.)
		Perirolandic subcortical WM
5 months	**Cerebral hemispheres**	
	Body of corpus callosum, most of	Splenium and posterior body of corpus callosum
	Genu of corpus callosum (beg.)	
	Occipital deep and subcortical WM	
	Frontal and parietal deep WM	

(continued)

Table 1:
Continued

Age	T1 Hyperintensity (Relative to Unmyelinated WM)**	T2 Hypointensity (Relative to Unmyelinated WM)**
6 months	**Cerebral hemispheres**	
	Globi pallidi becoming mildly hyperintense to striatal nuclei; continues through adulthood	(Ventrolateral thalamic nuclei hypointensity less marked compared to neonate)
		PLIC, entire
	Temporal deep WM	ALIC (beg.)
	Corpus callosum, entire	Genu of corpus callosum (beg.)
8 months	**Cerebral hemispheres**	
	Occipital fine arborization	ALIC, entire
	Frontal and parietal subcortical WM	Corpus callosum, entire
		Centrum semiovale
10 months	**Brainstem and Cerebellum**	
		Cerebellar subcortical WM
	Cerebral hemispheres	
	Temporal pole subcortical WM (beg.)	Occipital deep and subcortical WM
	Parietal fine arborization	Frontal and parietal deep WM
1 year	**Cerebral hemispheres**	
	Anterior inferior frontal fine arborization	Occipital fine arborization
	Subcortical myelination is nearly complete throughout brain on T1W images.	Frontal and parietal subcortical WM (beg.)
		Temporal deep WM
1 year 6 months	**Cerebral hemispheres**	
	Temporal pole fine arborization	Frontal and parietal fine arborization
		Temporal pole subcortical WM
2 years	**Cerebral hemispheres**	
		Subcortical myelination is nearly complete throughout brain on T2W images.
3 years	**Cerebral hemispheres**	
		Fine arborization of anterior and superior medial frontal lobes and anterior temporal lobes may continue to 3–4 years of age. Peritrigonal white matter may remain hyperintense into early adulthood.

*Structures expected to have myelin signal *present* at the specifed age, although myelination may be incomplete.

**Minor differences in signal conspicuity when comparing fast spin-echo and conventional spin-echo images, or 1.5T and 3T magnet systems, are taken into account.

beg. (beginning): indicates the structure may show only subtle changes of myelination, or myelin signal that is not yet well developed; GM, gray matter; WM, white matter; PLIC, posterior limb of internal capsule; ALIC, anterior limb of internal capsule healthy premature infant's brain *imaged at term-equivalent age* (e.g., 8-week-old infant born at 32 weeks gestation) can differ in significant ways from a term-born neonate's brain, especially for a very preterm infant (< 32 weeks), and is outside the scope of this atlas (9, 35, 36).

Cortical Folding and Sulcation

Cortical folding is a good indicator of early brain maturation. Visual assessment of the brain surfaces can be done to confirm GA and to detect major abnormalities of sulcation and gyration (37). Before 24 weeks GA, the brain is essentially smooth on fetal MRI, except for shallow, round-edged depressions of the Sylvian fissure, calcarine fissure, parietooccipital fissure, callosal sulcus, and cingulate sulcus (38). The general rules of gyration and sulcation are that with growth, sulci appear and gradually become deeper, the side walls become steeper, the distance between adjacent sulci narrows, and the sulci branch and become more complex. Most of the process of cortical folding occurs between 26 and 44 weeks GA (Fig. 1A and B) (39), with a surprising amount of change occurring in as little as every 2–4 weeks during this period. Gyral development is slowest in the frontal and anterior temporal lobes (10). It is important to not mistake a preterm infant's normally shallow sulci, smooth gyri, and wide Sylvian fissures for a malformation of cortical development.

Germinal Matrix

The germinal matrix, present in all very preterm infants, is identified by its shape and subependymal location, most prominently adjacent to the anterior and lateral margins of the lateral ventricles, but also found in the caudothalamic notch and posterior to the thalami at their junction with the optic radiations (11). Germinal matrix has moderately high signal on T1W images and low signal on T2W images due to its high cellularity. Hemorrhages in germinal matrix also show T1 and T2 shortening but are distinguished by irregular shape, asymmetry, and greater persistence (34). The normal germinal matrix gradually regresses between 26 and 34 weeks GA (30, 34), although small remnants may be identified at term (11).

Myelination and White Matter Maturation

Myelination in the very preterm infant between 25 and 28 weeks GA is most apparent on FSE T2W images as hypointense signal in multiple dorsal brainstem nuclei and white matter tracts, the cerebellar vermis, dentate nuclei, superior and inferior cerebellar peduncles, decussation of the superior cerebellar peduncles, inferior colliculi, subthalamic nuclei, medial geniculate nuclei, and ventrolateral thalamic nuclei (3). T1W images will show most, but not all, of these structures developing hyperintensity between 25 and 30 weeks GA.

Between 28 and 36 weeks GA, myelin increases in the same areas above but is not visualized at new sites. Ventral pontine signal is homogeneous and stands out as more hypointense on T1W images and more hyperintense on T2W images than the dorsal brainstem. The pallidal and subthalamic nuclei may be more hyperintense on T1W images than the thalamic ventrolateral nuclei at this stage, while on T2W images it is the ventrolateral nuclei that are more hypointense than the pallidal and subthalamic

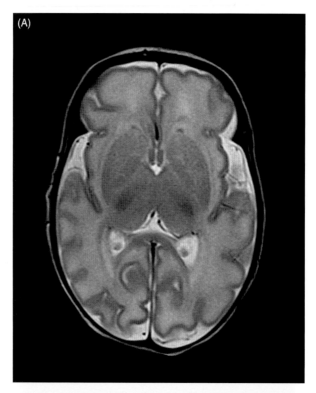

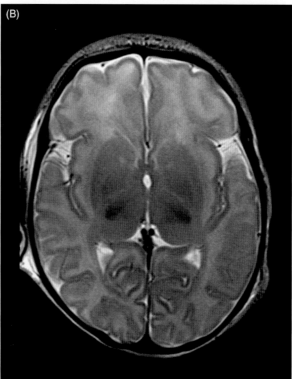

Fig. 1 Cortical folding and sulcal development, T2W images. **A.** Normal 31-week GA preterm infant, imaged at age 3 weeks of life (i.e., corrected age 34 weeks). Cerebral sulci are shallow and gyri are broad and relatively smooth at this age. Sylvian fissures are mildly prominent and the insular sulci and gyri have an immature appearance.

B. Normal 40-week GA infant, imaged at age 2 days of life. Notice the increased depth, narrowness, and complexity of sulci and the narrowing of gyri compared to A, especially evident in the posterior temporal and occipital lobes. The frontal lobes show less advanced gyral development. Further deepening of sulci and more complex branching of sulci and gyri will continue after term, reaching a mature pattern around age 3 months.

nuclei. At 36 to 37 weeks, T1 hyperintensity develops in the posterior one-third of the posterior limb of the internal capsule (PLIC), corona radiata, and the corticospinal tracts of the precentral and postcentral gyri (3).

The developing deep cerebral white matter of infants born at less than 30 weeks GA is overall hyperintense on T2W images and hypointense on T1W images (due to high water content), but on close inspection is seen to contain moderately distinct bands of alternating signal. These regions have been labeled "caps" around the frontal horns of the lateral ventricles and "arrowheads" around the posterior lateral ventricles (Fig. 2), and are thought to correspond to radial glial fibers and migrating glial cells (34, 37). Also known as "crossroads," these areas of regional, periventricular T2 high signal reflect healthy, immature white matter (40, 41). The visibility of these bands diminishes with increasing GA, although they may still be faintly visible at term.

Corpus Callosum

The corpus callosum is difficult to see in the preterm infant due to its extreme thinness and hypointensity to cortical gray matter on T1W images; accordingly, care must

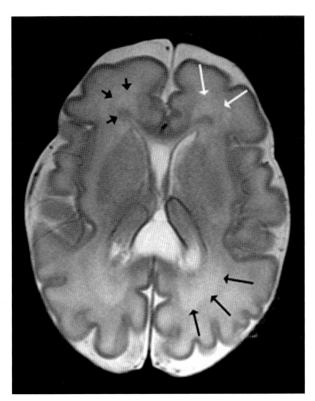

Fig. 2 Immature white matter in a normal 30-week GA preterm infant, imaged at corrected age 32 weeks. T2W image shows normal white matter "caps" (white arrows) of mild T2 hyperintensity around the frontal horns and "arrowheads" (black long arrows) around the posterior lateral ventricles, corresponding to developing white matter fibers. Darker bands within these areas (black short arrows) correspond to migrating cells, or remnants of, from the germinal matrix or subependymal layer. Note: This infant has a cystic dilatation of the velum interpositum.

be taken to avoid misdiagnosing callosal hypoplasia or atrophy. The presence of a corpus callosum can be confirmed by locating the cingulate gyri and sulci parallel to the expected callosal location (1). Despite being unmyelinated, the corpus callosum is of intermediate signal intensity on T2W images, similar to cerebral cortex.

Diffusion Weighted Imaging

Diffusion weighted images have a high contrast appearance in preterm neonates due to the large differences in ADC values between gray and white matter. On DWI, most of the cerebral white matter is very hypointense relative to cortical gray matter. On ADC maps, the cerebral white matter is hyperintense and the gray matter of the cerebral cortex, basal ganglia, and thalami is hypointense. The exceptions to this rule are the internal capsules (especially the posterior limbs), the corpus callosum, and the optic radiations, which display isointensity to slight hyperintensity to cortical gray matter on DWI and hypointensity on ADC maps compared to cerebral white matter (11, 42, 43). The anisotropy of diffusion in these structures occurs before the histological appearance of myelin, or of visible myelination signs on T1W or T2W images, and has been termed "premyelination" (44). Processes occurring in the immature brain that consist mainly of functional alterations of axons and oligodendrocytes are thought to be responsible for the naturally observed decreases in ADC (44, 45). Thus, the imaging characteristics of these specific white matter tracts in the preterm infant (internal capsules, corpus callosum, optic radiations) must not be confused with pathologically restricted diffusion.

The normal preterm (and term) brainstem contains areas of hypointense signal on ADC maps, mostly dorsally and in the central tegmentum of the midbrain. The vermis and dentate nuclei display slightly lower signal on ADC maps compared to the remainder of the cerebellum. On DWI, the signal in the brainstem and cerebellum is more homogenous.

Ventricles and Subarachnoid Spaces

Ventricular size is traditionally assessed at fetal ultrasound by measuring the width of the atria of the lateral ventricles, not including the ventricular walls. The normal measurement of ventricular width as <10 mm on ultrasound is also applicable to MRI and is generally quite stable throughout gestation (46, 47). On MRI, measurements can be made on a coronal slice parallel to the long axis of the brainstem at the level of the choroid plexi, using a line perpendicular to the major axis of the atrium (46). The occipital horns of the lateral ventricles are normally prominent in very preterm neonates (46, 48) and should not be included in this measurement. By 34–36 weeks, the ventricles are typically small (49). A cavum septi pellucidi is a normal developmental finding in a preterm infant, and may be accompanied by a cavum Vergae (50).

The subarachnoid spaces posterior to the parietooccipital lobes are noticeably enlarged in very preterm infants, not to be mistaken for cerebral atrophy or a gyral anomaly (Fig. 3A). The subarachnoid spaces anterior to the temporal and frontal poles are also relatively larger in premature infants compared to term newborns. These spaces, along with all pericerebral spaces, gradually diminish in size and are usually no longer prominent at term (Fig. 3B) (48). The anterior temporal and

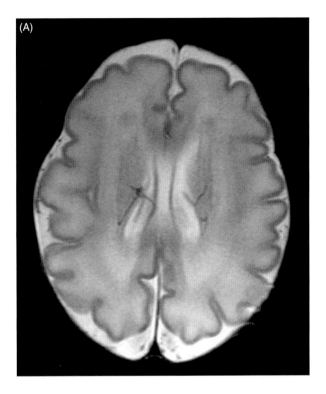

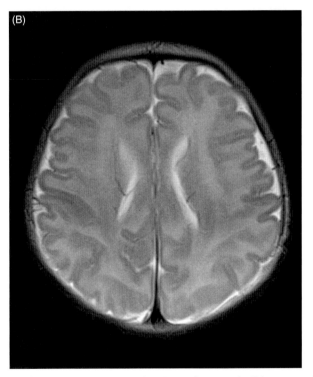

Fig. 3 Subarachnoid spaces, T2W images. **A.** Normal 30-week GA preterm infant, imaged at corrected age 32 weeks. The subarachnoid spaces in preterm infants are prominent, especially posterior to the parietal lobes and anterior to the frontal and temporal poles. Care must be taken to not mistake this for atrophy or a cortical malformation. **B.** Normal 42-week term infant. The pericerebral spaces are no longer prominent by term except anterior to the frontal and temporal lobes, where they may be 5–6 mm in width.

frontal lobe subarachnoid spaces, however, can be a bit conspicuous for several more months.

Pituitary Gland

The pituitary gland is diffusely hyperintense on T1W images in premature infants, as it is in fetuses and term-born neonates, a finding that has been attributed to intense synthetic secretory activity of the gland around the time of birth (51, 52). The anterior lobe of the pituitary gland then fades on T1W images to become isointense with cortical gray matter over approximately the next 8 weeks of life, regardless of GA at birth. In other words, if a very preterm infant is imaged near term-equivalent age (e.g., a 9-week-old infant born at 31 weeks GA), the anterior lobe will no longer be significantly hyperintense on T1W images (51, 53).

Term Infant to Age 4 Months

Cortical Folding and Sulcation

At term, the general pattern of cortical folding is similar to that of an adult brain. The sulci have all developed by 38 weeks and will continue to deepen and branch after birth. Most of the gyri, however, continue to be shorter, broader, and have more rounded edges than that of an older infant. The exception to this is the medial occipital and perirolandic cortices, which are the most advanced. At the other extreme are the anterior temporal gyri, which are still rounded and immature looking, most obvious on sagittal images. By 3 months of age, an approximately mature gyral and sulcal pattern is achieved (10), although sulcal and gyral complexity continues to increase well into the first year of life (54). Normal cortical thickness on MRI in the mature brain is 1 mm at the deepest part of a sulcus and 2–3 mm at the crown of a gyrus (55).

Germinal Matrix

Small T2 hypointense patches attributed to migrating glial cells can be seen within the center of the deep white matter anterior to the frontal horns at term (56), and may be faintly visible until around 1 month of age. Deep to these patches and directly bordering the tips of the frontal horns are small T2 hypointense areas of residual germinal matrix that may still be identified in term neonates (57, 58).

Myelination and White Matter Maturation

In the term newborn, unmyelinated cerebral white matter demonstrates high signal intensity on T2W images, low signal intensity on T1W images, and shows a regional gradation of signal intensity. From the deep white matter outward, the T2 hyperintense signal subtly fades as it reaches the subcortical white matter, although it is not completely uniform in every gyrus (Fig. 4A). The most hyperintense T2 signal is found in the periventricular white matter anterior, posterior, and just superior to the lateral ventricles. These are the same locations where "caps" and "arrowheads" were found in the preterm infant, but now those specific features are much less evident.

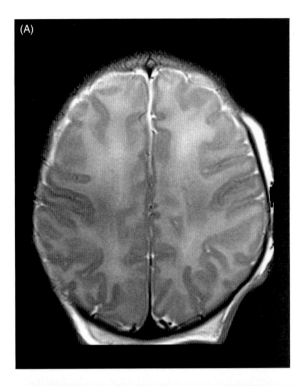

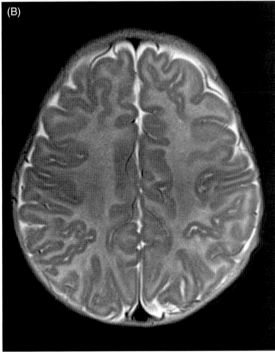

Fig. 4 Evolution of newborn white matter signal, T2W images. **A.** A 40-week GA infant displays the normal regional gradation in cerebral white matter signal, with the deep white matter showing mildly more T2 hyperintensity than the subcortical white matter. **B.** Normal 2-month-old. The deep white matter is no longer more T2 hyperintense than the subcortical white matter.

On T1W images, the signal gradation (more T1 hypointensity centrally than peripherally) is detected to a lesser degree. The gradation of white matter signal on both T1W and T2W images gradually disappears by 1–2 months of age (Fig. 4B).

A healthy term newborn will show evidence of myelination on T1W and T2W images in multiple dorsal brainstem nuclei and white matter tracts, most of the medulla, the inferior and superior cerebellar peduncles, cerebellar vermis and flocculi, dentate nuclei, deep cerebellar white matter (on T1W images), inferior colliculi, most of the midbrain, subthalamic nuclei, ventrolateral thalamic nuclei, and the optic nerves, chiasm, and tracts (1, 10). The beginnings of myelination signal in the optic radiations can be seen on T1W images in the first month of life.

Particular attention needs to be paid to the posterior limb of the internal capsule (PLIC) in a newborn, as this site is vulnerable to hypoxic-ischemic injury and abnormalities in this location are associated with poor neurological outcome (59–61). Starting at 36–37 weeks, T1W hyperintensity can be observed in the posterior one-third of the PLIC (Fig. 5), the contiguous white matter of the central corona radiata, and in the precentral and postcentral parasagittal areas (1, 3, 11). On T2W images, a discrete, short streak of hypointense signal is seen in the posterior portion of the PLIC at term, though it is smaller than the corresponding region of T1 hyperintensity. The perirolandic cortex shows a distinctive T1 hyperintensity and T2 hypointensity between 37 and 42 weeks, a finding probably due to tissue changes other than myelination (11).

By 3 months of age, both T1W and T2W images show myelin more completely in the middle cerebellar peduncles, peripheral cerebellar white matter, anterior corona radiata, pre- and postcentral subcortical white matter, and progressing anteriorly in the centrum semiovale. The entire PLIC is now hyperintense on T1W images. The anterior limb of the internal capsule appears myelinated on T1W images by 3–4 months, but not yet on T2W images. The occipital white matter around the calcarine fissure becomes hyperintense on T1W images by 3–4 months of age, approaching isointensity with the cortex. The entire pons is of approximately the same hyperintensity on T1W images and hypointensity on T2W images by age 3–4 months, having lost the marked signal contrast between the ventral and dorsal portions that was present in the newborn period.

Corpus Callosum

At term, the corpus callosum continues to be uniformly slender, slightly thicker than the preterm appearance, and without the enlargements of the genu or splenium that will develop later (Fig. 6). A common error is to label this as callosal hypoplasia, "thinning," or atrophy. The genu will start to show slight thickening at 2–3 months and the splenium follows, starting at approximately 3–4 months.

The signal intensity of the corpus callosum at term is close to that of cortical gray matter on T1W images. On T2W images, the corpus callosum should be of homogeneous, intermediate to low signal at birth, also close in signal to cortex. Tight packing of white matter fibers may partially explain the presence of callosal T2 shortening prior to the onset of myelination (11).

Myelination proceeds from posterior to anterior, appearing initially on T1W images in the splenium and posterior body by 3–4 months (1). At approximately the same time, callosal signal may become mildly hyperintense relative to cortex on T2W

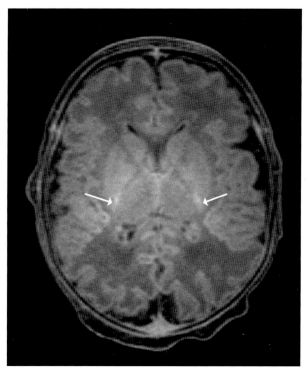

Fig. 5 Internal capsule myelination signal in a normal 38-week GA infant, 3DT1-weighted image. A strip of hyperintense signal in the posterior one-third of the posterior limb of the internal capsules (white arrows) should be visible on MRI in newborns of 36–37 weeks GA and older.

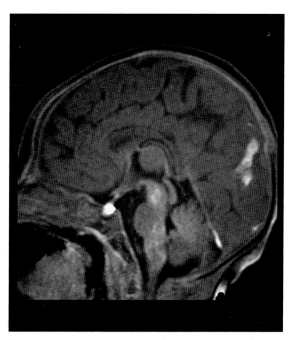

Fig. 6 Corpus callosum in a normal term infant, 3DT1-weighted image. The unmyelinated corpus callosum of newborns has a uniformly thin, tubular shape until approximately 3–4 months of age, when thickening of the genu and splenium should be evident. Note the presence of thin subdural hematomas, common in newborns, in the posterior interhemispheric fissure and tentorium.

images until the darker signal of myelination is apparent in the splenium by 6 months of age.

Basal Ganglia and Thalami

Because cerebral white matter volume increases greatly in the first 2 years of life compared to relatively little change in the basal ganglia and thalamic volumes, the deep gray nuclei appear large compared to the rest of the cerebral hemispheres in early infancy. They also undergo complex signal changes in the first weeks and months of life and so are among the most difficult areas of the neonatal brain to assess.

The basal ganglia and thalami contain a relatively high quantity of axons for gray matter structures, and some of these undergo early myelination. The T1 and T2 signal changes evolve fairly rapidly, and differently in different segments of these nuclei; therefore other maturational processes in addition to myelination likely influence the MR appearance (3). By term, the globi pallidi show diffuse T1 hyperintensity with indistinct margins (Fig. 7) and mild T2 hypointensity; the posterior putamina are comparatively less T1 hyperintense. Mild differences in T2 hypointensity between these nuclei fade by 1 month of age (2). The subthalamic nuclei are distinctly T1 hyperintense, T2 hypointense, and easy to identify in both preterm and term infants.

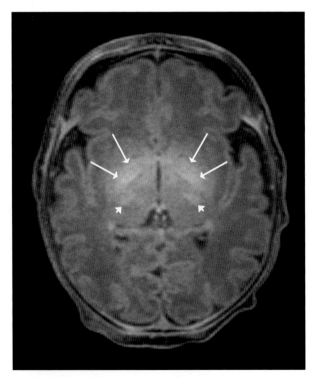

Fig. 7 Inferior basal ganglia and thalami in a normal 38-week GA infant. 3DT1-weighted image shows diffuse, ill defined hyperintensity in the globi pallidi (white long arrows) that is slightly brighter than the signal in the posterior putamina. The ventrolateral thalamic nuclei are also T1 hyperintense (white short arrows) in preterm and term neonates. The pallidal signal gradually fades on T1W images after the first postnatal month, while the ventrolateral thalamic signal fades over a longer period of time.

The ventrolateral thalamic nuclei are hyperintense with unsharp margins on T1W images at term (Fig. 7), and their T2 hypointensity is more marked than in either the pallidal nuclei or putamina. The pulvinar and more dorsal parts of the thalami possess homogeneous, intermediate T2 signal, comparable to that of the caudate nuclei, and are clearly more T2 hypointense than the nearby temporal lobe white matter. By 3 months of age, the signal intensity in the basal ganglia and thalami is more homogeneous on both T1W and T2W images, with the ventrolateral and subthalamic nuclei showing only mild persistence of T1 hyperintensity and T2 hypointensity.

The deep gray nuclei in neonates is vulnerable to hypoxic-ischemic insults and so it is imperative to be able to differentiate the normal areas of T1 hyperintensity from pathological T1 shortening that may be found in the subacute phase after injury (61–64).

Diffusion Weighted Imaging

By term birth, diffusion weighted images show a relative increase in signal intensity of the unmyelinated cerebral white matter compared to what is seen in premature infants, resulting in decreased contrast between cerebral cortex and white matter (42). As with preterm infants, normal diffusion restriction (i.e., higher signal on DWI) in term neonates precedes the onset of visible myelination signal changes on T1W and T2W images (44).

In newborns, the posterior limbs of the internal capsules, corpus callosum, corona radiata, and optic radiations are isointense to subtly hyperintense to cortical gray matter at a b-value of 1000 s/mm^2 (Fig. 8A) (11, 42, 43). If there is a question of abnormality, these areas should be compared with normal age-matched images and the ADC maps should be analyzed to prevent misdiagnosis of acute tissue injury. If b-values greater or lesser than 1000 s/mm^2 are used, the resulting images will show increased or decreased tissue contrast, respectively, and ADC values will also change (20). Physiologic diffusion restriction increases further during white matter maturation, and between about 2 and 5 months of age very little contrast is present between cerebral gray and white matter on DWI.

The ADC values of the normal neonatal brain decrease rapidly during the first 5 months of life and more slowly thereafter (45). Strong contrast between gray and white matter on ADC maps is present at birth, unlike the essentially equal ADC values for white and gray matter in adults. Neonatal white matter on ADC is hyperintense to gray matter except for the posterior limbs of the internal capsule, corona radiata, corpus callosum, optic radiations, middle cerebellar peduncles, mesencephalon, and the dorsal pons, all of which appear hypointense on ADC images (Fig. 8B). For most of the first year, the cerebellum as a whole can have a noticeably more hypointense appearance on ADC than the cerebral hemispheres, while on DWI it is isointense to subtly hyperintense to the cerebrum.

Ventricles and Subarachnoid Spaces

The ventricles in a term newborn are normally small (48). Mild right-left asymmetry in lateral ventricular size is normal. Cava septi pellucidi are present in the majority of newborns and usually disappear in the first months of life (65). The anterior temporal lobe and frontal lobe subarachnoid spaces may be mildly prominent early in infancy. The cisterns around the brainstem and cerebellum also remain proportionally large in

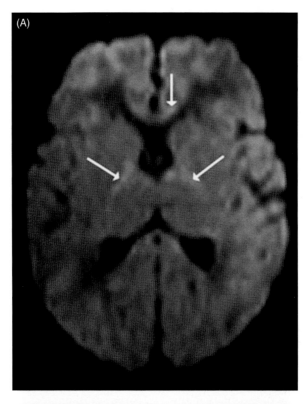

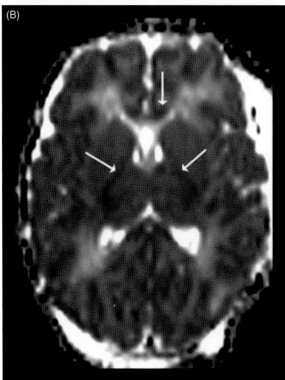

Fig. 8 DWI, b = 1000 **(A),** and ADC **(B)** images in a 40-week GA infant.
A. The entire posterior limb of the internal capsules and the corpus callosum (arrows) are isointense to subtly hyperintense to cerebral cortex. **B.** ADC image shows corresponding low signal intensity (arrows) in the same areas, reflecting reduced water motion. Normal diffusion restriction in preterm and term neonates precedes the onset of visible myelination signal change on T1W and T2W images. Note also the strong contrast between gray and white matter on ADC images **(B)** that is present in the first few months of life.

young infants, and should not be misinterpreted as indicating hypoplasia or atrophy of the brainstem, vermis, or cerebellar hemispheres.

Pituitary Gland

In the term neonate, as in the fetus and the infant born prematurely, the anterior lobe of the pituitary gland is hyperintense on T1W images (Fig. 9) (51, 52). The anterior lobe then fades to isointensity with cortical gray matter on T1W images over approximately the next 8 weeks of life. The posterior lobe is markedly bright on T1W images in neonates and then becomes less intensely bright after about 2 months. The shape of the pituitary gland also changes in the first months of life, showing a convex superior margin from term up to about 2 months, then tending to be flat or convex throughout the rest of childhood (52, 66). The normal range of pituitary gland height on MRI throughout childhood is approximately 2–6 mm (66).

Age 4 Months to 3 Years

Myelination and White Matter Maturation

By 4 months of age, gray matter and incompletely myelinated white matter are almost equal in signal intensity on T1W images, rendering cortical differentiation poor (11). At 6 months, the central white matter of the frontal, parietal, and temporal lobes shows myelination on T1W images. The occipital white matter is more advanced, showing both deep and subcortical white matter myelination at this time.

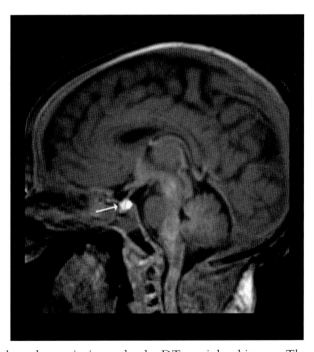

Fig. 9 Normal newborn pituitary gland, 3DT1-weighted image. The anterior lobe of the pituitary gland (arrow) is hyperintense on T1W images and has a convex superior margin for approximately two months after birth. The posterior lobe is also markedly bright on T1W images in neonates.

The entire PLIC, which displays hyperintensity on T1W images at 3 months, becomes T2 hypointense by 6–7 months, although the change on T2W images may be evident earlier, particularly with fast spin-echo imaging at 3T. The anterior limb of the internal capsule (ALIC), which becomes hyperintense on T1W images by 3–4 months, develops T2 hypointensity to match the PLIC between about 6 and 10 months, although this too may develop earlier.

Cerebellar subcortical white matter myelination is visible on T1W images by age 3 months and on T2W images by age 3–4 months. It continues to progress on T2W images, appearing as finely arborized hypointense signal throughout the cerebellar hemispheres during the first year of life, reaching an adult appearance at approximately 15–18 months of age (1).

Throughout the second half of the first year, peripheral white matter in the cerebral hemispheres becomes progressively more hyperintense on T1W images, assuming the appearance of fine arborization. This occurs at age 7–8 months in the occipital lobes and at approximately 8–11 months in the frontal, and then temporal lobes (1, 11). Prior to the completion of this process, and chiefly between ages 4 and 8 months, the subcortical white matter in various areas of the brain passes through periods of isointensity with cortex on T1W images, giving the false appearance of excessive cortical thickness (Fig. 10A). Examination of the T2W images of infants in this age group will provide a truer estimation of cortical thickness (Fig. 10B), especially up to 6–7 months of age. After that time and into the beginning of the second year of life, cortical gray-white matter differentiation on T2W images can be patchy and poorly defined as the maturing subcortical white matter changes from hyperintensity to hypointensity relative to gray matter. By 12–15 months, myelination essentially reaches an adult appearance on T1W images, with minimal further T1 shortening occurring in subcortical U-fibers until approximately 18 months of age (4, 11).

On T2W images, the same process of peripheral white matter myelination is visible later: between about 9–12 months in the occipital lobes, 11–14 months in the frontal lobes, and 16–18 months in the temporal lobes (11). By 2 years of age, subcortical white matter myelination is nearly complete on T2W images (2, 11). Beyond that time, the very last subcortical white matter areas to myelinate (i.e., true "terminal zones") are found in the anterior and superior medial frontal lobes (Fig. 11A) and the anterior medial temporal lobes (Fig. 11B). In these locations, small areas of T2 (and FLAIR) hyperintensity near the cortex may still be apparent at 3–4 years of age (67, 68).

The description of "terminal zones of myelination" on MRI initially referred to the deep white matter superior and posterior to the trigones of the lateral ventricles that can normally remain mildly hyperintense on T2W images into early adulthood. The T2 and FLAIR hyperintense signal commonly present in these areas has indistinct margins, is usually bilaterally symmetric, is peripheral to a zone of myelinated white matter immediately bordering the lateral ventricles, and is not associated with ventricular enlargement or callosal thinning (1, 69). The etiology of this normally occurring signal change remains unclear (11, 67).

A more diffuse deep cerebral white matter slight hyperintensity, apart from the peritrigonal changes described earlier, has been reported as a normal finding on

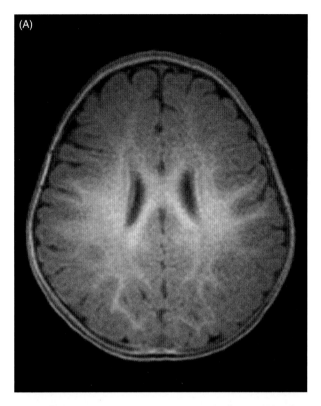

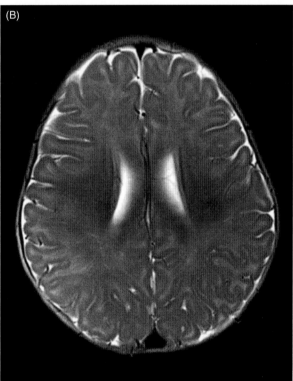

Fig. 10 Appearance of cerebral cortex on T1W **(A)** versus T2W **(B)** images in a normal 6-month-old. **A.** Note the "pseudo-thickening" of cerebral cortex and lack of sharp demarcation between cortex and subcortical white matter. Evaluation of the cortex for malformations and other abnormalities on T1W sequences is difficult between approximately 4–8 months of age due to incomplete myelination of the subcortical white matter. T2W images **(B)** at this age, however, depict the cortical ribbon more accurately.

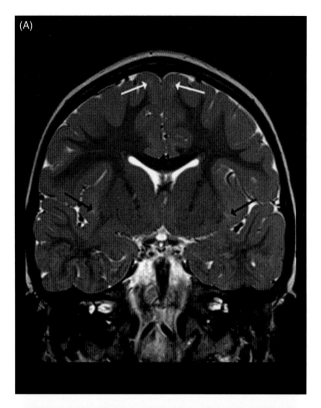

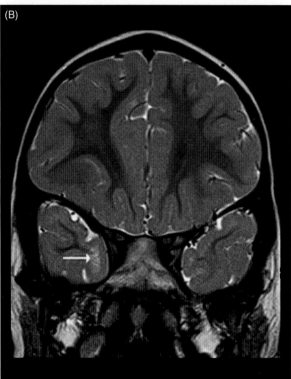

Fig. 11 Final subcortical areas to myelinate, coronal T2W images. **A.** Normal 2-year 6-month-old. **B.** Normal 3-year-old. The anterior and superior medial frontal lobes (**A**, white arrows) and anterior medial temporal lobes (**B**, white arrow) in very young children may show persistent, small areas of juxtacortical T2 and FLAIR hyperintensity, often with a finely striated appearance. This may also be seen in the insular white matter (**A**, black arrows).

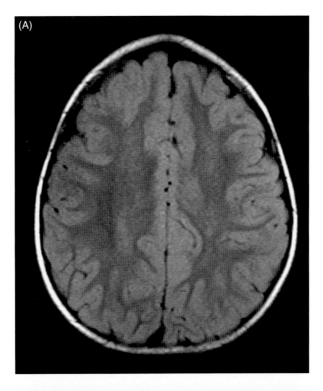

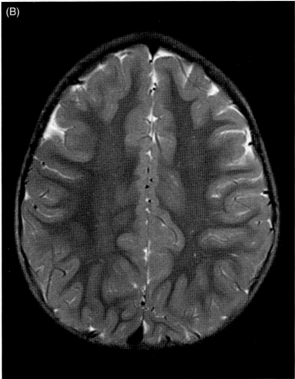

Fig. 12 Deep white matter signal on 3T imaging in a normal 2-year 6-month-old.
A. Notice the hazy, mildly increased FLAIR signal in the centrum semiovale
bilaterally. This is generally most apparent at 3T imaging, may persist to a lesser
degree into adulthood, and should not be mistaken for pathology. **B.** TSE T2W
image in the same subject. The same finding is more subtle, or may be unapparent,
on T2W images.

3T with FLAIR imaging in healthy adults (70). This appearance can also be observed on 3T FLAIR images in children (Fig. 12A) and may be subtly present on corresponding T2W images (Fig. 12B).

Corpus Callosum

Between 4 and 6 months of age, myelination progresses from the splenium and posterior body of the corpus callosum more anteriorly into the body and genu on T1W images. On T2W images, the splenium becomes hypointense by about 6 months, while the body and genu show milder degrees of hypointensity. By about 8 months, the genu should be nearly the same T2 hypointensity as the splenium (10).

There is progressive thickening of the splenium and genu from infancy until 3 years of age, at which time the corpus callosum reaches a relatively adult morphology (71). Callosal growth is rapid during the first 3 years, and the length continues to increase subtly through adolescence (71). The length of the corpus callosum has some correlation with head shape, and in brachycephalic patients the splenium may have a sharply vertical orientation. Focal thinning of the posterior body of the corpus callosum at the junction with the splenium (i.e., the isthmus), when found in isolation, is most likely a normal variant (72).

Basal Ganglia and Thalami

The volume of the basal ganglia and thalami appears to decrease relative to cerebral white matter after age 6 months due to rapid growth of the latter. Between 4 and 8–11 months of age, the globi pallidi are mildly hyperintense on T2W images compared to the putamina (Fig. 13), after which time the lentiform nuclei become isointense with each other (1). Between 10 and 12 months of age, the basal ganglia start to lose their previously distinctive T2 hypointensity as the surrounding white matter myelinates. On T1W images, the globi pallidi are mildly and homogenously hyperintense compared to the striatal nuclei, a subtle difference that increases throughout childhood.

Diffusion Weighted Imaging

On DWI, gray and white matter show increasing contrast to each other in the second half of the first year, with the cerebral white matter eventually becoming hypointense to cortex and remaining so throughout childhood. On ADC maps, however, the previously hyperintense white matter which showed strong contrast with gray matter in the neonate and young infant, gradually decreases in ADC value so that cerebral gray and white matter approach isointensity after approximately 1 year of age. The peritrigonal regions and some subcortical white matter may remain hyperintense on ADC maps.

T2 FLAIR

The progression of normal myelination on FLAIR images in infants and young children has been studied by some authors (5, 24, 73, 74), although it is not widely used clinically. This atlas includes FLAIR images starting at age 1 year. Between 1 and

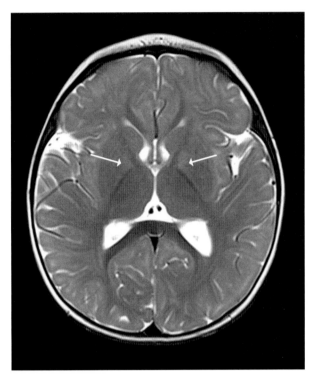

Fig. 13 Globus pallidus signal on T2W images, normal 11 month-old. The globi pallidi (arrows) may be slightly hyperintense to the rest of the basal ganglia on T2W images from after the newborn period up until approximately 1 year of age.

2 years of age, progressive myelination leads to the development of hypointensity on FLAIR images in the deep and then the subcortical white matter; this follows the same pattern as on standard T2W images but lags behind by several months. The extended timeframe on FLAIR images is probably due to the T1-weighting that is inherent in the FLAIR technique, even though image contrast in FLAIR is based primarily on T2 relaxation differences (24). In other words, the presence of some T1 relaxation effect in FLAIR imaging serves to dampen the T2 effect that causes signal to become hypointense as myelin matures.

By age 12 months, white matter areas that have attained hypointensity on FLAIR include the entire internal capsule and corpus callosum, the perirolandic centrum semiovale and subcortical white matter, optic radiations, occipital deep white matter, cerebral peduncles, ventral pons, middle cerebellar peduncles, and the deep and subcortical cerebellar white matter (24). By 14 to 18 months, the subcortical white matter of the occipital lobes develops hypointensity and the frontal deep white matter becomes hypointense. By 20 to 24 months, frontal subcortical white matter hypointensity is evident on FLAIR, and temporal deep white matter is becoming hypointense. Note that these time points on FLAIR imaging all occur later than the corresponding changes on T2W images by at least several months. Accordingly, the subcortical U-fibers of the anterior frontal and temporal lobes, as the last areas to myelinate, may remain mildly hyperintense to isointense with cortex on FLAIR after age 24 months (5, 24, 73).

Summary

Knowledge of the timing and sequence of brain myelination is essential for anyone reporting on MR examinations in pediatric patients. In clinical practice, imaging assessment of brain maturation can be reliably done using standard MR sequences complemented by the informed use of age-matched, normal comparison images and myelination milestone tables. This same approach will facilitate early identification of subtle, diffuse, or symmetric lesions due to white matter disorders, congenital malformations, or other disease processes that can affect the developing brain.

References

1. Barkovich AJ, Mukherjee P. Normal development of the neonatal and infant brain, skull, and spine. In: Barkovich AJ, Raybaud C, eds. *Pediatric neuroimaging.* 5th ed. Philadelphia, PA: Wolters Kluwer Health/Lippincott Williams & Wilkins; 2012:21–80.

2. Griffiths P. *Atlas of fetal and postnatal brain MR.* 1st ed. Philadelphia, PA: Mosby/Elsevier; 2010:266.

3. Counsell SJ, Maalouf EF, Fletcher AM, et al. MR imaging assessment of myelination in the very preterm brain. *AJNR Am J Neuroradiol.* 2002;23(5):872–881.

4. Parazzini C, Bianchini E, Triulzi F. Myelination. In: Tortori-Donati P, Rossi A, Biancheri R, eds. *Pediatric neuroradiology.* Berlin and Heidelberg, Germany: Springer-Verlag; 2005:21–40.

5. Welker KM, Patton A. Assessment of normal myelination with magnetic resonance imaging. *Semin Neurol.* 2012;32(1):15–28. doi: 10.1055/s-0032-1306382; 10.1055/s-0032-1306382.

6. Branson HM. Normal myelination: a practical pictorial review. *Neuroimaging Clin N Am.* 2013;23(2):183–195. doi: 10.1016/j.nic.2012.12.001; 10.1016/j.nic.2012.12.001.

7. Hintz SR, O'Shea M. Neuroimaging and neurodevelopmental outcomes in preterm infants. *Semin Perinatol.* 2008;32(1):11–19. doi: 10.1053/j.semperi.2007.12.010; 10.1053/j.semperi.2007.12.010.

8. Kapellou O, Counsell SJ, Kennea N, et al. Abnormal cortical development after premature birth shown by altered allometric scaling of brain growth. *PLoS Med.* 2006;3(8):e265. doi: 10.1371/journal.pmed.0030265.

9. Ajayi-Obe M, Saeed N, Cowan FM, Rutherford MA, Edwards AD. Reduced development of cerebral cortex in extremely preterm infants. *Lancet.* 2000;356(9236):1162–1163.

10. van der Knaap MS, Valk J. Myelination and retarded myelination. In: van der Knaap MS, Valk J, eds. *Magnetic resonance of myelination and myelin disorders.* 3rd ed. Berlin and Heidelberg, Germany: Springer; 2005:37–65.

11. Cowan FM. Magnetic resonance imaging of the normal infant brain: term to 2 years. In: Rutherford MA, ed. *MRI of the neonatal brain.* London, UK; New York, NY: W. B. Saunders; 2002:51–81.

12. Hess CP, Barkovich AJ. Techniques and methods in pediatric neuroimaging. In: Barkovich AJ, Raybaud C, eds. *Pediatric neuroimaging.* 5th ed. Philadelphia, PA: Wolters Kluwer Health/Lippincott Williams & Wilkins; 2012:1–19.

13. Deoni SC, Mercure E, Blasi A, et al. Mapping infant brain myelination with magnetic resonance imaging. *J Neurosci.* 2011;31(2):784–791. doi: 10.1523/JNEUROSCI.2106-10.2011 [doi].

14. Knickmeyer RC, Gouttard S, Kang C, et al. A structural MRI study of human brain development from birth to 2 years. *J Neurosci.* 2008;28(47):12176–12182. doi: 10.1523/JNEUROSCI.3479-08.2008.

15. Laule C, Vavasour IM, Kolind SH, et al. Magnetic resonance imaging of myelin. *Neurotherapeutics.* 2007;4(3):460–484. doi: S1933-7213(07)00088-8 [pii].

16. Sarikaya B, McKinney AM, Spilseth B, Truwit CL. Comparison of spin-echo T1- and T2-weighted and gradient-echo T1-weighted images at 3T in evaluating very preterm neonates at term-equivalent age. *AJNR Am J Neuroradiol.* 2013;34(5):1098–1103. doi: 10.3174/ajnr.A3323; 10.3174/ajnr.A3323.

17. Shaw DW, Weinberger E, Astley SJ, Tsuruda JS. Quantitative comparison of conventional spin echo and fast spin echo during brain myelination. *J Comput Assist Tomogr.* 1997;21(6):867–871.

18. Dagia C, Ditchfield M. 3T MRI in paediatrics: challenges and clinical applications. *Eur J Radiol.* 2008;68(2):309–319. doi: 10.1016/j.ejrad.2008.05.019.

19. van Wezel-Meijler G, Leijser LM, de Bruine FT, Steggerda SJ, van der Grond J, Walther FJ. Magnetic resonance imaging of the brain in newborn infants: practical aspects. *Early Hum Dev.* 2009;85(2):85–92. doi: 10.1016/j.earlhumdev.2008.11.009.

20. Dudink J, Larkman DJ, Kapellou O, et al. High b-value diffusion tensor imaging of the neonatal brain at 3T. *AJNR Am J Neuroradiol.* 2008;29(10):1966–1972. doi: 10.3174/ajnr.A1241.

21. Shroff MM, Soares-Fernandes JP, Whyte H, Raybaud C. MR imaging for diagnostic evaluation of encephalopathy in the newborn. *Radiographics.* 2010;30(3):763–780. doi: 10.1148/rg.303095126.

22. Huppi PS, Dubois J. Diffusion tensor imaging of brain development. *Semin Fetal Neonatal Med.* 2006;11(6):489–497. doi: S1744-165X(06)00074-6 [pii].

23. Rodrigues K, Ellen Grant P. Diffusion-weighted imaging in neonates. *Neuroimaging Clin N Am.* 2011;21(1):127–151, viii. doi: 10.1016/j.nic.2011.01.012.

24. Kizildag B, Dusunceli E, Fitoz S, Erden I. The role of classic spin echo and FLAIR sequences for the evaluation of myelination in MR imaging. *Diagn Interv Radiol.* 2005;11(3):130–136.

25. Gawne-Cain ML, O'Riordan JI, Thompson AJ, Moseley IF, Miller DH. Multiple sclerosis lesion detection in the brain: a comparison of fast fluid-attenuated inversion recovery and conventional T2-weighted dual spin echo. *Neurology.* 1997;49(2):364–370.

26. Stevenson VL, Gawne-Cain ML, Barker GJ, Thompson AJ, Miller DH. Imaging of the spinal cord and brain in multiple sclerosis: a comparative study between fast FLAIR and fast spin echo. *J Neurol.* 1997;244(2):119–124.

27. Baumann N, Pham-Dinh D. Biology of oligodendrocyte and myelin in the mammalian central nervous system. *Physiol Rev.* 2001;81(2):871–927.

28. Kinney HC, Brody BA, Kloman AS, Gilles FH. Sequence of central nervous system myelination in human infancy. II. patterns of myelination in autopsied infants. *J Neuropathol Exp Neurol.* 1988;47(3):217–234.

29. Barkovich AJ. Concepts of myelin and myelination in neuroradiology. *AJNR Am J Neuroradiol.* 2000;21(6):1099–1109.

30. Arthur R. Magnetic resonance imaging in preterm infants. *Pediatr Radiol.* 2006;36(7):593–607. doi: 10.1007/s00247-006-0154-x.

31. Barkovich AJ, Kjos BO, Jackson DE,Jr, Norman D. Normal maturation of the neonatal and infant brain: MR imaging at 1.5 T. *Radiology.* 1988;166(1 Pt 1):173–180.

32. McArdle CB, Richardson CJ, Nicholas DA, Mirfakhraee M, Hayden CK, Amparo EG. Developmental features of the neonatal brain: MR imaging. part I. gray-white matter differentiation and myelination. *Radiology.* 1987;162(1 Pt 1):223–229.

33. Bird CR, Hedberg M, Drayer BP, Keller PJ, Flom RA, Hodak JA. MR assessment of myelination in infants and children: usefulness of marker sites. *AJNR Am J Neuroradiol.* 1989;10(4):731–740.

34. Battin MR, Maalouf EF, Counsell SJ, et al. Magnetic resonance imaging of the brain in very preterm infants: visualization of the germinal matrix, early myelination, and cortical folding. *Pediatrics.* 1998;101(6):957–962.

35. Ramenghi LA, Mosca F, Counsell S, Rutherford MA. Magnetic resonance imaging of the brain in preterm infants. In: Tortori-Donati P, Rossi A, Biancheri R, eds. *Pediatric neuroradiology.* Berlin and Heidelberg, Germany: Springer-Verlag; 2005:199–234.

36. Hart AR, Whitby EW, Griffiths PD, Smith MF. Magnetic resonance imaging and developmental outcome following preterm birth: review of current evidence. *Dev Med Child Neurol.* 2008;50(9):655–663. doi: 10.1111/j.1469-8749.2008.03050.x.

37. Battin M, Rutherford MA. Magnetic resonance imaging of the brain in preterm infants: 24 weeks' gestation to term. In: Rutherford MA, ed. *MRI of the neonatal brain.* London, UK; New York, NY: W. B. Saunders; 2002:25–49.

38. Garel C, Chantrel E, Brisse H, et al. Fetal cerebral cortex: normal gestational landmarks identified using prenatal MR imaging. *AJNR Am J Neuroradiol.* 2001;22(1):184–189.

39. Chi JG, Dooling EC, Gilles FH. Gyral development of the human brain. *Ann Neurol.* 1977;1(1):86–93. doi: 10.1002/ana.410010109.

40. Judas M, Rados M, Jovanov-Milosevic N, Hrabac P, Stern-Padovan R, Kostovic I. Structural, immunocytochemical, and MR imaging properties of periventricular crossroads of growing cortical pathways in preterm infants. *AJNR Am J Neuroradiol.* 2005;26(10):2671–2684.

41. Kidokoro H, Anderson PJ, Doyle LW, Neil JJ, Inder TE. High signal intensity on T2-weighted MR imaging at term-equivalent age in preterm infants does not predict 2-year neurodevelopmental outcomes. *AJNR Am J Neuroradiol.* 2011;32(11):2005–2010. doi: 10.3174/ajnr.A2703; 10.3174/ajnr.A2703.

42. Tanner SF, Ramenghi LA, Ridgway JP, et al. Quantitative comparison of intrabrain diffusion in adults and preterm and term neonates and infants. *AJR Am J Roentgenol.* 2000;174(6):1643–1649.

43. Martin-Fiori E, Huisman TAGM. Diffusion-weighted, perfusion-weighted,and functional MR imaging. In: Tortori-Donati P, Rossi A, Biancheri R, eds. *Pediatric neuroradiology.* Berlin and Heidelberg, Germany: Springer-Verlag; 2005:1073–1114.

44. Prayer D, Barkovich AJ, Kirschner DA, et al. Visualization of nonstructural changes in early white matter development on diffusion-weighted MR images: evidence supporting premyelination anisotropy. *AJNR Am J Neuroradiol.* 2001;22(8):1572–1576.

45. Engelbrecht V, Scherer A, Rassek M, Witsack HJ, Modder U. Diffusion-weighted MR imaging in the brain in children: findings in the normal brain and in the brain with white matter diseases. *Radiology.* 2002;222(2):410–418.

46. Garel C. *MRI of the fetal brain: normal development and cerebral pathologies.* Berlin, Germany; New York, NY: Springer; 2004:267.

47. Filly RA, Goldstein RB. The fetal ventricular atrium: fourth down and 10 mm to go. *Radiology.* 1994;193(2):315–317.

48. McArdle CB, Richardson CJ, Nicholas DA, Mirfakhraee M, Hayden CK, Amparo EG. Developmental features of the neonatal brain: MR imaging. part II. ventricular size and extracerebral space. *Radiology.* 1987;162(1 Pt 1):230–234.

49. Gerard N, Huisman TAGM. Fetal magnetic resonance imaging of the central nervous system. In: Tortori-Donati P, Rossi A, Biancheri R, eds. *Pediatric neuroradiology*. Berlin and Heidelberg, Germany: Springer-Verlag; 2005:1219–1253.

50. Jou HJ, Shyu MK, Wu SC, Chen SM, Su CH, Hsieh FJ. Ultrasound measurement of the fetal cavum septi pellucidi. *Ultrasound Obstet Gynecol*. 1998;12(6):419–421. doi: 10.1046/j.1469-0705.1998.12060419.x.

51. Argyropoulou MI, Xydis V, Kiortsis DN, et al. Pituitary gland signal in pre-term infants during the first year of life: an MRI study. *Neuroradiology*. 2004;46(12):1031–1035. doi: 10.1007/s00234-004-1285-0.

52. Dietrich RB, Lis LE, Greensite FS, Pitt D. Normal MR appearance of the pituitary gland in the first 2 years of life. *AJNR Am J Neuroradiol*. 1995;16(7):1413–1419.

53. Kitamura E, Miki Y, Kawai M, et al. T1 signal intensity and height of the anterior pituitary in neonates: correlation with postnatal time. *AJNR Am J Neuroradiol*. 2008;29(7):1257–1260. doi: 10.3174/ajnr.A1094.

54. Nie J, Li G, Wang L, Gilmore JH, Lin W, Shen D. A computational growth model for measuring dynamic cortical development in the first year of life. *Cereb Cortex*. 2012;22 (10) 2272–2284 first published online November 2, 2011; doi: 10.1093/cercor/bhr293.

55. Raybaud C, Widjaja E. Development and dysgenesis of the cerebral cortex: malformations of cortical development. *Neuroimaging Clin N Am*. 2011;21(3):483–543, vii. doi: 10.1016/j.nic.2011.05.014.

56. Childs AM, Ramenghi LA, Evans DJ, et al. MR features of developing periventricular white matter in preterm infants: evidence of glial cell migration. *AJNR Am J Neuroradiol*. 1998;19(5):971–976.

57. Evans DJ, Childs AM, Ramenghi LA, Arthur RJ, Levene MI. Magnetic-resonance imaging of the brain of premature infants. *Lancet*. 1997;350(9076):522. doi: S0140–6736(05)63118-2 [pii].

58. van Wezel-Meijler G, van der Knaap MS, Sie LT, et al. Magnetic resonance imaging of the brain in premature infants during the neonatal period. Normal phenomena and reflection of mild ultrasound abnormalities. *Neuropediatrics*. 1998;29(2):89–96. doi: 10.1055/s-2007-973541.

59. Goergen SK, Ang H, Wong F, et al. Early MRI in term infants with perinatal hypoxic-ischaemic brain injury: interobserver agreement and MRI predictors of outcome at 2 years. *Clin Radiol*. 2014;69(1):72–81. doi: 10.1016/j.crad.2013.09.001.

60. Liauw L, van der Grond J, van den Berg-Huysmans AA, Laan LA, van Buchem MA, van Wezel-Meijler G. Is there a way to predict outcome in (near) term neonates with hypoxic-ischemic encephalopathy based on MR imaging? *AJNR Am J Neuroradiol*. 2008;29(9):1789–1794. doi: 10.3174/ajnr.A1188.

61. Martinez-Biarge M, Diez-Sebastian J, Kapellou O, et al. Predicting motor outcome and death in term hypoxic-ischemic encephalopathy. *Neurology*. 2011;76(24):2055–2061. doi: 10.1212/WNL.0b013e31821f442d.

62. Schwartz ES, Barkovich AJ. Brain and spine injuries in infancy and childhood. In: Barkovich AJ, Raybaud C, eds. *Pediatric neuroimaging*. 5th ed. Philadelphia, PA: Wolters Kluwer Health/Lippincott Williams & Wilkins; 2012:240–366.

63. Rutherford MA. The asphyxiated term infant. In: Rutherford MA, ed. *MRI of the neonatal brain*. London, UK; New York, NY: W. B. Saunders; 2002:99–128.

64. Liauw L, Palm-Meinders IH, van der Grond J, et al. Differentiating normal myelination from hypoxic-ischemic encephalopathy on T1-weighted MR images: a new approach. *AJNR Am J Neuroradiol.* 2007;28(4):660–665. doi: 28/4/660 [pii].

65. Schwidde JT. Incidence of cavum septi pellucidi and cavum vergae in 1,032 human brains. *AMA Arch Neurol Psychiatry.* 1952;67(5):625–632.

66. Elster AD. Modern imaging of the pituitary. *Radiology.* 1993;187(1):1–14.

67. Parazzini C, Baldoli C, Scotti G, Triulzi F. Terminal zones of myelination: MR evaluation of children aged 20–40 months. *AJNR Am J Neuroradiol.* 2002;23(10):1669–1673.

68. Maricich SM, Azizi P, Jones JY, et al. Myelination as assessed by conventional MR imaging is normal in young children with idiopathic developmental delay. *AJNR Am J Neuroradiol.* 2007;28(8):1602–1605. doi: 10.3174/ajnr.A0602.

69. Liauw L, van der Grond J, Slooff V, et al. Differentiation between peritrigonal terminal zones and hypoxic-ischemic white matter injury on MRI. *Eur J Radiol.* 2008;65(3):395–401. doi: 10.1016/j.ejrad.2007.04.016.

70. Neema M, Guss ZD, Stankiewicz JM, Arora A, Healy BC, Bakshi R. Normal findings on brain fluid-attenuated inversion recovery MR images at 3T. *AJNR Am J Neuroradiol.* 2009;30(5):911–916. doi: 10.3174/ajnr.A1514.

71. Garel C, Cont I, Alberti C, Josserand E, Moutard ML, Ducou le Pointe H. Biometry of the corpus callosum in children: MR imaging reference data. *AJNR Am J Neuroradiol.* 2011;32(8):1436–1443. doi: 10.3174/ajnr.A2542; 10.3174/ajnr.A2542.

72. McLeod NA, Williams JP, Machen B, Lum GB. Normal and abnormal morphology of the corpus callosum. *Neurology.* 1987;37(7):1240–1242.

73. Murakami JW, Weinberger E, Shaw DW. Normal myelination of the pediatric brain imaged with fluid-attenuated inversion-recovery (FLAIR) MR imaging. *AJNR Am J Neuroradiol.* 1999;20(8):1406–1411.

74. Ashikaga R, Araki Y, Ono Y, Nishimura Y, Ishida O. Appearance of normal brain maturation on fluid-attenuated inversion-recovery (FLAIR) MR images. *AJNR Am J Neuroradiol.* 1999;20(3):427–431.

75. Pujol J, Lopez-Sala A, Sebastian-Galles N, et al. Delayed myelination in children with developmental delay detected by volumetric MRI. *Neuroimage.* 2004;22(2):897–903. doi: 10.1016/j.neuroimage.2004.01.029.

76. Schiffmann R, van der Knaap MS. Invited article: An MRI-based approach to the diagnosis of white matter disorders. *Neurology.* 2009;72(8):750–759. doi: 10.1212/01.wnl.0000343049.00540.c8; 10.1212/01.wnl.0000343049.00540.c8.

Normal Brain Maturation Images

32 Weeks, Axial T1

Between ~30–35 wks GA, no new sites of myelination are seen on MRI and only a subtle increase in myelin signal at the sites already myelinated by 30 wks GA occurs. White matter development, reflected by "caps," "arrowheads," and "bands," continues during this period prior to visible T1 or T2 shortening.

Meanwhile, gyral and sulcal development is proceeding, signal changes in the basal ganglia and thalami are evolving, and the germinal matrix continues to involute.

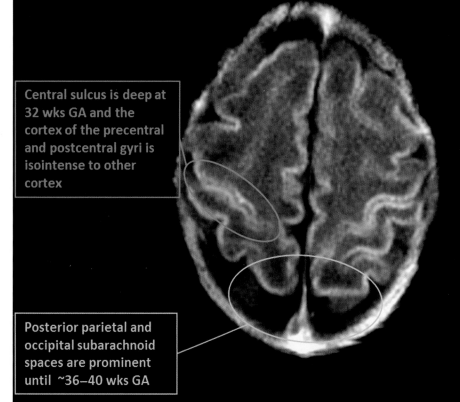

Central sulcus is deep at 32 wks GA and the cortex of the precentral and postcentral gyri is isointense to other cortex

Posterior parietal and occipital subarachnoid spaces are prominent until ~36–40 wks GA

Cerebral white matter in preterm infants has a high water content and is hypointense on T1W images and hyperintense on T2W images

32 Weeks, Axial T1 Images 1-10

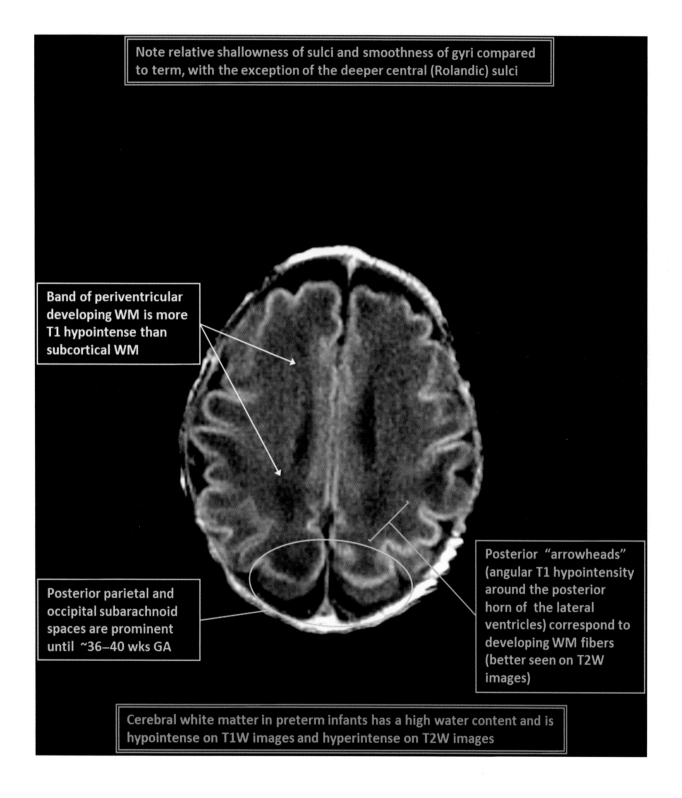

Note relative shallowness of sulci and smoothness of gyri compared to term, with the exception of the deeper central (Rolandic) sulci

Band of periventricular developing WM is more T1 hypointense than subcortical WM

Posterior parietal and occipital subarachnoid spaces are prominent until ~36–40 wks GA

Posterior "arrowheads" (angular T1 hypointensity around the posterior horn of the lateral ventricles) correspond to developing WM fibers (better seen on T2W images)

Cerebral white matter in preterm infants has a high water content and is hypointense on T1W images and hyperintense on T2W images

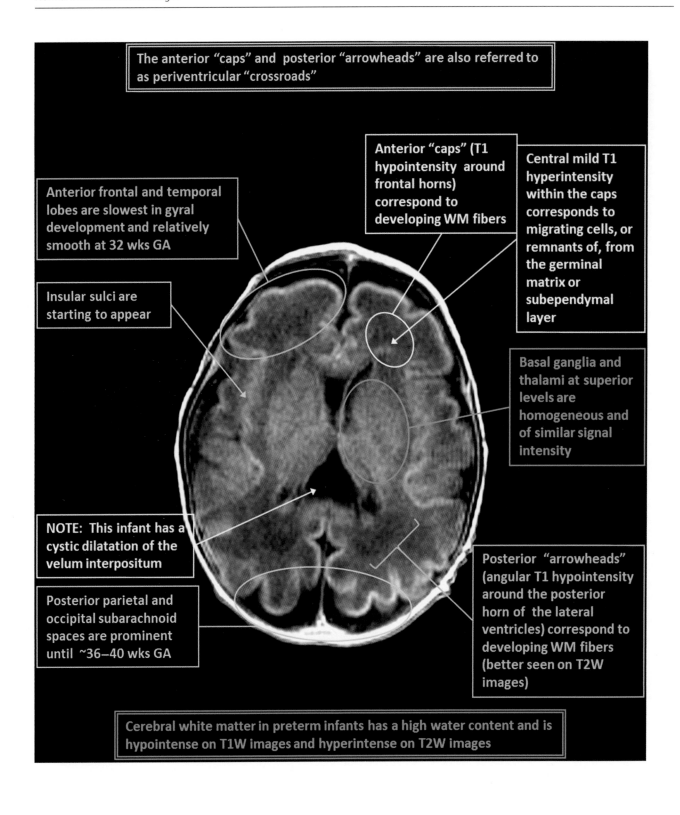

The anterior "caps" and posterior "arrowheads" are also referred to as periventricular "crossroads"

Anterior "caps" (T1 hypointensity around frontal horns) correspond to developing WM fibers

Central mild T1 hyperintensity within the caps corresponds to migrating cells, or remnants of, from the germinal matrix or subependymal layer

Anterior frontal and temporal lobes are slowest in gyral development and relatively smooth at 32 wks GA

Insular sulci are starting to appear

Basal ganglia and thalami at superior levels are homogeneous and of similar signal intensity

NOTE: This infant has a cystic dilatation of the velum interpositum

Posterior parietal and occipital subarachnoid spaces are prominent until ~36–40 wks GA

Posterior "arrowheads" (angular T1 hypointensity around the posterior horn of the lateral ventricles) correspond to developing WM fibers (better seen on T2W images)

Cerebral white matter in preterm infants has a high water content and is hypointense on T1W images and hyperintense on T2W images

The anterior "caps" and posterior "arrowheads" are also referred to as periventricular "crossroads"

Anterior "caps" (T1 hypointensity around frontal horns) correspond to developing WM fibers

Central mild T1 hyperintensity within the caps corresponds to migrating cells, or remnants of, from the germinal matrix or subependymal layer

Anterior frontal and temporal lobes are slowest in gyral development and relatively smooth at 32 wks GA

Insular sulci are starting to appear; Sylvian fissures are prominent

Claustrum

Internal capsules are unmyelinated on T1 until ~36–37 wks GA

NOTE: This infant has a cystic dilatation of the velum interpositum

Posterior parietal and occipital subarachnoid spaces are prominent until ~36–40 wks GA

Globi pallidi are T1 hyperintense and brighter than posterolateral putamina

Ventrolateral thalamic nuclei become T1 hyperintense at ~28 wks GA (although are better seen on T2)

Corpus callosum is thin and of intermediate signal intensity, not yet myelinated

Cerebral white matter in preterm infants has a high water content and is hypointense on T1W images and hyperintense on T2W images

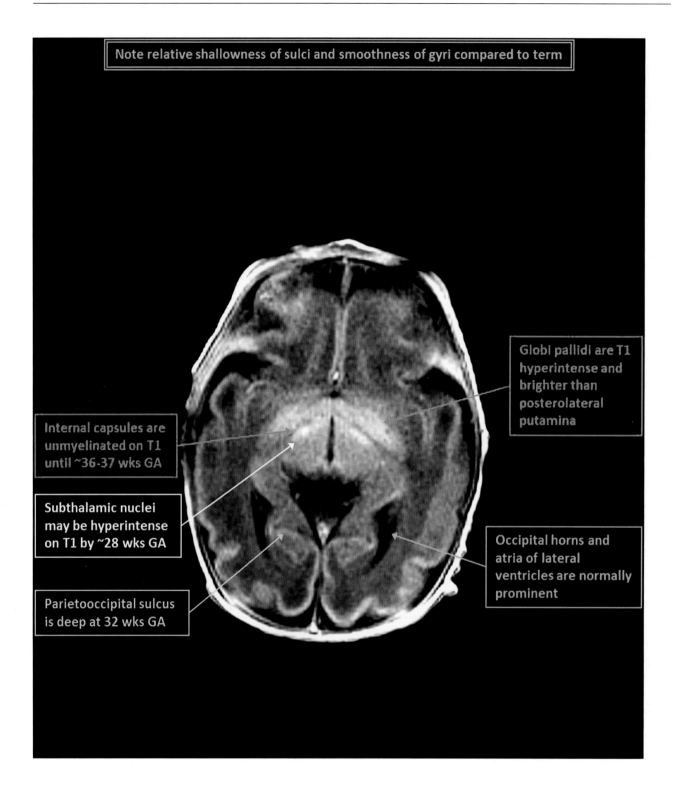

Note relative shallowness of sulci and smoothness of gyri compared to term

Internal capsules are unmyelinated on T1 until ~36-37 wks GA

Subthalamic nuclei may be hyperintense on T1 by ~28 wks GA

Parietooccipital sulcus is deep at 32 wks GA

Globi pallidi are T1 hyperintense and brighter than posterolateral putamina

Occipital horns and atria of lateral ventricles are normally prominent

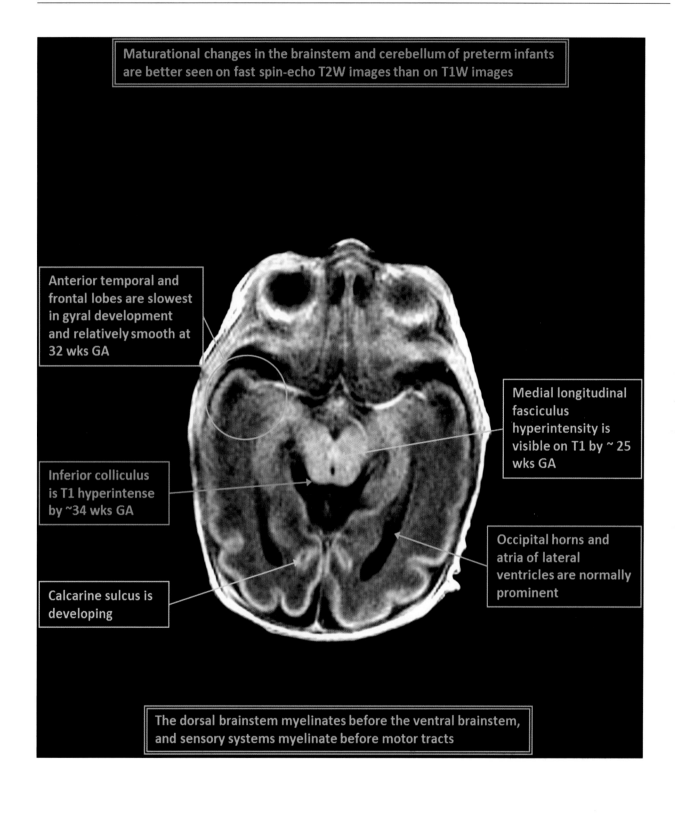

Maturational changes in the brainstem and cerebellum of preterm infants are better seen on fast spin-echo T2W images than on T1W images

Anterior temporal and frontal lobes are slowest in gyral development and relatively smooth at 32 wks GA

Medial longitudinal fasciculus hyperintensity is visible on T1 by ~ 25 wks GA

Inferior colliculus is T1 hyperintense by ~34 wks GA

Occipital horns and atria of lateral ventricles are normally prominent

Calcarine sulcus is developing

The dorsal brainstem myelinates before the ventral brainstem, and sensory systems myelinate before motor tracts

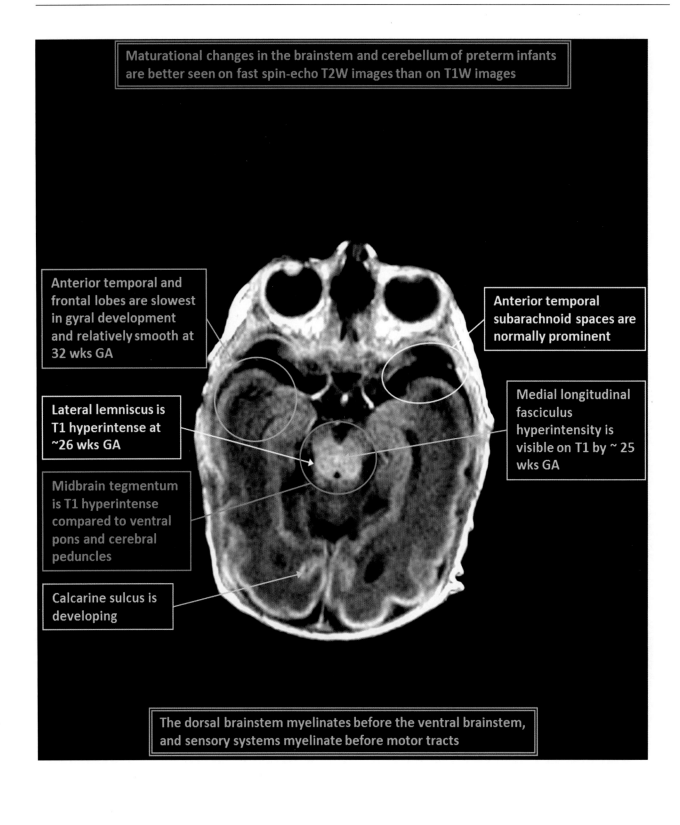

Maturational changes in the brainstem and cerebellum of preterm infants are better seen on fast spin-echo T2W images than on T1W images

Anterior temporal and frontal lobes are slowest in gyral development and relatively smooth at 32 wks GA

Anterior temporal subarachnoid spaces are normally prominent

Lateral lemniscus is T1 hyperintense at ~26 wks GA

Medial longitudinal fasciculus hyperintensity is visible on T1 by ~ 25 wks GA

Midbrain tegmentum is T1 hyperintense compared to ventral pons and cerebral peduncles

Calcarine sulcus is developing

The dorsal brainstem myelinates before the ventral brainstem, and sensory systems myelinate before motor tracts

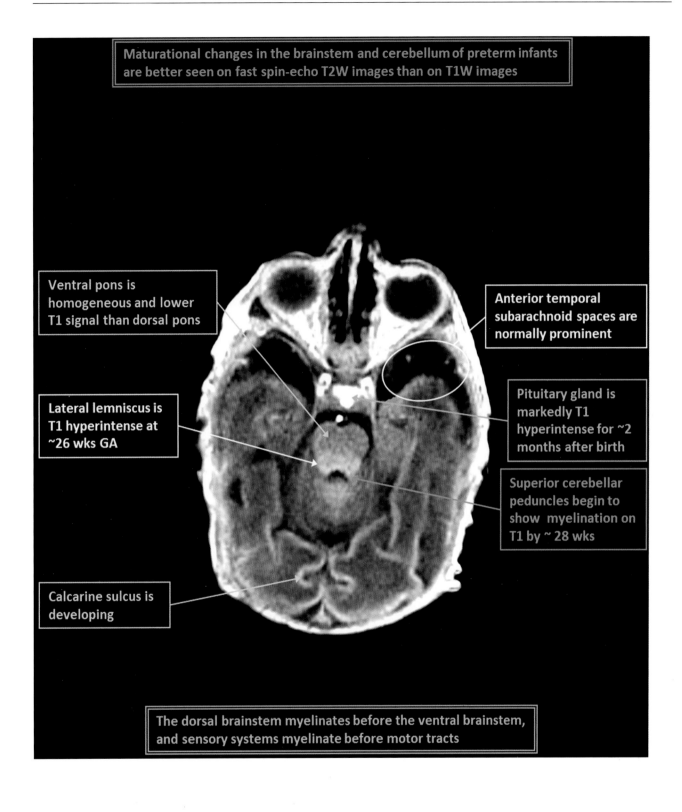

Maturational changes in the brainstem and cerebellum of preterm infants are better seen on fast spin-echo T2W images than on T1W images

Ventral pons is homogeneous and lower T1 signal than dorsal pons

Anterior temporal subarachnoid spaces are normally prominent

Lateral lemniscus is T1 hyperintense at ~26 wks GA

Pituitary gland is markedly T1 hyperintense for ~2 months after birth

Superior cerebellar peduncles begin to show myelination on T1 by ~ 28 wks

Calcarine sulcus is developing

The dorsal brainstem myelinates before the ventral brainstem, and sensory systems myelinate before motor tracts

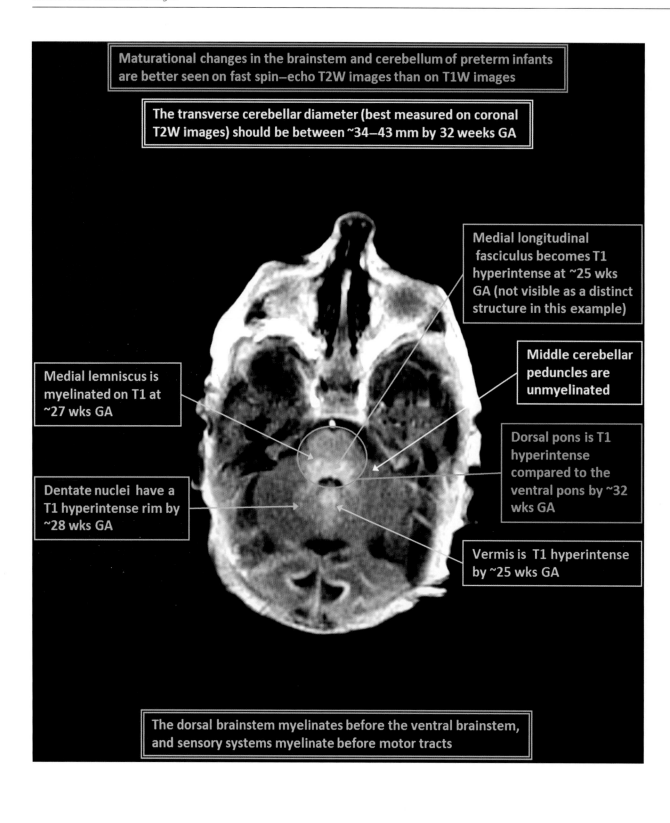

Maturational changes in the brainstem and cerebellum of preterm infants are better seen on fast spin–echo T2W images than on T1W images

The transverse cerebellar diameter (best measured on coronal T2W images) should be between ~34–43 mm by 32 weeks GA

Medial longitudinal fasciculus becomes T1 hyperintense at ~25 wks GA (not visible as a distinct structure in this example)

Middle cerebellar peduncles are unmyelinated

Medial lemniscus is myelinated on T1 at ~27 wks GA

Dorsal pons is T1 hyperintense compared to the ventral pons by ~32 wks GA

Dentate nuclei have a T1 hyperintense rim by ~28 wks GA

Vermis is T1 hyperintense by ~25 wks GA

The dorsal brainstem myelinates before the ventral brainstem, and sensory systems myelinate before motor tracts

Maturational changes in the brainstem and cerebellum of preterm infants are better seen on fast spin–echo T2W images than on T1W images

The transverse cerebellar diameter (best measured on coronal T2W images) should be between ~34–43 mm by 32 weeks GA

Flocculus cerebelli are myelinated before term

Inferior cerebellar peduncles appear hyperintense on T1 as early as ~28 wks GA

Dentate nuclei have a T1 hyperintense rim by ~28 wks GA

Dorsal pons and medulla show myelination in some gray matter nuclei and white matter tracts as early as ~25 wks GA on T1

The dorsal brainstem myelinates before the ventral brainstem, and sensory systems myelinate before motor tracts

32 Weeks, Axial TSE T2

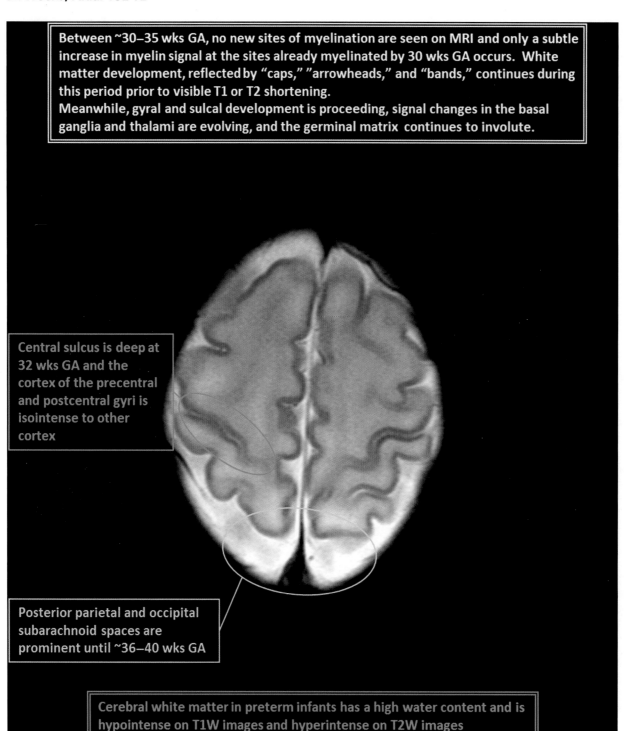

Between ~30–35 wks GA, no new sites of myelination are seen on MRI and only a subtle increase in myelin signal at the sites already myelinated by 30 wks GA occurs. White matter development, reflected by "caps," "arrowheads," and "bands," continues during this period prior to visible T1 or T2 shortening.
Meanwhile, gyral and sulcal development is proceeding, signal changes in the basal ganglia and thalami are evolving, and the germinal matrix continues to involute.

Central sulcus is deep at 32 wks GA and the cortex of the precentral and postcentral gyri is isointense to other cortex

Posterior parietal and occipital subarachnoid spaces are prominent until ~36–40 wks GA

Cerebral white matter in preterm infants has a high water content and is hypointense on T1W images and hyperintense on T2W images

32 Weeks, Axial TSE T2 Images 1–10

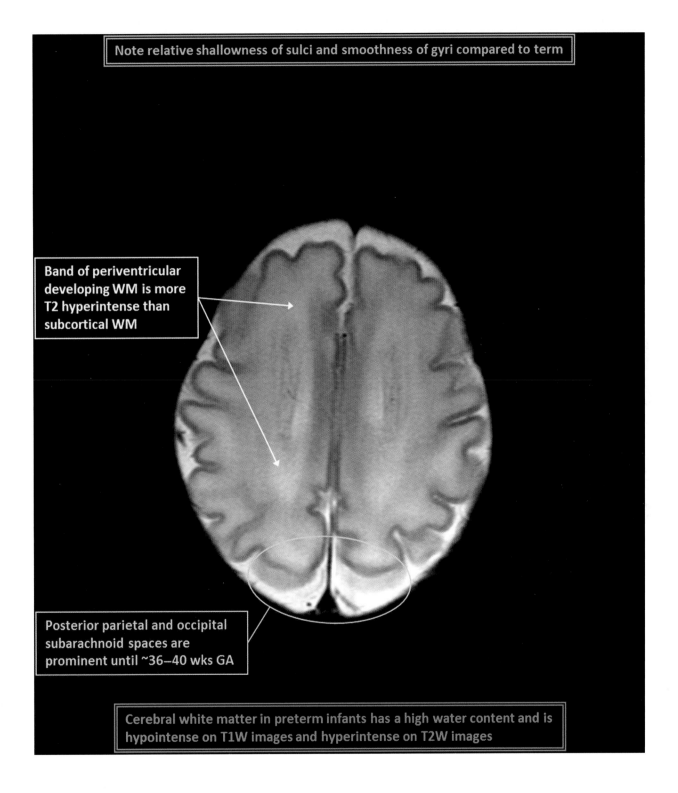

Note relative shallowness of sulci and smoothness of gyri compared to term

Band of periventricular developing WM is more T2 hyperintense than subcortical WM

Posterior parietal and occipital subarachnoid spaces are prominent until ~36–40 wks GA

Cerebral white matter in preterm infants has a high water content and is hypointense on T1W images and hyperintense on T2W images

Note relative shallowness of sulci and smoothness of gyri compared to term

Anterior "caps" (mild T2 hyperintensity around frontal horns) correspond to developing WM fibers

Central mild T2 hypointensity within the caps corresponds to migrating cells, or remnants of, from the germinal matrix or subependymal layer

Anterior frontal and temporal lobes are slowest in gyral development and relatively smooth at 32 wks GA

Insular sulci are starting to appear

Basal ganglia at mid and superior levels are homogeneous and of similar signal intensity as posterior thalami

Intermediate zone of migrating cells is faintly visible as T2 hypointensity between the periventricular and subcortical WM

Posterior parietal and occipital subarachnoid spaces are prominent until ~36–40 wks GA

Posterior "arrowheads" (angular T2 hyperintensity around the posterior horn of the lateral ventricles) correspond to developing WM fibers

The anterior "caps" and posterior "arrowheads" are also referred to as periventricular "crossroads"

Note relative shallowness of sulci and smoothness of gyri compared to term

Anterior "caps" (mild T2 hyperintensity around frontal horns) correspond to developing WM fibers

Central mild T2 hypointensity within the caps corresponds to migrating cells, or remnants of, from the germinal matrix or subependymal layer

Residual germinal matrix (mild T2 hypointensity) at tips of frontal horns

Insular sulci are starting to appear; Sylvian fissures are prominent

Claustrum

Putamina are more T2 hypointense laterally than medially

Internal capsules are unmyelinated on T2 until ~term

Ventrolateral thalamic nuclei become T2 hypointense at ~25 wks GA

NOTE: This infant has a cystic dilatation of the velum interpositum

Intermediate zone of migrating cells (subtle T2 hypointensity)

Posterior parietal and occipital subarachnoid spaces are prominent until ~36–40 wks GA

Corpus callosum is thin and of intermediate signal intensity, not yet myelinated

The anterior "caps" and posterior "arrowheads" are also referred to as periventricular "crossroads"

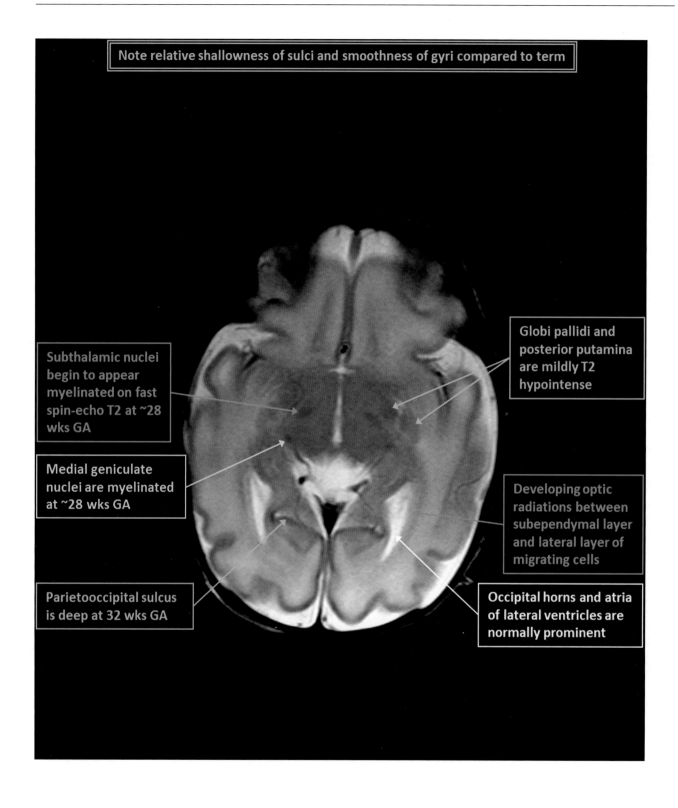

Note relative shallowness of sulci and smoothness of gyri compared to term

Subthalamic nuclei begin to appear myelinated on fast spin-echo T2 at ~28 wks GA

Medial geniculate nuclei are myelinated at ~28 wks GA

Parietooccipital sulcus is deep at 32 wks GA

Globi pallidi and posterior putamina are mildly T2 hypointense

Developing optic radiations between subependymal layer and lateral layer of migrating cells

Occipital horns and atria of lateral ventricles are normally prominent

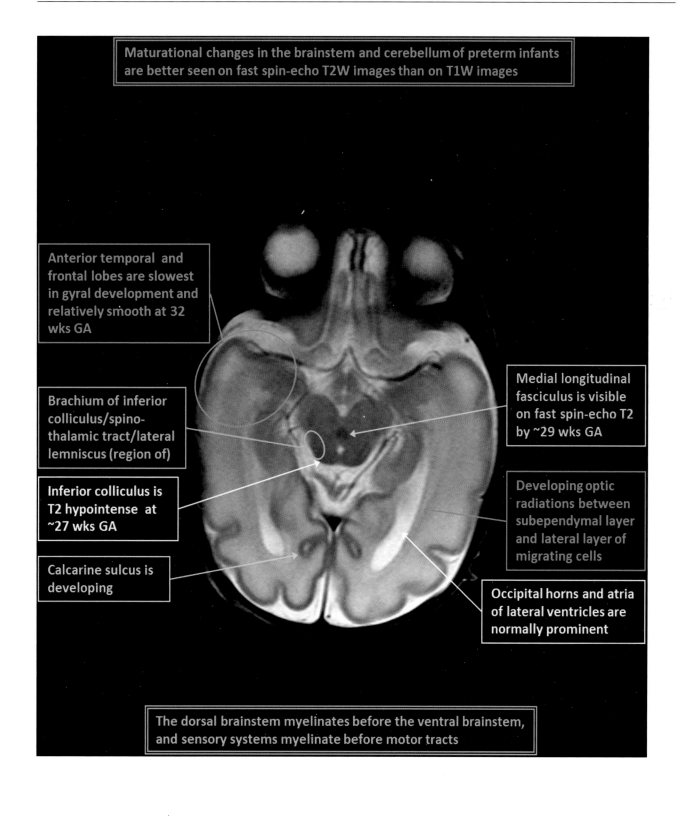

Maturational changes in the brainstem and cerebellum of preterm infants are better seen on fast spin-echo T2W images than on T1W images

Anterior temporal and frontal lobes are slowest in gyral development and relatively smooth at 32 wks GA

Brachium of inferior colliculus/spino-thalamic tract/lateral lemniscus (region of)

Inferior colliculus is T2 hypointense at ~27 wks GA

Calcarine sulcus is developing

Medial longitudinal fasciculus is visible on fast spin-echo T2 by ~29 wks GA

Developing optic radiations between subependymal layer and lateral layer of migrating cells

Occipital horns and atria of lateral ventricles are normally prominent

The dorsal brainstem myelinates before the ventral brainstem, and sensory systems myelinate before motor tracts

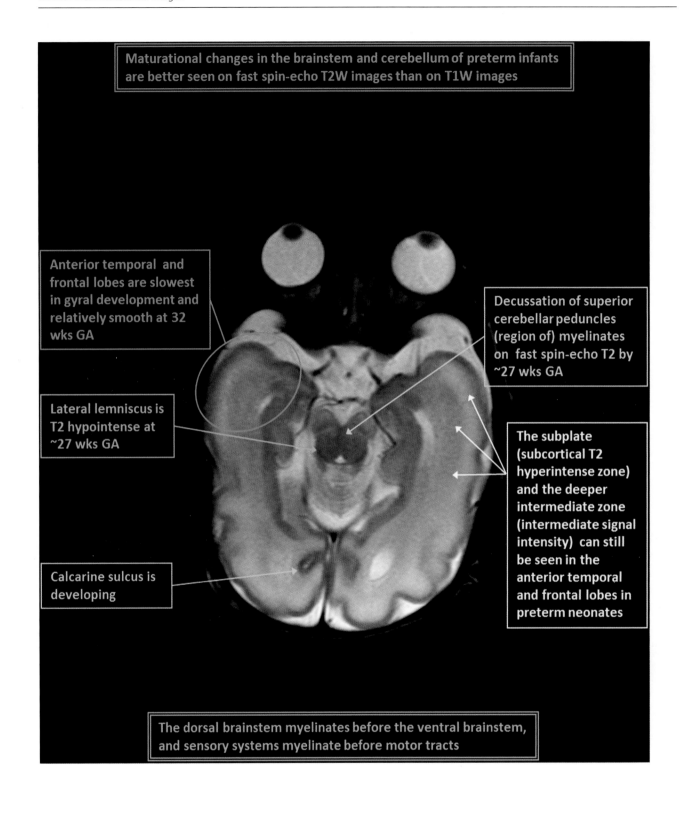

Maturational changes in the brainstem and cerebellum of preterm infants are better seen on fast spin-echo T2W images than on T1W images

Anterior temporal and frontal lobes are slowest in gyral development and relatively smooth at 32 wks GA

Decussation of superior cerebellar peduncles (region of) myelinates on fast spin-echo T2 by ~27 wks GA

Lateral lemniscus is T2 hypointense at ~27 wks GA

The subplate (subcortical T2 hyperintense zone) and the deeper intermediate zone (intermediate signal intensity) can still be seen in the anterior temporal and frontal lobes in preterm neonates

Calcarine sulcus is developing

The dorsal brainstem myelinates before the ventral brainstem, and sensory systems myelinate before motor tracts

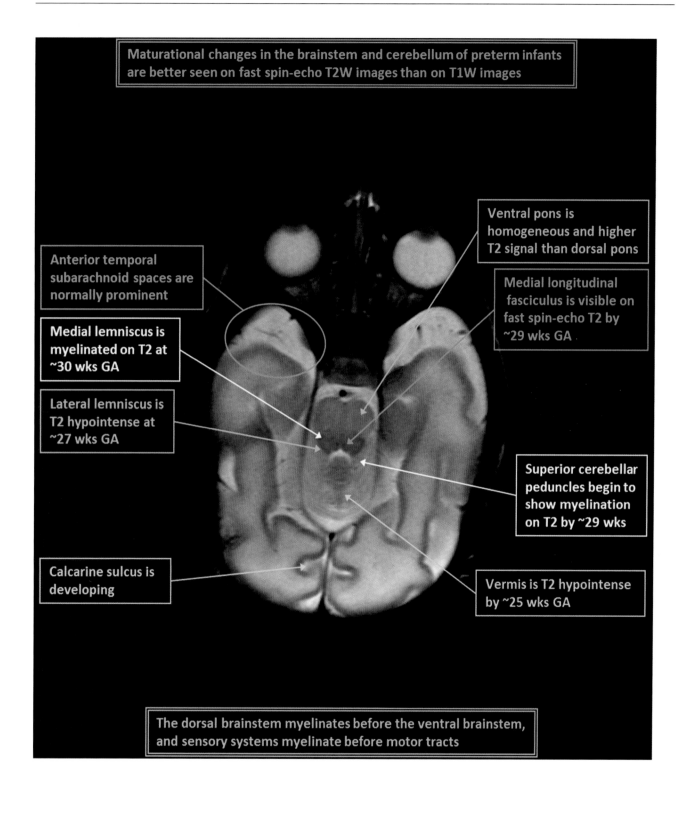

Maturational changes in the brainstem and cerebellum of preterm infants are better seen on fast spin-echo T2W images than on T1W images

Ventral pons is homogeneous and higher T2 signal than dorsal pons

Anterior temporal subarachnoid spaces are normally prominent

Medial longitudinal fasciculus is visible on fast spin-echo T2 by ~29 wks GA

Medial lemniscus is myelinated on T2 at ~30 wks GA

Lateral lemniscus is T2 hypointense at ~27 wks GA

Superior cerebellar peduncles begin to show myelination on T2 by ~29 wks

Calcarine sulcus is developing

Vermis is T2 hypointense by ~25 wks GA

The dorsal brainstem myelinates before the ventral brainstem, and sensory systems myelinate before motor tracts

Maturational changes in the brainstem and cerebellum of preterm infants are better seen on fast spin–echo T2W images than on T1W images

The transverse cerebellar diameter (best measured on coronal T2W images) should be between ~34–43 mm by 32 weeks GA

Ventral pons is homogeneous and higher T2 signal than dorsal pons

Medial lemniscus is myelinated on T2 at ~30 wks GA (also region of trapezoid body/auditory fibers)

Medial longitudinal fasciculus is visible on fast spin-echo T2 by ~29 wks GA

Cranial nerve V fascicle

Middle cerebellar peduncles are unmyelinated

Region of nuclei of CN VII, VIII and spinal nucleus of CN V

Dorsal pons shows myelination in some gray matter nuclei and white matter tracts as early as ~25 wks GA on fast spin–echo T2

Dentate nuclei have a T2 hypointense rim by ~25 wks GA

Vermis is T2 hypointense by ~25 wks GA

The T2 hypointensity of gray matter nuclei is likely due to a combination of myelination, increased cellular density, and other complex changes that reduce free water content

Maturational changes in the brainstem and cerebellum of preterm infants are better seen on fast spin–echo T2W images than on T1W images

The transverse cerebellar diameter (best measured on coronal T2W images) should be between ~34–43 mm by 32 weeks GA

Medial longitudinal fasciculus is visible on fast spin–echo T2 by ~29 wks GA

Flocculus cerebelli are myelinated by term

Vestibular nuclei are T2 hypointense by ~25 wks GA

Dentate nuclei have a T2 hypointense rim by ~25 wks GA

CSF spaces around the brainstem and cerebellum are relatively large in infancy

Dorsal pons and medulla show myelination in some gray matter nuclei and white matter tracts as early as ~25 wks GA on fast spin-echo T2

Vermis is T2 hypointense by ~25 wks GA

The T2 hypointensity of gray matter nuclei is likely due to a combination of myelination, increased cellular density, and other complex changes that reduce free water content

32 Weeks, Diffusion Weighted Imaging (DWI) (b=1000 s/mm²)

In premature and term neonates, diffusion weighted images have a high contrast appearance due to the increased rate of diffusion in white matter compared to gray matter. As a result, most of the cerebral hemispheric white matter is hypointense compared to the brighter cerebral cortex, basal ganglia, and thalami.

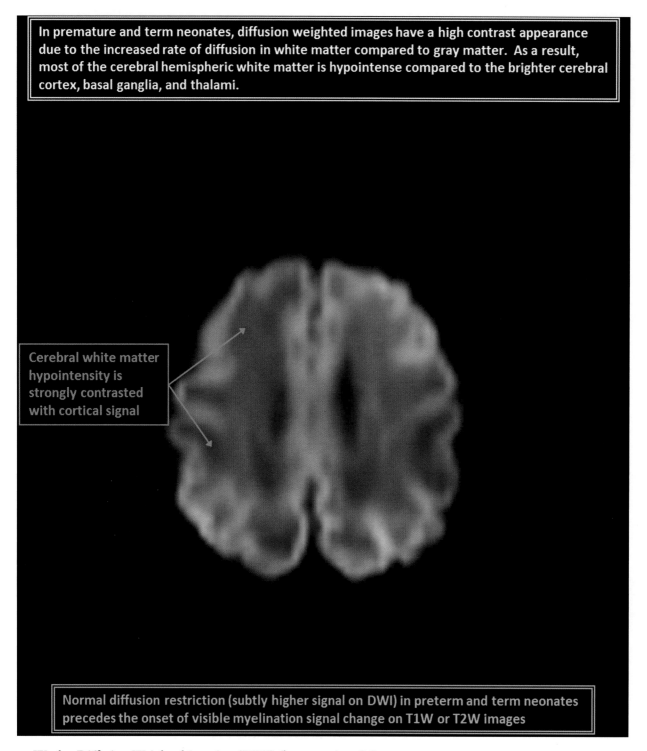

Cerebral white matter hypointensity is strongly contrasted with cortical signal

Normal diffusion restriction (subtly higher signal on DWI) in preterm and term neonates precedes the onset of visible myelination signal change on T1W or T2W images

32 Weeks, Diffusion Weighted Imaging (DWI) (b=1000 s/mm²) Images 1-5

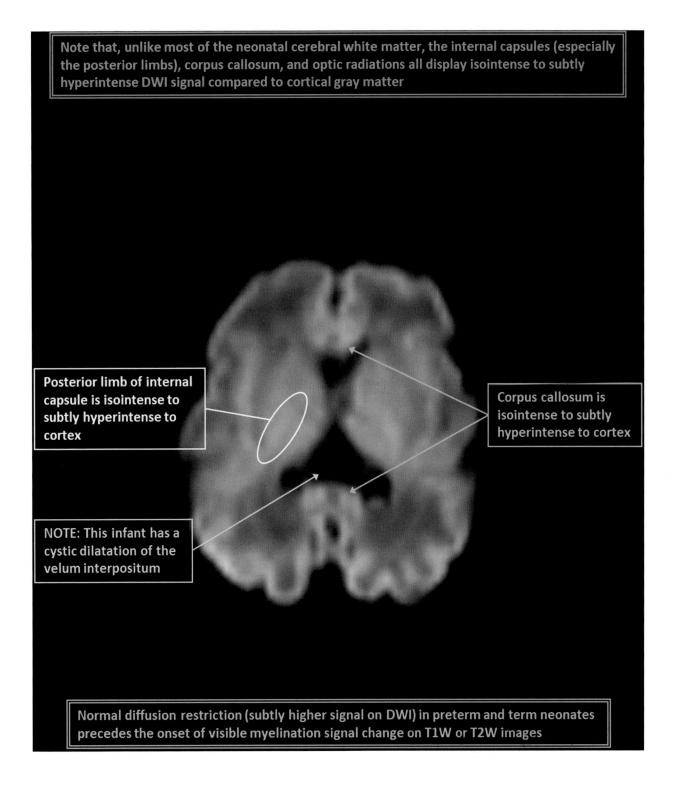

Note that, unlike most of the neonatal cerebral white matter, the internal capsules (especially the posterior limbs), corpus callosum, and optic radiations all display isointense to subtly hyperintense DWI signal compared to cortical gray matter

Posterior limb of internal capsule is isointense to subtly hyperintense to cortex

Corpus callosum is isointense to subtly hyperintense to cortex

NOTE: This infant has a cystic dilatation of the velum interpositum

Normal diffusion restriction (subtly higher signal on DWI) in preterm and term neonates precedes the onset of visible myelination signal change on T1W or T2W images

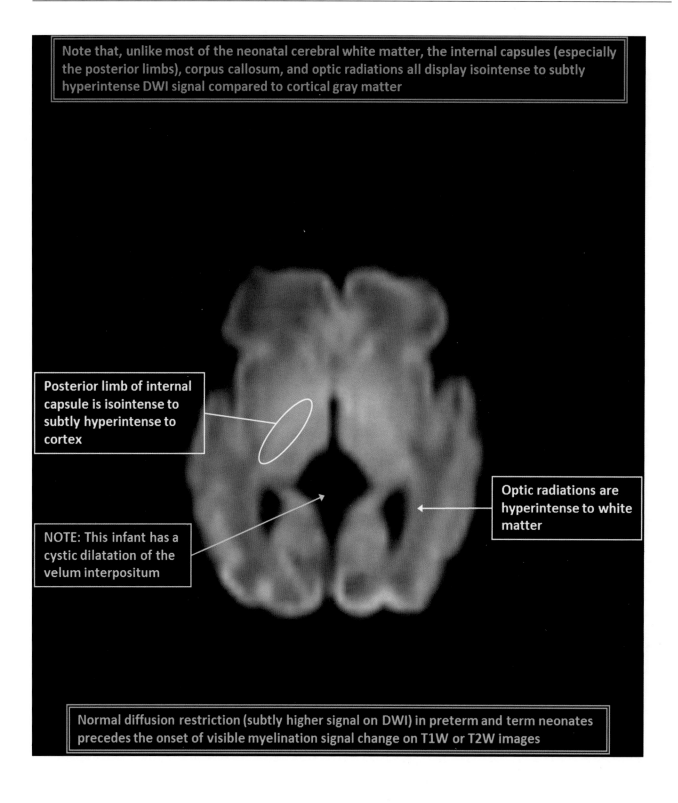

Note that, unlike most of the neonatal cerebral white matter, the internal capsules (especially the posterior limbs), corpus callosum, and optic radiations all display isointense to subtly hyperintense DWI signal compared to cortical gray matter

Posterior limb of internal capsule is isointense to subtly hyperintense to cortex

Optic radiations are hyperintense to white matter

NOTE: This infant has a cystic dilatation of the velum interpositum

Normal diffusion restriction (subtly higher signal on DWI) in preterm and term neonates precedes the onset of visible myelination signal change on T1W or T2W images

Note that, unlike most of the neonatal cerebral white matter, the internal capsules (especially the posterior limbs), corpus callosum, and optic radiations all display isointense to subtly hyperintense DWI signal compared to cortical gray matter

Normal diffusion restriction (subtly higher signal on DWI) in preterm and term neonates precedes the onset of visible myelination signal change on T1W or T2W images

For most of the first year of life, the cerebellum as a whole can have a noticeably more hypointense appearance on ADC than the cerebral hemispheres, while on DWI it is isointense to subtly hyperintense to the cerebrum

Slightly brighter DWI signal in the vermis and dentate nuclei compared to remainder of cerebellum

Normal diffusion restriction (subtly higher signal on DWI) in preterm and term neonates precedes the onset of visible myelination signal change on T1W or T2W images

32 Weeks, Apparent Diffusion Coefficient (ADC) Map

In premature and term neonates, ADC images have a high contrast appearance due to the increased rate of diffusion in white matter compared to gray matter. As a result, most of the cerebral hemispheric white matter is hyperintense compared to the darker cerebral cortex, basal ganglia, and thalami.

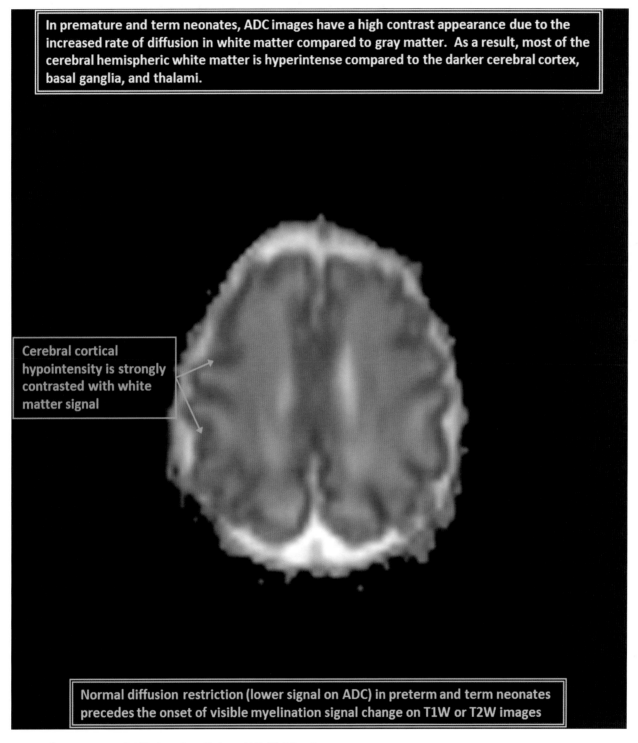

Cerebral cortical hypointensity is strongly contrasted with white matter signal

Normal diffusion restriction (lower signal on ADC) in preterm and term neonates precedes the onset of visible myelination signal change on T1W or T2W images

32 Weeks, Apparent Diffusion Coefficient (ADC) Map Images 1–5

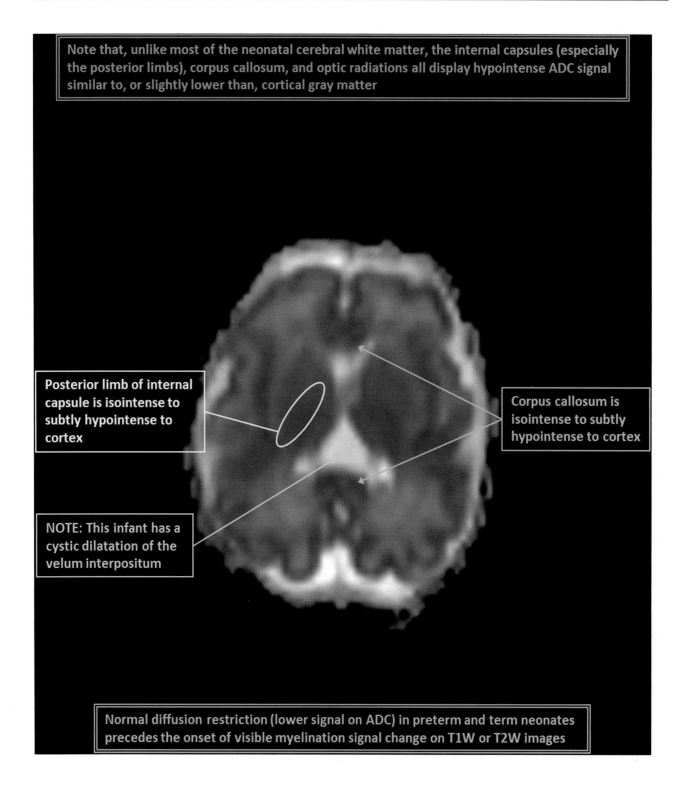

Note that, unlike most of the neonatal cerebral white matter, the internal capsules (especially the posterior limbs), corpus callosum, and optic radiations all display hypointense ADC signal similar to, or slightly lower than, cortical gray matter

Posterior limb of internal capsule is isointense to subtly hypointense to cortex

Corpus callosum is isointense to subtly hypointense to cortex

NOTE: This infant has a cystic dilatation of the velum interpositum

Normal diffusion restriction (lower signal on ADC) in preterm and term neonates precedes the onset of visible myelination signal change on T1W or T2W images

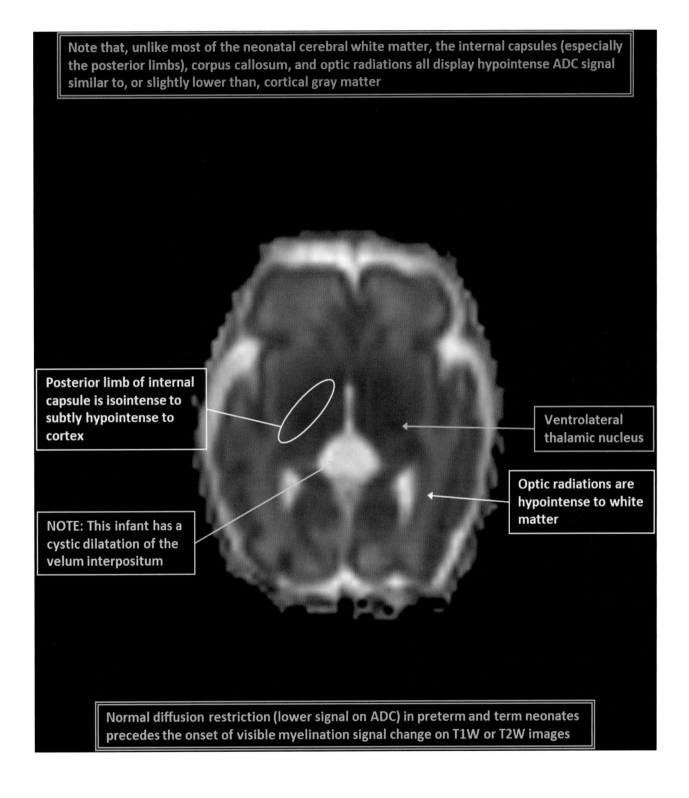

Note that, unlike most of the neonatal cerebral white matter, the internal capsules (especially the posterior limbs), corpus callosum, and optic radiations all display hypointense ADC signal similar to, or slightly lower than, cortical gray matter

Posterior limb of internal capsule is isointense to subtly hypointense to cortex

Ventrolateral thalamic nucleus

Optic radiations are hypointense to white matter

NOTE: This infant has a cystic dilatation of the velum interpositum

Normal diffusion restriction (lower signal on ADC) in preterm and term neonates precedes the onset of visible myelination signal change on T1W or T2W images

Note that, unlike most of the neonatal cerebral white matter, the internal capsules (especially the posterior limbs), corpus callosum, and optic radiations all display hypointense ADC signal similar to, or slightly lower than, cortical gray matter

The normal premature and term infant brainstem has areas of mildly more hypointense signal on ADC, mainly dorsally and in the central tegmentum of the midbrain

For most of the first year of life, the cerebellum as a whole can have a noticeably more hypointense appearance on ADC than the cerebral hemispheres, while on DWI it is isointense to subtly hyperintense to the cerebrum

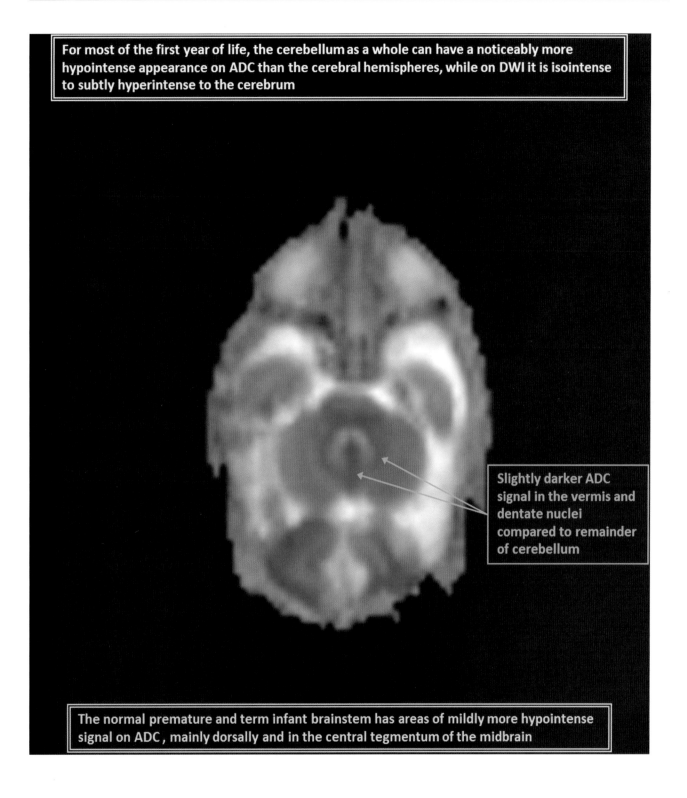

Slightly darker ADC signal in the vermis and dentate nuclei compared to remainder of cerebellum

The normal premature and term infant brainstem has areas of mildly more hypointense signal on ADC, mainly dorsally and in the central tegmentum of the midbrain

32 Weeks, Sagittal T1

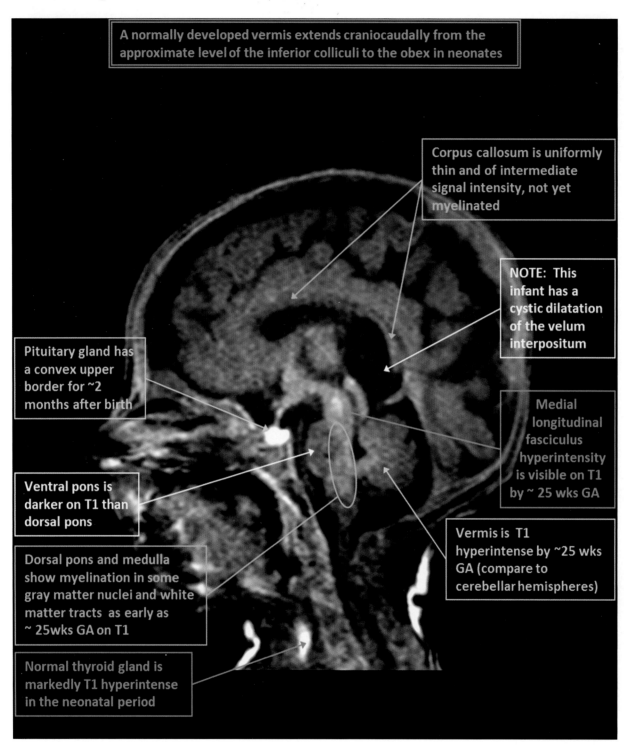

A normally developed vermis extends craniocaudally from the approximate level of the inferior colliculi to the obex in neonates

Corpus callosum is uniformly thin and of intermediate signal intensity, not yet myelinated

NOTE: This infant has a cystic dilatation of the velum interpositum

Pituitary gland has a convex upper border for ~2 months after birth

Medial longitudinal fasciculus hyperintensity is visible on T1 by ~ 25 wks GA

Ventral pons is darker on T1 than dorsal pons

Vermis is T1 hyperintense by ~25 wks GA (compare to cerebellar hemispheres)

Dorsal pons and medulla show myelination in some gray matter nuclei and white matter tracts as early as ~ 25wks GA on T1

Normal thyroid gland is markedly T1 hyperintense in the neonatal period

32 Weeks, Sagittal T1 Images 1–4

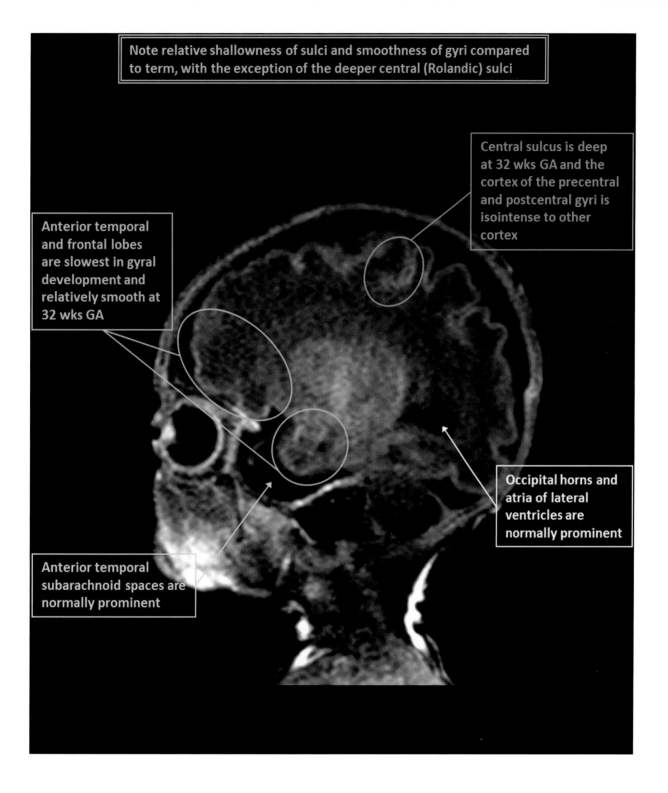

Note relative shallowness of sulci and smoothness of gyri compared to term, with the exception of the deeper central (Rolandic) sulci

Central sulcus is deep at 32 wks GA and the cortex of the precentral and postcentral gyri is isointense to other cortex

Anterior temporal and frontal lobes are slowest in gyral development and relatively smooth at 32 wks GA

Occipital horns and atria of lateral ventricles are normally prominent

Anterior temporal subarachnoid spaces are normally prominent

32 Weeks, Coronal TSE T2

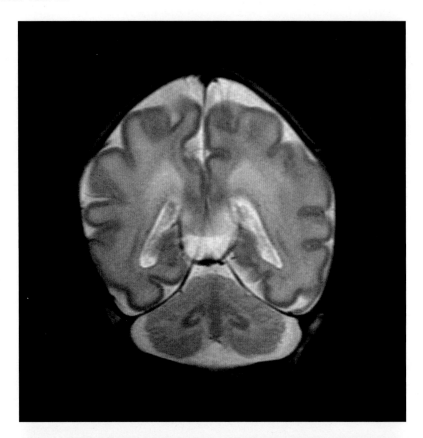

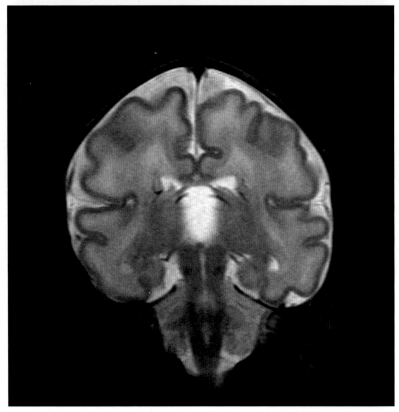

32 Weeks, Coronal TSE T2 Images 1–4

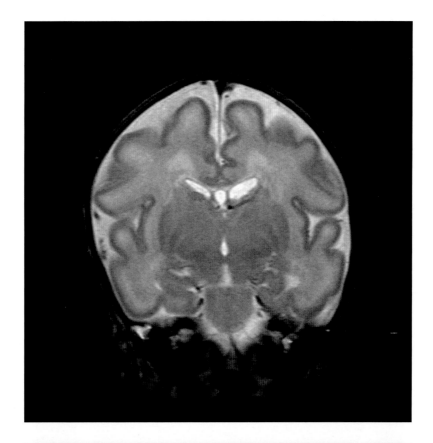

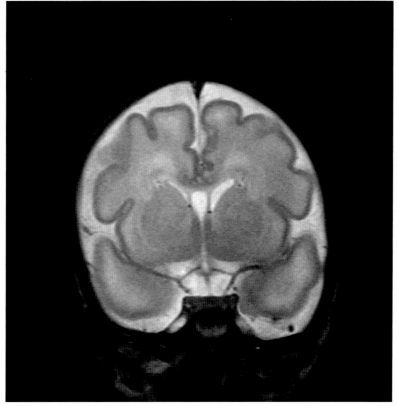

35 Weeks, Axial T1

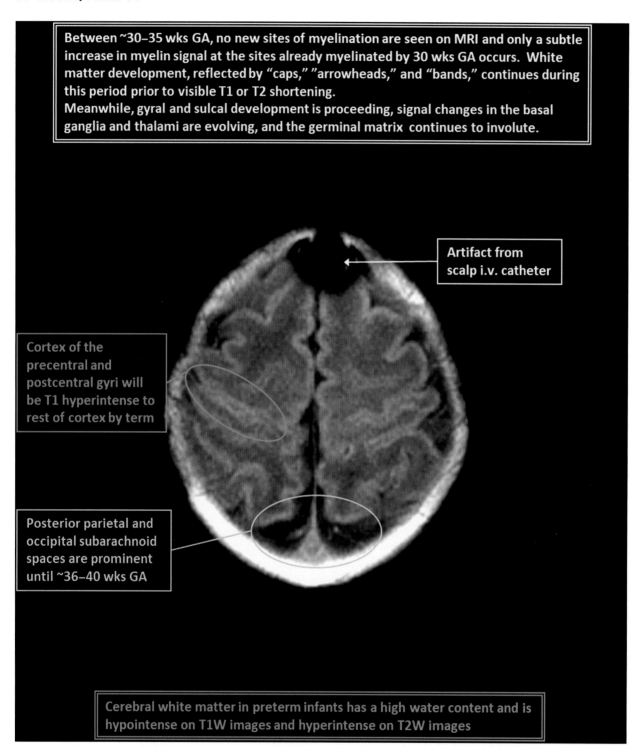

Between ~30–35 wks GA, no new sites of myelination are seen on MRI and only a subtle increase in myelin signal at the sites already myelinated by 30 wks GA occurs. White matter development, reflected by "caps," "arrowheads," and "bands," continues during this period prior to visible T1 or T2 shortening.

Meanwhile, gyral and sulcal development is proceeding, signal changes in the basal ganglia and thalami are evolving, and the germinal matrix continues to involute.

Artifact from scalp i.v. catheter

Cortex of the precentral and postcentral gyri will be T1 hyperintense to rest of cortex by term

Posterior parietal and occipital subarachnoid spaces are prominent until ~36–40 wks GA

Cerebral white matter in preterm infants has a high water content and is hypointense on T1W images and hyperintense on T2W images

35 Weeks, Axial T1 Images 1–10

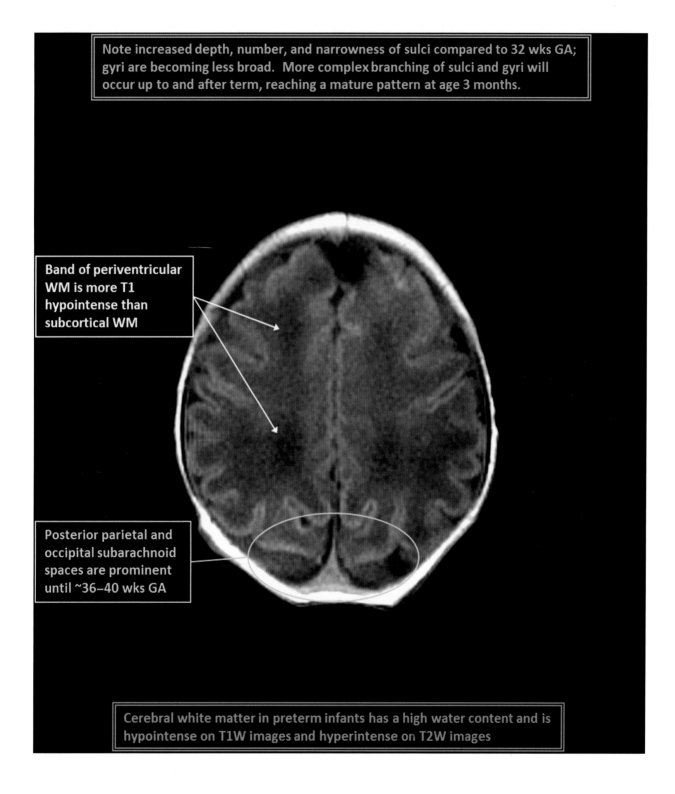

Note increased depth, number, and narrowness of sulci compared to 32 wks GA; gyri are becoming less broad. More complex branching of sulci and gyri will occur up to and after term, reaching a mature pattern at age 3 months.

Band of periventricular WM is more T1 hypointense than subcortical WM

Posterior parietal and occipital subarachnoid spaces are prominent until ~36–40 wks GA

Cerebral white matter in preterm infants has a high water content and is hypointense on T1W images and hyperintense on T2W images

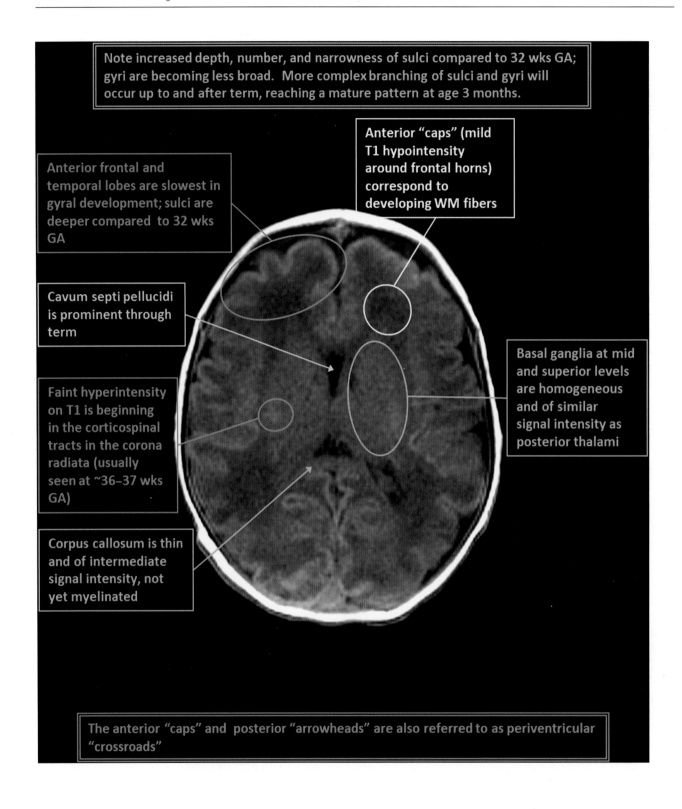

Note increased depth, number, and narrowness of sulci compared to 32 wks GA; gyri are becoming less broad. More complex branching of sulci and gyri will occur up to and after term, reaching a mature pattern at age 3 months.

Anterior "caps" (mild T1 hypointensity around frontal horns) correspond to developing WM fibers

Anterior frontal and temporal lobes are slowest in gyral development; sulci are deeper compared to 32 wks GA

Cavum septi pellucidi is prominent through term

Basal ganglia at mid and superior levels are homogeneous and of similar signal intensity as posterior thalami

Faint hyperintensity on T1 is beginning in the corticospinal tracts in the corona radiata (usually seen at ~36–37 wks GA)

Corpus callosum is thin and of intermediate signal intensity, not yet myelinated

The anterior "caps" and posterior "arrowheads" are also referred to as periventricular "crossroads"

Note increased depth, number, and narrowness of sulci compared to 32 wks GA; gyri are becoming less broad. More complex branching of sulci and gyri will occur up to and after term, reaching a mature pattern at age 3 months.

Anterior "caps" (mild T1 hypointensity around frontal horns) correspond to developing WM fibers

Central mild T1 hyperintensity within the caps corresponds to migrating cells, or remnants of, from the germinal matrix or subependymal layer

Cavum septi pellucidi is prominent through term

Caudate and anterior putamen at mid and superior levels are homogeneous

Posterior 1/3 of the PLIC is isointense with the lentiform nuclei in this 35 wk infant ; it typically becomes T1 hyperintense at ~36–37 wks GA

Ventrolateral thalamic nuclei are T1 hyperintense (although better seen on T2)

Parietooccipital sulci are increasingly complex compared to 32 wks GA

Posterior thalami are homogeneous and of intermediate T1 signal intensity

The anterior "caps" and posterior "arrowheads" are also referred to as periventricular "crossroads"

Note increased depth, number, and narrowness of sulci compared to 32 wks GA; gyri are becoming less broad. More complex branching of sulci and gyri will occur up to and after term, reaching a mature pattern at age 3 months.

Anterior "caps" (mild T1 hypointensity around frontal horns) correspond to developing WM fibers

Central mild T1 hyperintensity within the caps corresponds to migrating cells, or remnants of, from the germinal matrix or subependymal layer

ALIC is hypointense

Globi pallidi are diffusely T1 hyperintense by ~35 wks GA and more so than posterior inferior putamina

Caudate and anterior putamen are homogeneous

Posterior 1/3 of the PLIC is isointense with the lentiform nuclei in this 35 wk infant ; it typically becomes T1 hyperintense at ~36–37 wks GA

Ventrolateral thalamic nuclei are T1 hyperintense (although better seen on T2)

Occipital sulci are more complex compared to 32 wks GA

Posterior thalami are homogeneous and of intermediate T1 signal intensity

The anterior "caps" and posterior "arrowheads" are also referred to as periventricular "crossroads"

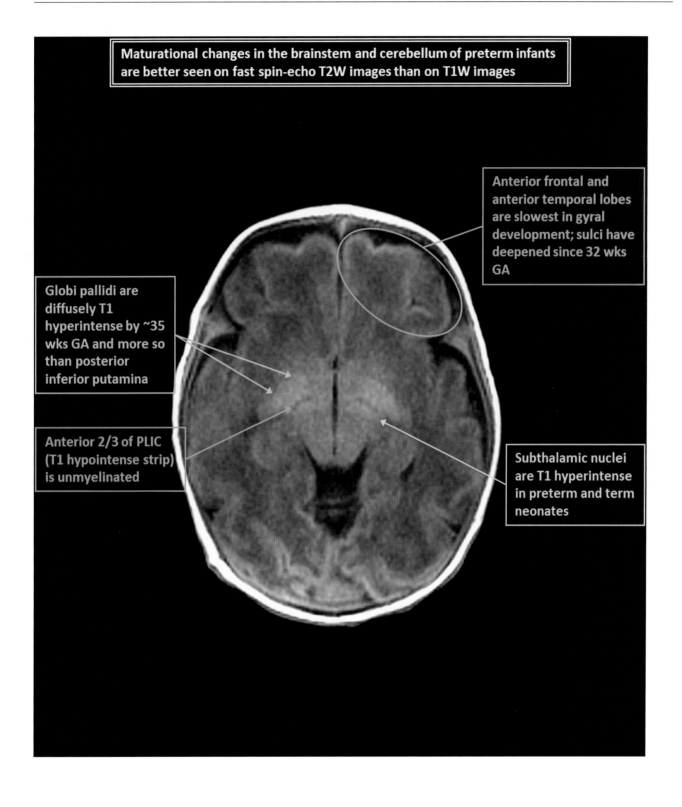

Maturational changes in the brainstem and cerebellum of preterm infants are better seen on fast spin-echo T2W images than on T1W images

Anterior frontal and anterior temporal lobes are slowest in gyral development; sulci have deepened since 32 wks GA

Globi pallidi are diffusely T1 hyperintense by ~35 wks GA and more so than posterior inferior putamina

Anterior 2/3 of PLIC (T1 hypointense strip) is unmyelinated

Subthalamic nuclei are T1 hyperintense in preterm and term neonates

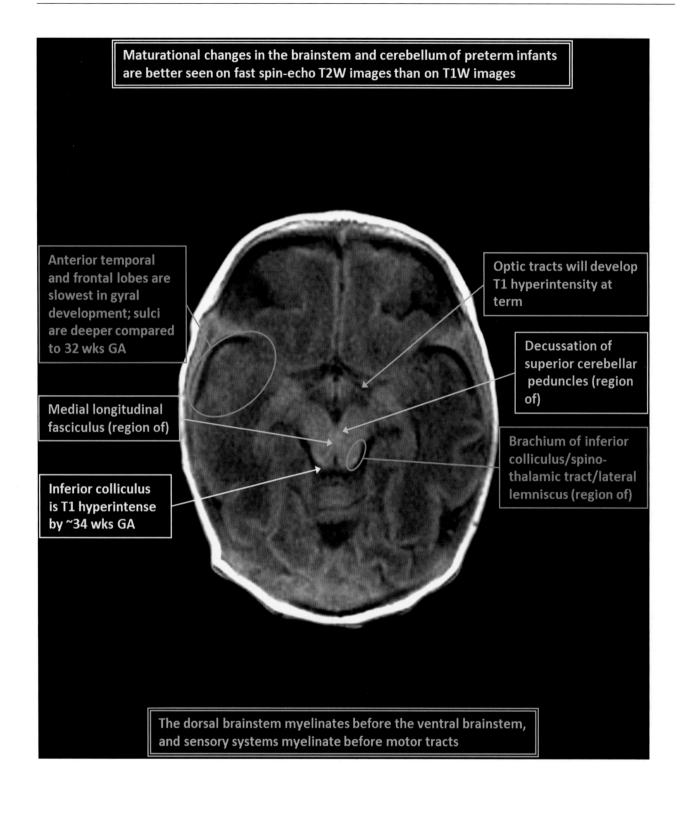

Maturational changes in the brainstem and cerebellum of preterm infants are better seen on fast spin-echo T2W images than on T1W images

Anterior temporal and frontal lobes are slowest in gyral development; sulci are deeper compared to 32 wks GA

Optic tracts will develop T1 hyperintensity at term

Decussation of superior cerebellar peduncles (region of)

Medial longitudinal fasciculus (region of)

Brachium of inferior colliculus/spino-thalamic tract/lateral lemniscus (region of)

Inferior colliculus is T1 hyperintense by ~34 wks GA

The dorsal brainstem myelinates before the ventral brainstem, and sensory systems myelinate before motor tracts

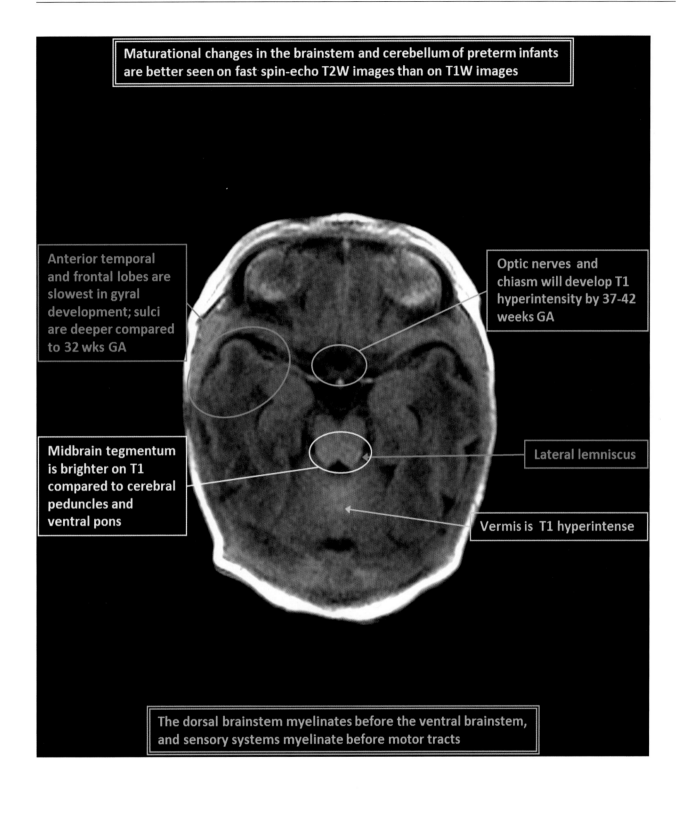

Maturational changes in the brainstem and cerebellum of preterm infants are better seen on fast spin-echo T2W images than on T1W images

Anterior temporal and frontal lobes are slowest in gyral development; sulci are deeper compared to 32 wks GA

Optic nerves and chiasm will develop T1 hyperintensity by 37-42 weeks GA

Midbrain tegmentum is brighter on T1 compared to cerebral peduncles and ventral pons

Lateral lemniscus

Vermis is T1 hyperintense

The dorsal brainstem myelinates before the ventral brainstem, and sensory systems myelinate before motor tracts

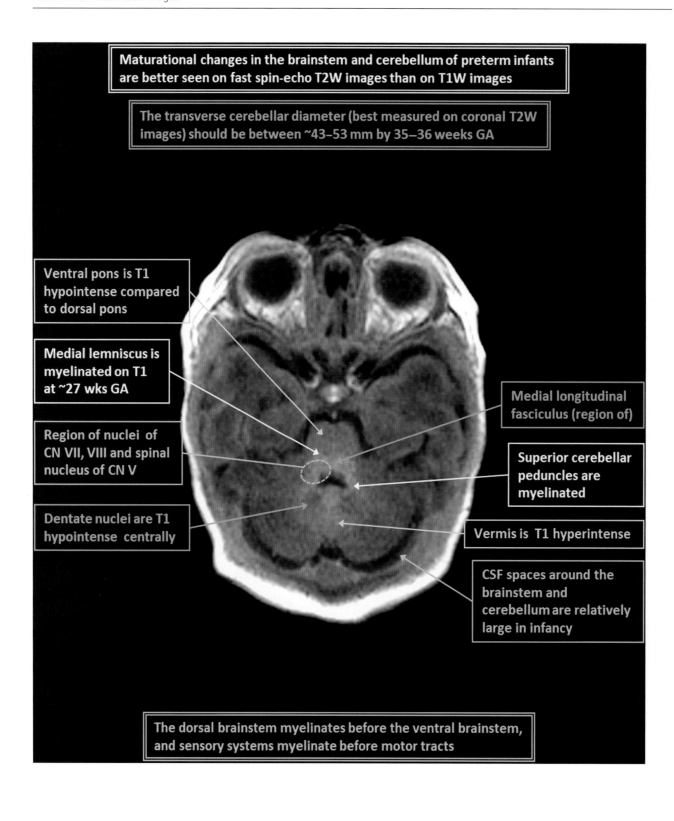

Maturational changes in the brainstem and cerebellum of preterm infants are better seen on fast spin-echo T2W images than on T1W images

The transverse cerebellar diameter (best measured on coronal T2W images) should be between ~43–53 mm by 35–36 weeks GA

Ventral pons is T1 hypointense compared to dorsal pons

Medial lemniscus is myelinated on T1 at ~27 wks GA

Region of nuclei of CN VII, VIII and spinal nucleus of CN V

Dentate nuclei are T1 hypointense centrally

Medial longitudinal fasciculus (region of)

Superior cerebellar peduncles are myelinated

Vermis is T1 hyperintense

CSF spaces around the brainstem and cerebellum are relatively large in infancy

The dorsal brainstem myelinates before the ventral brainstem, and sensory systems myelinate before motor tracts

Maturational changes in the brainstem and cerebellum of preterm infants are better seen on fast spin-echo T2W images than on T1W images

The transverse cerebellar diameter (best measured on coronal T2W images) should be between ~43–53 mm by 35–36 weeks GA

Medial lemniscus is myelinated on T1 at ~27 wks GA

Flocculus cerebelli are myelinated by term

Dorsal pons and medulla are T1 hyperintense by 32 wks due to myelination in some gray matter nuclei and white matter tracts

Medial longitudinal fasciculus (region of)

CSF spaces around the brainstem and cerebellum are relatively large in infancy

The dorsal brainstem myelinates before the ventral brainstem, and sensory systems myelinate before motor tracts

35 Weeks, Axial TSE T2

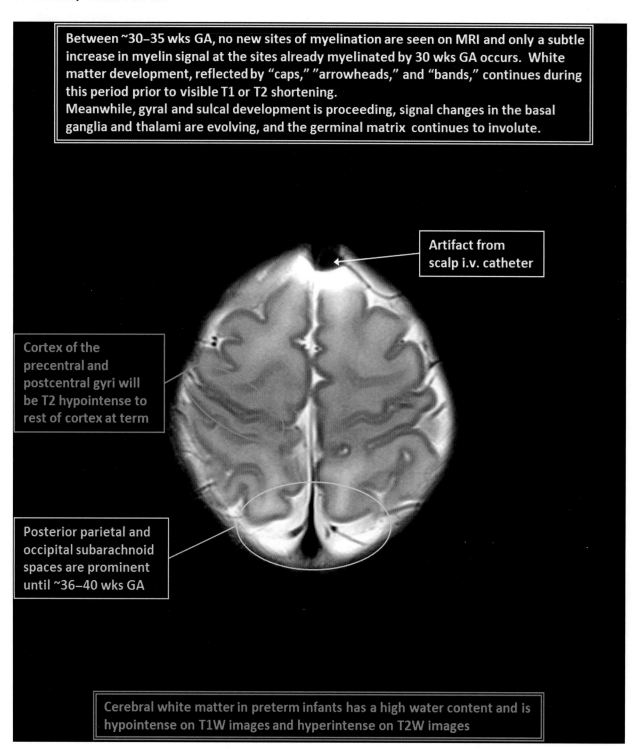

Between ~30–35 wks GA, no new sites of myelination are seen on MRI and only a subtle increase in myelin signal at the sites already myelinated by 30 wks GA occurs. White matter development, reflected by "caps," "arrowheads," and "bands," continues during this period prior to visible T1 or T2 shortening.

Meanwhile, gyral and sulcal development is proceeding, signal changes in the basal ganglia and thalami are evolving, and the germinal matrix continues to involute.

Artifact from scalp i.v. catheter

Cortex of the precentral and postcentral gyri will be T2 hypointense to rest of cortex at term

Posterior parietal and occipital subarachnoid spaces are prominent until ~36–40 wks GA

Cerebral white matter in preterm infants has a high water content and is hypointense on T1W images and hyperintense on T2W images

35 Weeks, Axial TSE T2 Images 1–10

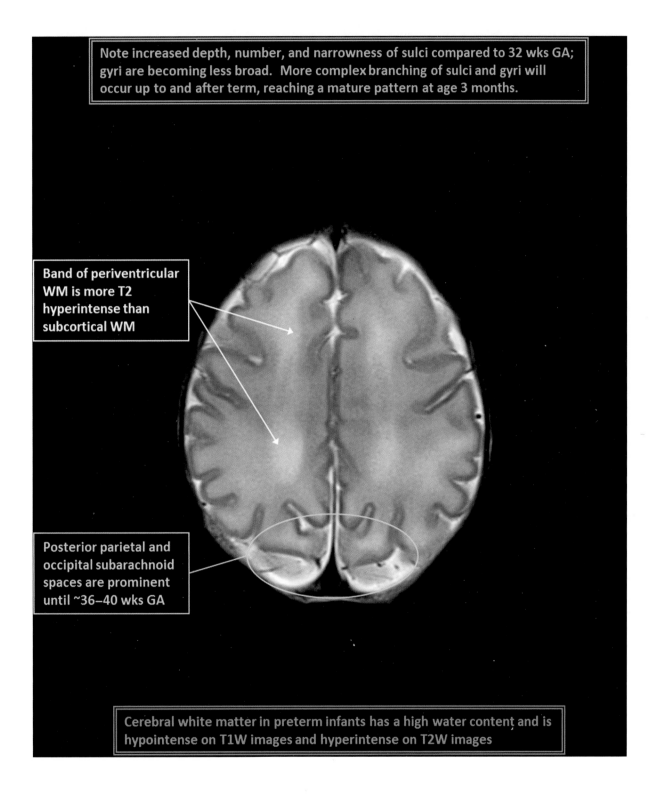

Note increased depth, number, and narrowness of sulci compared to 32 wks GA; gyri are becoming less broad. More complex branching of sulci and gyri will occur up to and after term, reaching a mature pattern at age 3 months.

Band of periventricular WM is more T2 hyperintense than subcortical WM

Posterior parietal and occipital subarachnoid spaces are prominent until ~36–40 wks GA

Cerebral white matter in preterm infants has a high water content and is hypointense on T1W images and hyperintense on T2W images

Note increased depth, number, and narrowness of sulci compared to 32 wks GA; gyri are becoming less broad. More complex branching of sulci and gyri will occur up to and after term, reaching a mature pattern at age 3 months.

Anterior "caps" (mild T2 hyperintensity around frontal horns) correspond to developing WM fibers

Anterior frontal and temporal lobes are slowest in gyral development; sulci are deeper compared to 32 wks GA

Cavum septi pellucidi is prominent through term

Subtle hypointensity in the corticospinal tracts in the corona radiata can be detected in this 35 wk GA infant

Basal ganglia at mid and superior levels are homogeneous and of similar signal intensity as posterior thalami

Corpus callosum is thin and of intermediate signal intensity, not yet myelinated

The anterior "caps" and posterior "arrowheads" are also referred to as periventricular "crossroads"

Note increased depth, number, and narrowness of sulci compared to 32 wks GA; gyri are becoming less broad. More complex branching of sulci and gyri will occur up to and after term, reaching a mature pattern at age 3 months.

Anterior "caps" (mild T2 hyperintensity around frontal horns) correspond to developing WM fibers

Central mild T2 hypointensity within the caps corresponds to migrating cells, or remnants of, from the germinal matrix or subependymal layer

Anterior limb of internal capsule is mildly T2 hyperintense

Insular sulci are more developed compared to 32 wks GA

Short strip of T2 hypointense myelin in posterior 1/3 of PLIC is present at term; its visibility in this 35 wk GA infant is likely due to fast spin-echo technique

Parietooccipital sulci are increasingly complex compared to 32 wks GA

Putamina are more T2 hypointense laterally than medially

Ventrolateral thalamic nuclei are distinctly T2 hypointense

Posterior thalami are homogeneous and of intermediate T2 signal intensity

Medial occipital lobe and Rolandic area gyral development is more advanced at all ages compared to other areas

The anterior "caps" and posterior "arrowheads" are also referred to as periventricular "crossroads"

Note increased depth, number, and narrowness of sulci compared to 32 wks GA; gyri are becoming less broad. More complex branching of sulci and gyri will occur up to and after term, reaching a mature pattern at age 3 months.

Anterior "caps" (mild T2 hyperintensity around frontal horns) correspond to developing WM fibers

Central mild T2 hypointensity within the caps corresponds to migrating cells, or remnants of, from the germinal matrix or subependymal layer

Residual germinal matrix (moderate T2 hypointensity) at tips of frontal horns

Insular sulci are more developed compared to 32 wks GA; Sylvian fissures remain prominent

Claustrum

Globi pallidi and posterior putamina are moderately T2 hypointense

Posterior 1/3 of PLIC does not consistently show myelination on T2 until term

Ventrolateral thalamic nuclei are distinctly T2 hypointense

Occipital sulci are more complex compared to 32 wks GA

Developing optic radiations are mildly hypointense on T2

The anterior "caps" and posterior "arrowheads" are also referred to as periventricular "crossroads"

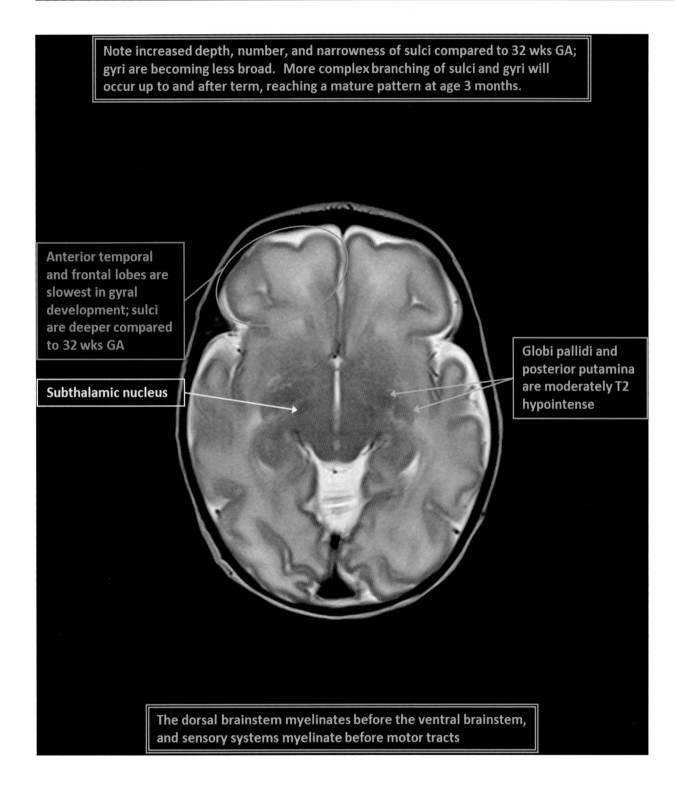

Note increased depth, number, and narrowness of sulci compared to 32 wks GA; gyri are becoming less broad. More complex branching of sulci and gyri will occur up to and after term, reaching a mature pattern at age 3 months.

Anterior temporal and frontal lobes are slowest in gyral development; sulci are deeper compared to 32 wks GA

Subthalamic nucleus

Globi pallidi and posterior putamina are moderately T2 hypointense

The dorsal brainstem myelinates before the ventral brainstem, and sensory systems myelinate before motor tracts

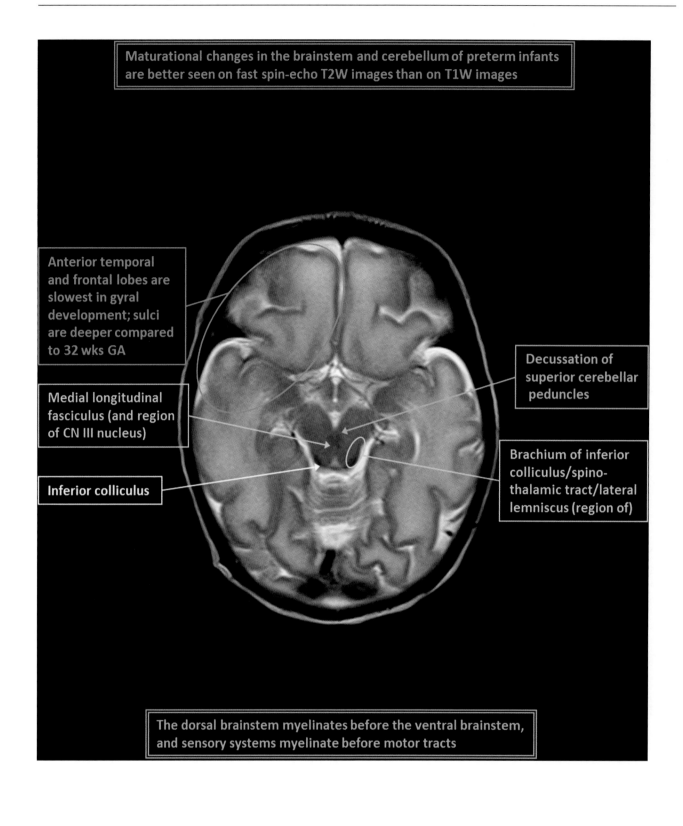

Maturational changes in the brainstem and cerebellum of preterm infants are better seen on fast spin-echo T2W images than on T1W images

Anterior temporal and frontal lobes are slowest in gyral development; sulci are deeper compared to 32 wks GA

Medial longitudinal fasciculus (and region of CN III nucleus)

Inferior colliculus

Decussation of superior cerebellar peduncles

Brachium of inferior colliculus/spino-thalamic tract/lateral lemniscus (region of)

The dorsal brainstem myelinates before the ventral brainstem, and sensory systems myelinate before motor tracts

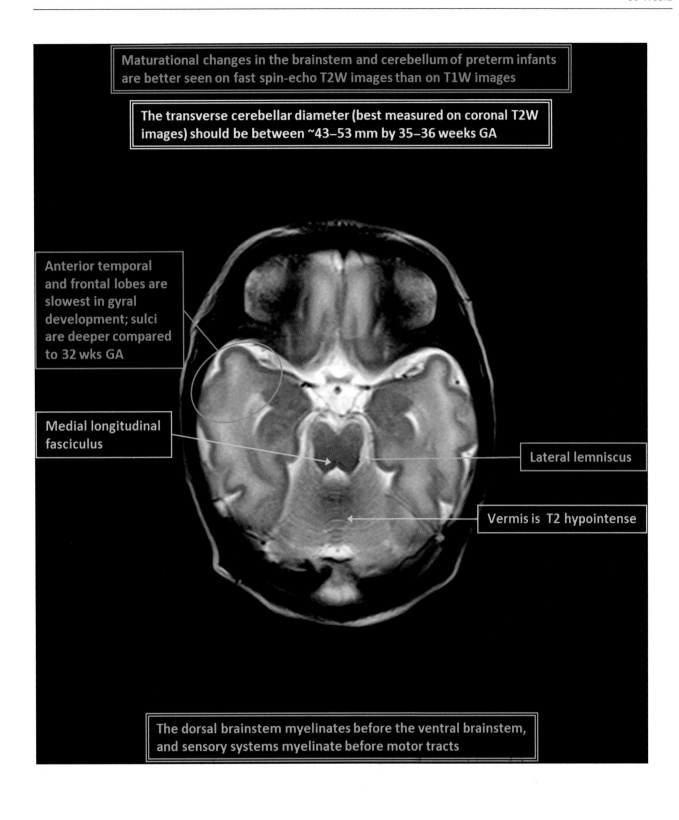

Maturational changes in the brainstem and cerebellum of preterm infants are better seen on fast spin-echo T2W images than on T1W images

The transverse cerebellar diameter (best measured on coronal T2W images) should be between ~43–53 mm by 35–36 weeks GA

Anterior temporal and frontal lobes are slowest in gyral development; sulci are deeper compared to 32 wks GA

Medial longitudinal fasciculus

Lateral lemniscus

Vermis is T2 hypointense

The dorsal brainstem myelinates before the ventral brainstem, and sensory systems myelinate before motor tracts

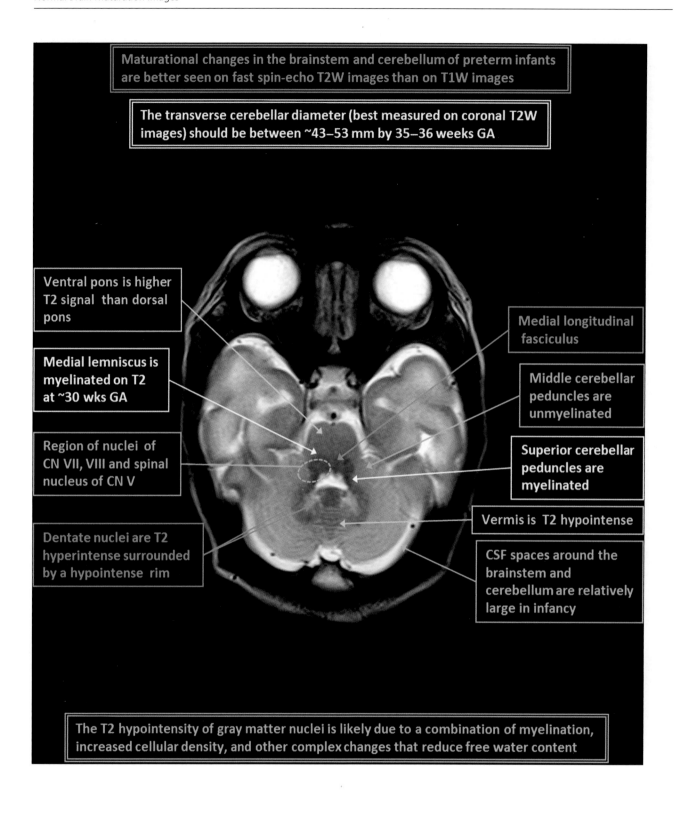

Maturational changes in the brainstem and cerebellum of preterm infants are better seen on fast spin-echo T2W images than on T1W images

The transverse cerebellar diameter (best measured on coronal T2W images) should be between ~43–53 mm by 35–36 weeks GA

Ventral pons is higher T2 signal than dorsal pons

Medial lemniscus is myelinated on T2 at ~30 wks GA

Region of nuclei of CN VII, VIII and spinal nucleus of CN V

Dentate nuclei are T2 hyperintense surrounded by a hypointense rim

Medial longitudinal fasciculus

Middle cerebellar peduncles are unmyelinated

Superior cerebellar peduncles are myelinated

Vermis is T2 hypointense

CSF spaces around the brainstem and cerebellum are relatively large in infancy

The T2 hypointensity of gray matter nuclei is likely due to a combination of myelination, increased cellular density, and other complex changes that reduce free water content

Maturational changes in the brainstem and cerebellum of preterm infants are better seen on fast spin-echo T2W images than on T1W images

The transverse cerebellar diameter (best measured on coronal T2W images) should be between ~43–53 mm by 35–36 weeks GA

Medial longitudinal fasciculus

Medial lemniscus is myelinated on T2 at ~30 wks GA

Vestibular nuclei

Flocculus cerebelli are myelinated by term

Dorsal pons and medulla are T2 hypointense due to myelination in some gray matter nuclei and white matter tracts

CSF spaces around the brainstem and cerebellum are relatively large in infancy

The T2 hypointensity of gray matter nuclei is likely due to a combination of myelination, increased cellular density, and other complex changes that reduce free water content

35 Weeks, Sagittal T1

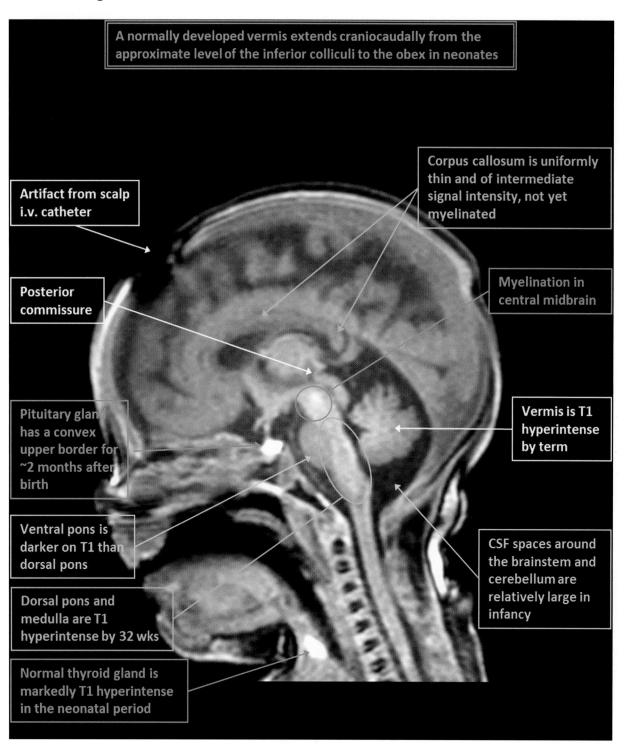

A normally developed vermis extends craniocaudally from the approximate level of the inferior colliculi to the obex in neonates

Artifact from scalp i.v. catheter

Posterior commissure

Pituitary gland has a convex upper border for ~2 months after birth

Ventral pons is darker on T1 than dorsal pons

Dorsal pons and medulla are T1 hyperintense by 32 wks

Normal thyroid gland is markedly T1 hyperintense in the neonatal period

Corpus callosum is uniformly thin and of intermediate signal intensity, not yet myelinated

Myelination in central midbrain

Vermis is T1 hyperintense by term

CSF spaces around the brainstem and cerebellum are relatively large in infancy

35 Weeks, Sagittal T1 Images 1-4

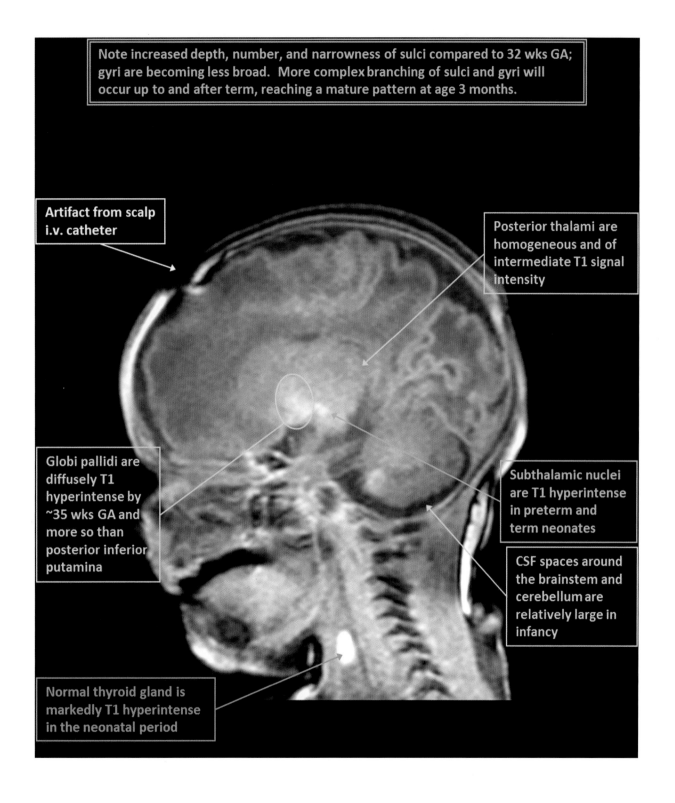

Note increased depth, number, and narrowness of sulci compared to 32 wks GA; gyri are becoming less broad. More complex branching of sulci and gyri will occur up to and after term, reaching a mature pattern at age 3 months.

Artifact from scalp i.v. catheter

Posterior thalami are homogeneous and of intermediate T1 signal intensity

Globi pallidi are diffusely T1 hyperintense by ~35 wks GA and more so than posterior inferior putamina

Subthalamic nuclei are T1 hyperintense in preterm and term neonates

CSF spaces around the brainstem and cerebellum are relatively large in infancy

Normal thyroid gland is markedly T1 hyperintense in the neonatal period

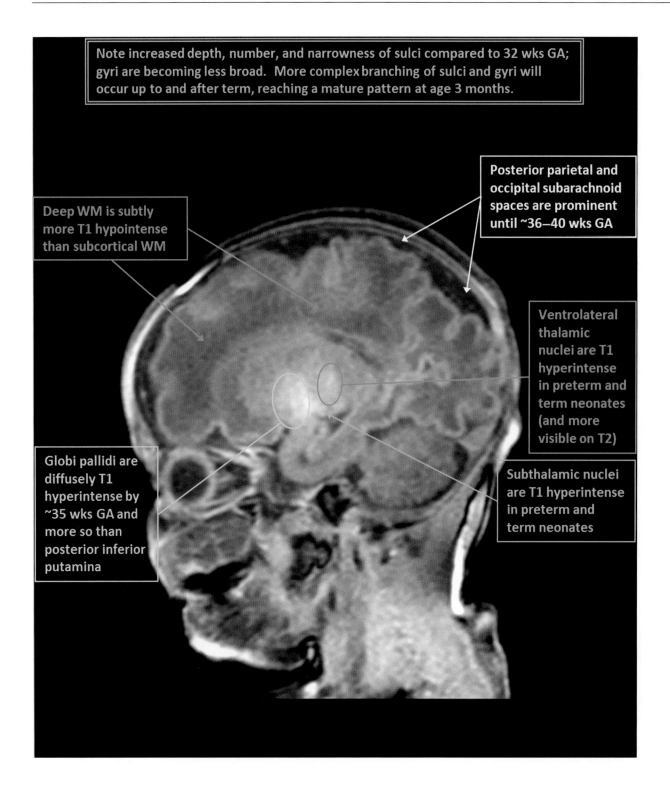

Note increased depth, number, and narrowness of sulci compared to 32 wks GA; gyri are becoming less broad. More complex branching of sulci and gyri will occur up to and after term, reaching a mature pattern at age 3 months.

Posterior parietal and occipital subarachnoid spaces are prominent until ~36–40 wks GA

Deep WM is subtly more T1 hypointense than subcortical WM

Ventrolateral thalamic nuclei are T1 hyperintense in preterm and term neonates (and more visible on T2)

Globi pallidi are diffusely T1 hyperintense by ~35 wks GA and more so than posterior inferior putamina

Subthalamic nuclei are T1 hyperintense in preterm and term neonates

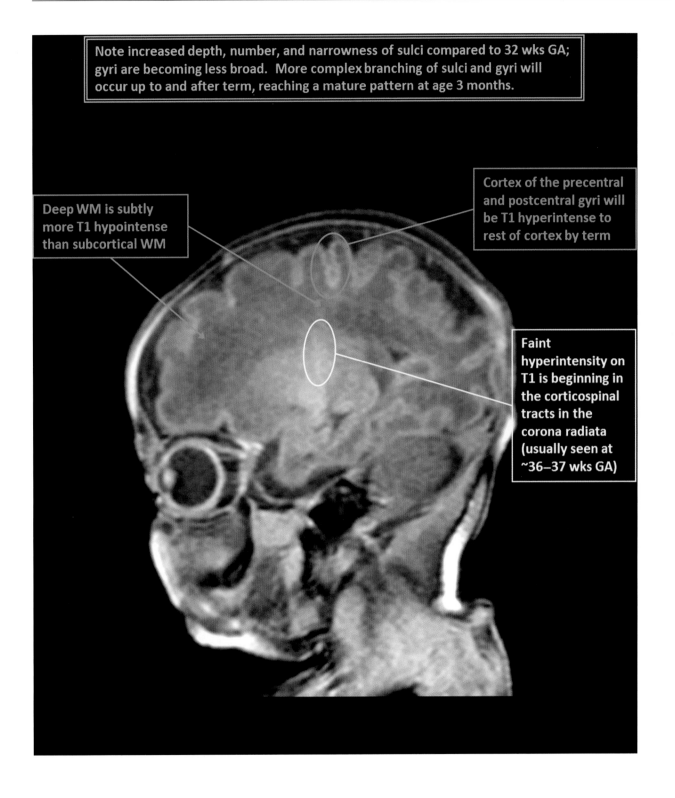

Note increased depth, number, and narrowness of sulci compared to 32 wks GA; gyri are becoming less broad. More complex branching of sulci and gyri will occur up to and after term, reaching a mature pattern at age 3 months.

Cortex of the precentral and postcentral gyri will be T1 hyperintense to rest of cortex by term

Deep WM is subtly more T1 hypointense than subcortical WM

Faint hyperintensity on T1 is beginning in the corticospinal tracts in the corona radiata (usually seen at ~36–37 wks GA)

35 Weeks, Coronal TSE T2

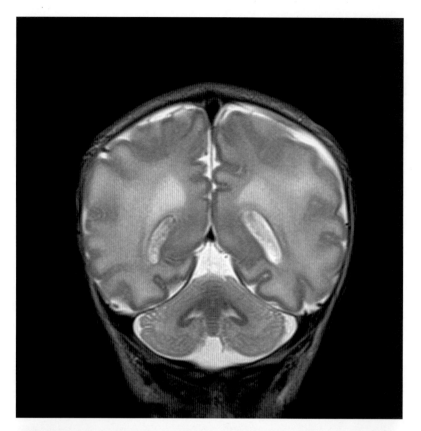

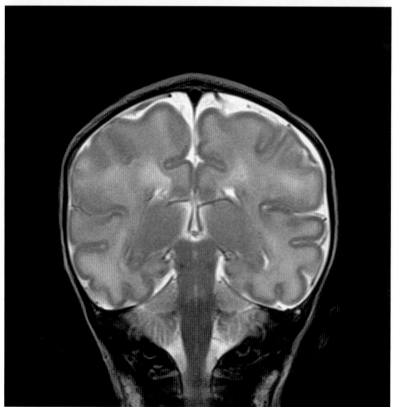

35 Weeks, Coronal TSE T2 Images 1–4

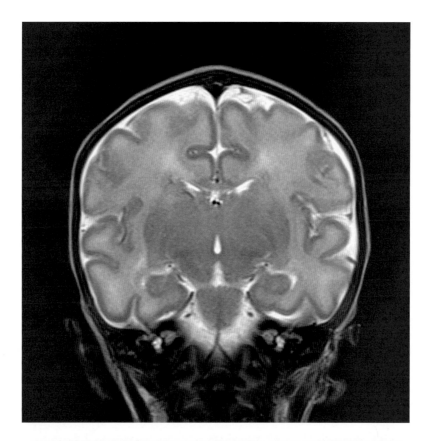

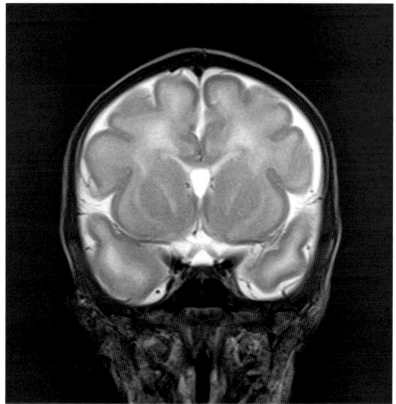

40 Weeks, Axial T1

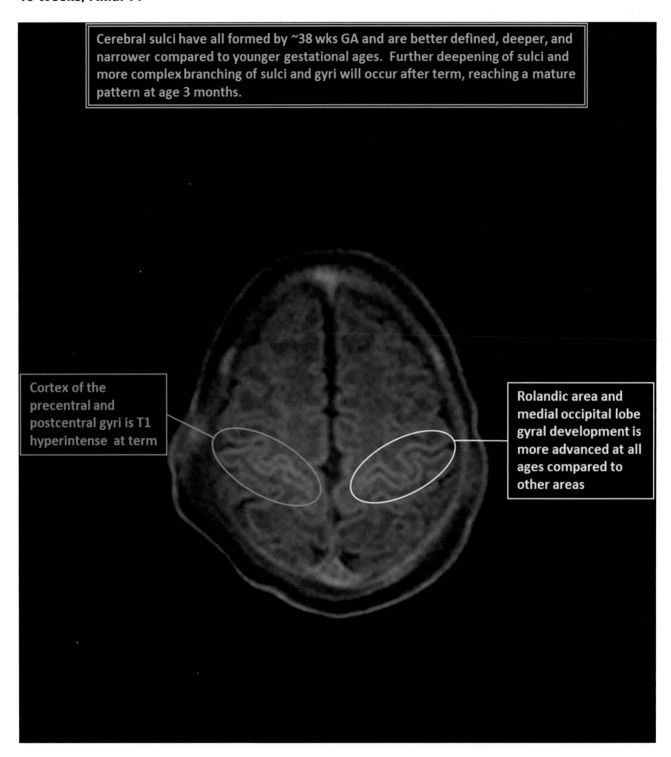

Cerebral sulci have all formed by ~38 wks GA and are better defined, deeper, and narrower compared to younger gestational ages. Further deepening of sulci and more complex branching of sulci and gyri will occur after term, reaching a mature pattern at age 3 months.

Cortex of the precentral and postcentral gyri is T1 hyperintense at term

Rolandic area and medial occipital lobe gyral development is more advanced at all ages compared to other areas

40 Weeks, Axial T1 Images 1–12

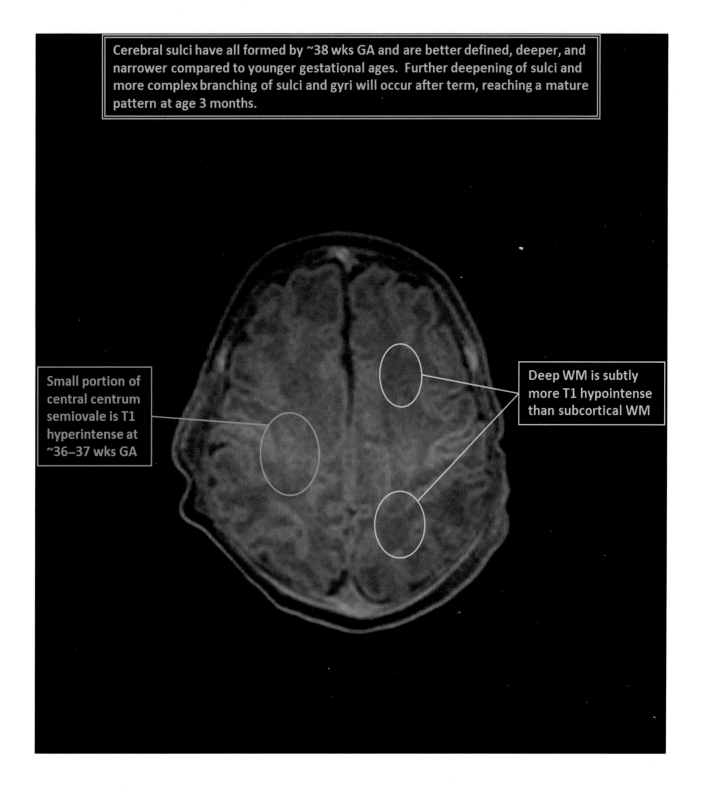

Cerebral sulci have all formed by ~38 wks GA and are better defined, deeper, and narrower compared to younger gestational ages. Further deepening of sulci and more complex branching of sulci and gyri will occur after term, reaching a mature pattern at age 3 months.

Small portion of central centrum semiovale is T1 hyperintense at ~36–37 wks GA

Deep WM is subtly more T1 hypointense than subcortical WM

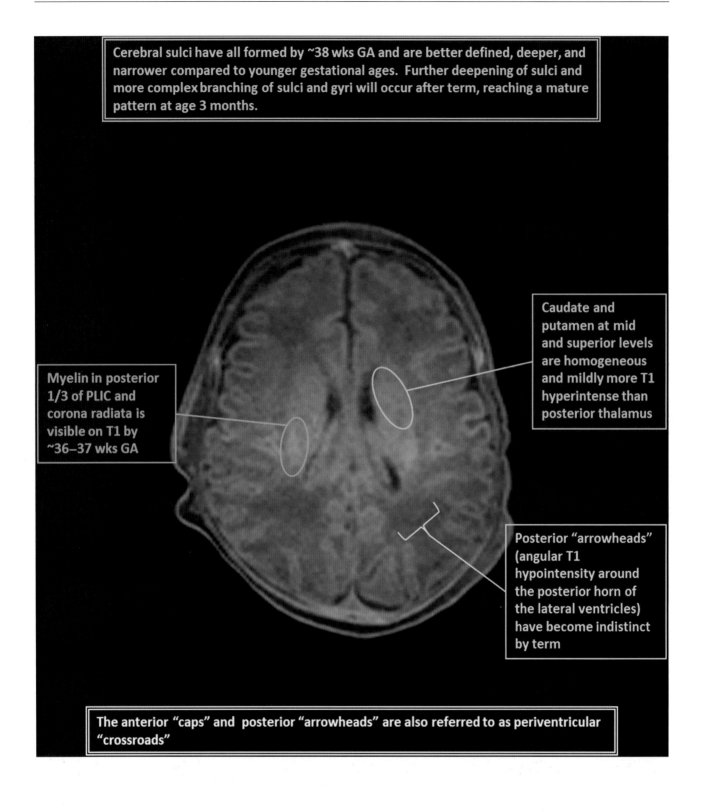

Cerebral sulci have all formed by ~38 wks GA and are better defined, deeper, and narrower compared to younger gestational ages. Further deepening of sulci and more complex branching of sulci and gyri will occur after term, reaching a mature pattern at age 3 months.

Caudate and putamen at mid and superior levels are homogeneous and mildly more T1 hyperintense than posterior thalamus

Myelin in posterior 1/3 of PLIC and corona radiata is visible on T1 by ~36–37 wks GA

Posterior "arrowheads" (angular T1 hypointensity around the posterior horn of the lateral ventricles) have become indistinct by term

The anterior "caps" and posterior "arrowheads" are also referred to as periventricular "crossroads"

The basal ganglia and thalami are relatively large at term compared to the rest of the cerebral hemispheres

Anterior temporal and frontal lobes are slowest in gyral development; sulci are deeper and more branched compared to 35 wks GA

Globi pallidi are diffusely T1 hyperintense by ~35 wks GA and more so than posterior inferior putamina

Caudate and putamen at mid and superior levels are homogeneous and mildly more T1 hyperintense than posterior thalamus

Anterior 2/3 of PLIC (T1 hypointense strip) remains unmyelinated at term

Ventrolateral thalamic nuclei are T1 hyperintense in preterm and term neonates (and more visible on T2)

Medial occipital (and rolandic area) gyral development is more advanced compared to other areas

Posterior, superior, and medial thalami are homogeneous and hypointense compared to the basal ganglia

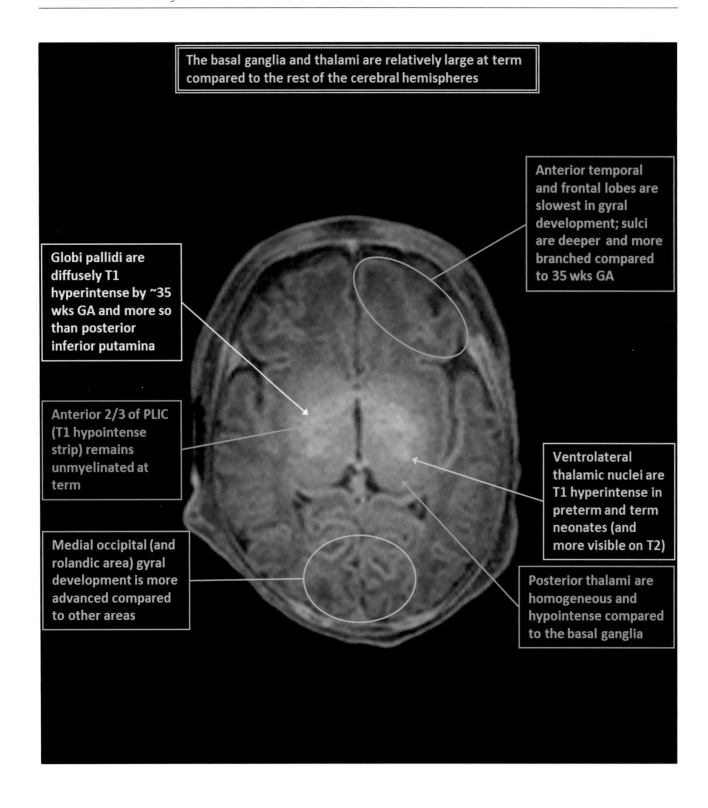

The basal ganglia and thalami are relatively large at term compared to the rest of the cerebral hemispheres

Anterior temporal and frontal lobes are slowest in gyral development; sulci are deeper and more branched compared to 35 wks GA

Globi pallidi are diffusely T1 hyperintense by ~35 wks GA and more so than posterior inferior putamina

Anterior 2/3 of PLIC (T1 hypointense strip) remains unmyelinated at term

Ventrolateral thalamic nuclei are T1 hyperintense in preterm and term neonates (and more visible on T2)

Medial occipital (and rolandic area) gyral development is more advanced compared to other areas

Posterior thalami are homogeneous and hypointense compared to the basal ganglia

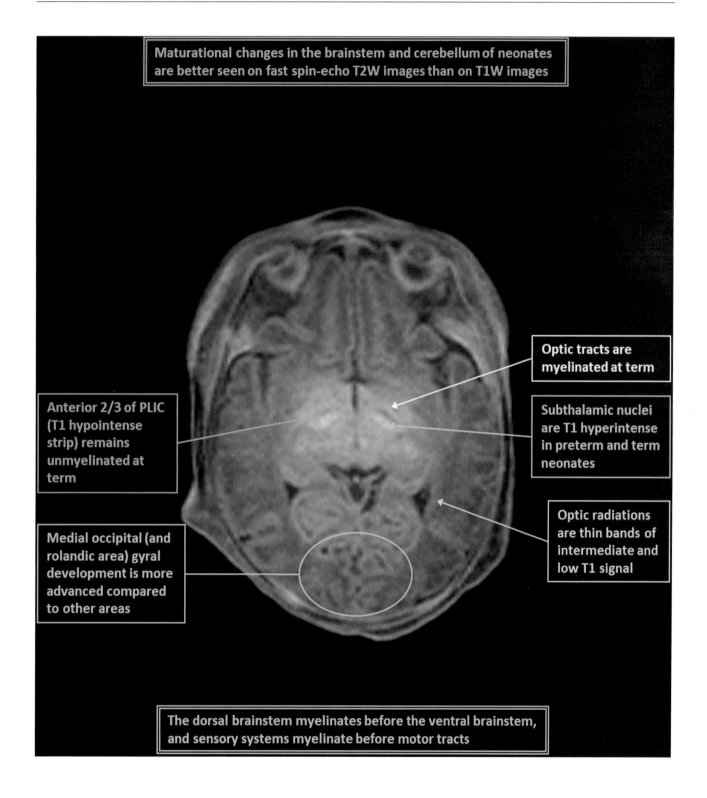

Maturational changes in the brainstem and cerebellum of neonates are better seen on fast spin-echo T2W images than on T1W images

Optic tracts are myelinated at term

Anterior 2/3 of PLIC (T1 hypointense strip) remains unmyelinated at term

Subthalamic nuclei are T1 hyperintense in preterm and term neonates

Optic radiations are thin bands of intermediate and low T1 signal

Medial occipital (and rolandic area) gyral development is more advanced compared to other areas

The dorsal brainstem myelinates before the ventral brainstem, and sensory systems myelinate before motor tracts

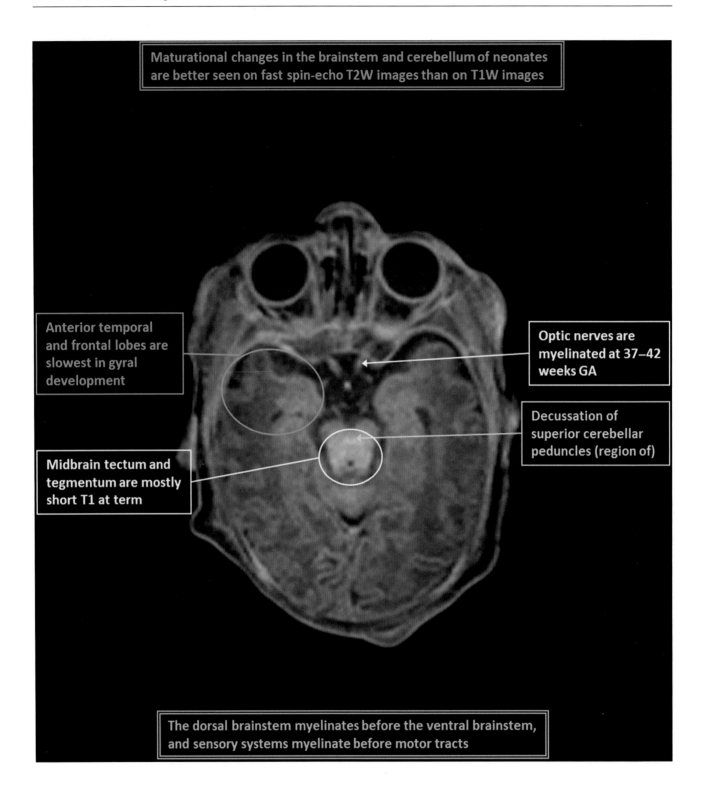

Maturational changes in the brainstem and cerebellum of neonates are better seen on fast spin-echo T2W images than on T1W images

Anterior temporal and frontal lobes are slowest in gyral development

Optic nerves are myelinated at 37–42 weeks GA

Decussation of superior cerebellar peduncles (region of)

Midbrain tectum and tegmentum are mostly short T1 at term

The dorsal brainstem myelinates before the ventral brainstem, and sensory systems myelinate before motor tracts

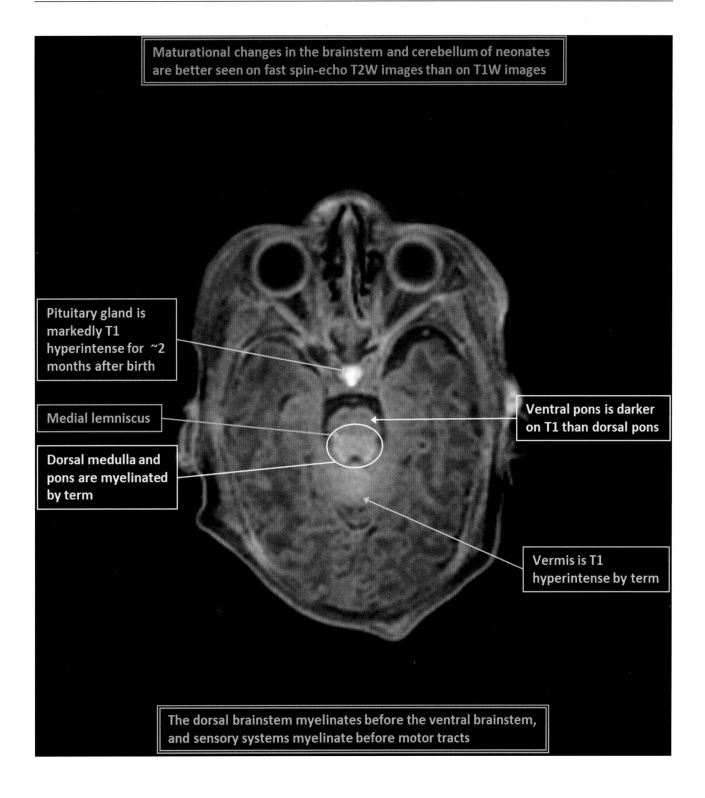

Maturational changes in the brainstem and cerebellum of neonates are better seen on fast spin-echo T2W images than on T1W images

Pituitary gland is markedly T1 hyperintense for ~2 months after birth

Medial lemniscus

Dorsal medulla and pons are myelinated by term

Ventral pons is darker on T1 than dorsal pons

Vermis is T1 hyperintense by term

The dorsal brainstem myelinates before the ventral brainstem, and sensory systems myelinate before motor tracts

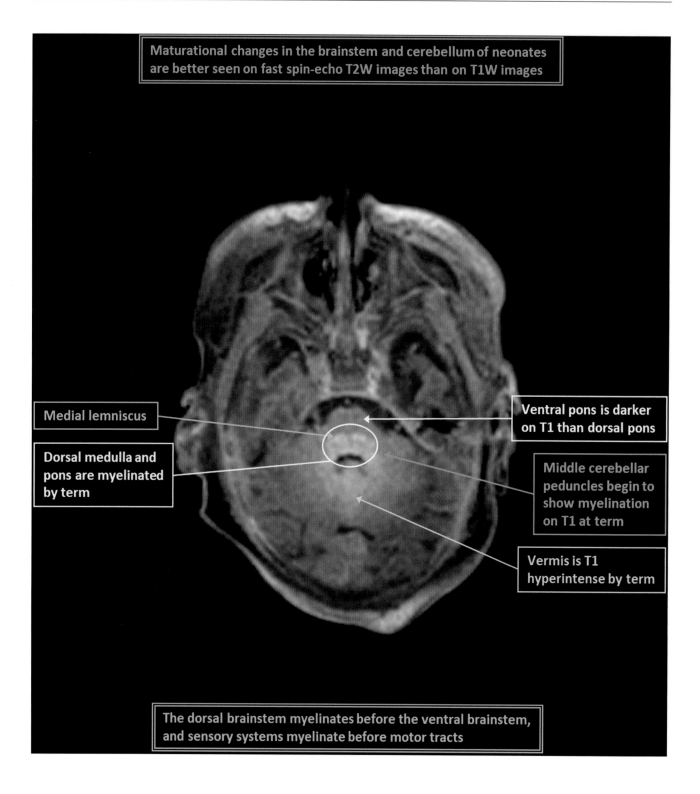

Maturational changes in the brainstem and cerebellum of neonates are better seen on fast spin-echo T2W images than on T1W images

Medial lemniscus

Dorsal medulla and pons are myelinated by term

Ventral pons is darker on T1 than dorsal pons

Middle cerebellar peduncles begin to show myelination on T1 at term

Vermis is T1 hyperintense by term

The dorsal brainstem myelinates before the ventral brainstem, and sensory systems myelinate before motor tracts

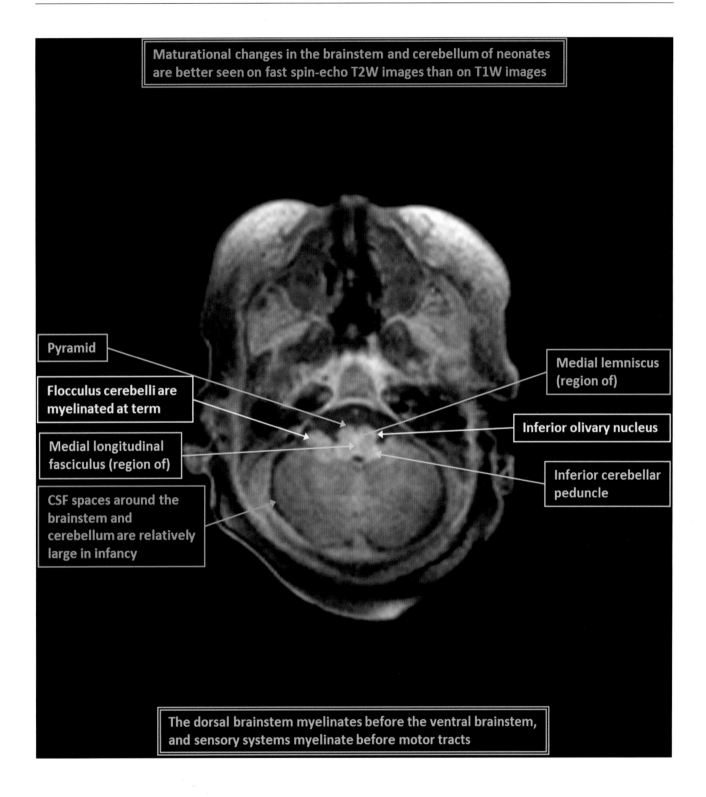

Maturational changes in the brainstem and cerebellum of neonates are better seen on fast spin-echo T2W images than on T1W images

Pyramid

Flocculus cerebelli are myelinated at term

Medial longitudinal fasciculus (region of)

CSF spaces around the brainstem and cerebellum are relatively large in infancy

Medial lemniscus (region of)

Inferior olivary nucleus

Inferior cerebellar peduncle

The dorsal brainstem myelinates before the ventral brainstem, and sensory systems myelinate before motor tracts

40 Weeks, Axial TSE T2

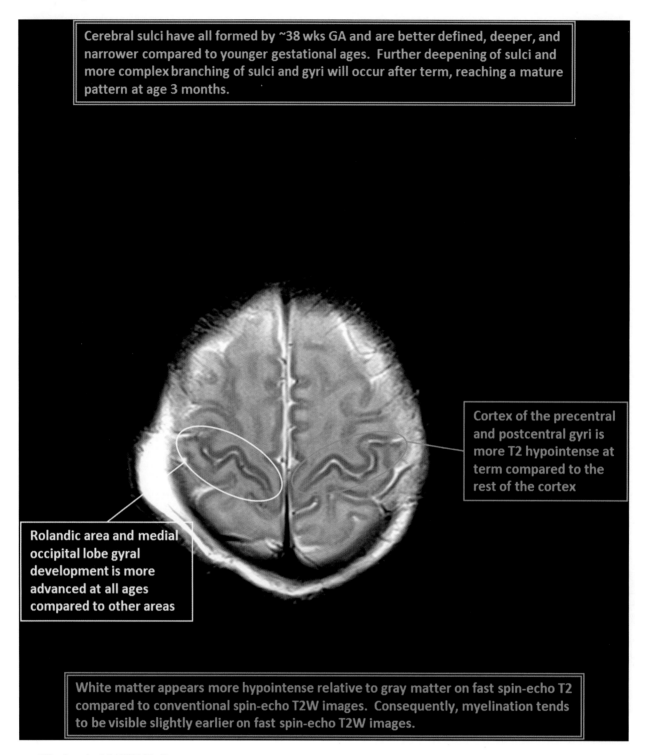

Cerebral sulci have all formed by ~38 wks GA and are better defined, deeper, and narrower compared to younger gestational ages. Further deepening of sulci and more complex branching of sulci and gyri will occur after term, reaching a mature pattern at age 3 months.

Cortex of the precentral and postcentral gyri is more T2 hypointense at term compared to the rest of the cortex

Rolandic area and medial occipital lobe gyral development is more advanced at all ages compared to other areas

White matter appears more hypointense relative to gray matter on fast spin-echo T2 compared to conventional spin-echo T2W images. Consequently, myelination tends to be visible slightly earlier on fast spin-echo T2W images.

40 Weeks, Axial TSE T2 Images 1–12

Cerebral sulci have all formed by ~38 wks GA and are better defined, deeper, and narrower compared to younger gestational ages. Further deepening of sulci and more complex branching of sulci and gyri will occur after term, reaching a mature pattern at age 3 months.

Cerebral white matter in newborns should be highest in T2 signal intensity in the deep and periventricular regions, and diminish in intensity as it nears the cortex

Small portion of central centrum semiovale is T2 hypointense at 40 wks

Rolandic area and medial occipital lobe gyral development is more advanced at all ages compared to other areas

White matter appears more hypointense relative to gray matter on fast spin-echo T2 compared to conventional spin-echo T2W images. Consequently, myelination tends to be visible slightly earlier on fast spin-echo T2W images.

Cerebral sulci have all formed by ~38 wks GA and are better defined, deeper, and narrower compared to younger gestational ages. Further deepening of sulci and more complex branching of sulci and gyri will occur after term, reaching a mature pattern at age 3 months.

Cerebral white matter in newborns should be highest in T2 signal intensity in the deep and periventricular regions, and diminish in intensity as it nears the cortex

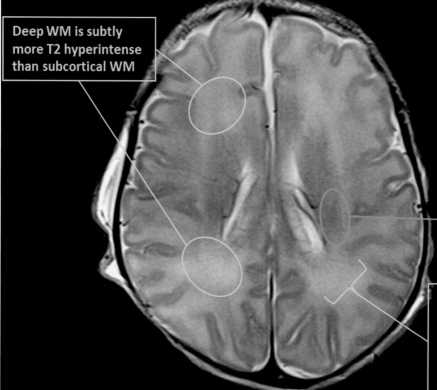

Deep WM is subtly more T2 hyperintense than subcortical WM

Myelin in posterior 1/3 of PLIC and corona radiata is visible on T2 at 40 wks

Posterior "arrowheads" (angular T2 hyperintensity around the posterior horn of the lateral ventricles) have become indistinct by term

White matter appears more hypointense relative to gray matter on fast spin-echo T2 compared to conventional spin-echo T2W images. Consequently, myelination tends to be visible slightly earlier on fast spin-echo T2W images.

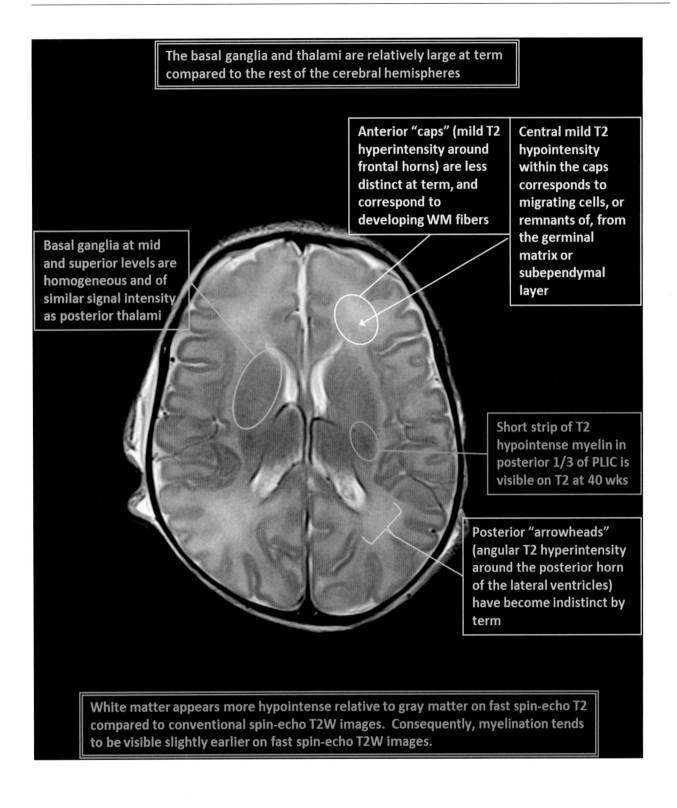

The basal ganglia and thalami are relatively large at term compared to the rest of the cerebral hemispheres

Anterior "caps" (mild T2 hyperintensity around frontal horns) are less distinct at term, and correspond to developing WM fibers

Central mild T2 hypointensity within the caps corresponds to migrating cells, or remnants of, from the germinal matrix or subependymal layer

Basal ganglia at mid and superior levels are homogeneous and of similar signal intensity as posterior thalami

Short strip of T2 hypointense myelin in posterior 1/3 of PLIC is visible on T2 at 40 wks

Posterior "arrowheads" (angular T2 hyperintensity around the posterior horn of the lateral ventricles) have become indistinct by term

White matter appears more hypointense relative to gray matter on fast spin-echo T2 compared to conventional spin-echo T2W images. Consequently, myelination tends to be visible slightly earlier on fast spin-echo T2W images.

The basal ganglia and thalami are relatively large at term compared to the rest of the cerebral hemispheres

Corpus callosum is thin and of intermediate T2 signal intensity, not yet myelinated

Basal ganglia at mid and superior levels are homogeneous and of similar signal intensity as posterior thalami

Anterior "caps" (mild T2 hyperintensity around frontal horns) are less distinct at term, and correspond to developing WM fibers

Central mild T2 hypointensity within the caps corresponds to migrating cells, or remnants of, from the germinal matrix or subependymal layer

Remnants of germinal matrix at tips of frontal horns (mild T2 hypointensity) will disappear by ~44 wks GA

Ventrolateral thalamic nuclei are distinctly T2 hypointense at term

Short strip of T2 hypointense myelin in posterior 1/3 of PLIC is visible on T2 at 40 wks, surrounded by mild T2 hyperintensity

Posterior thalami are homogeneous and of intermediate T2 signal intensity

Corpus callosum is thin and of intermediate signal intensity, not yet myelinated; tight packing of WM fibers may partially explain the T2 shortening before myelination

Note how the normally hypointense cortex contrasts with hyperintense white matter throughout the cerebral hemispheres on T2W images

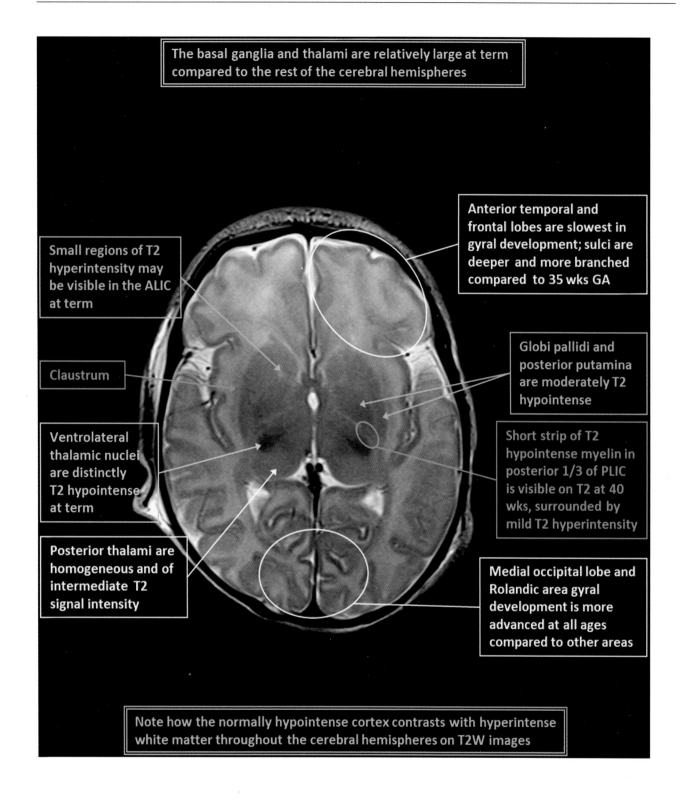

The basal ganglia and thalami are relatively large at term compared to the rest of the cerebral hemispheres

Anterior temporal and frontal lobes are slowest in gyral development; sulci are deeper and more branched compared to 35 wks GA

Small regions of T2 hyperintensity may be visible in the ALIC at term

Globi pallidi and posterior putamina are moderately T2 hypointense

Claustrum

Short strip of T2 hypointense myelin in posterior 1/3 of PLIC is visible on T2 at 40 wks, surrounded by mild T2 hyperintensity

Ventrolateral thalamic nuclei are distinctly T2 hypointense at term

Posterior thalami are homogeneous and of intermediate T2 signal intensity

Medial occipital lobe and Rolandic area gyral development is more advanced at all ages compared to other areas

Note how the normally hypointense cortex contrasts with hyperintense white matter throughout the cerebral hemispheres on T2W images

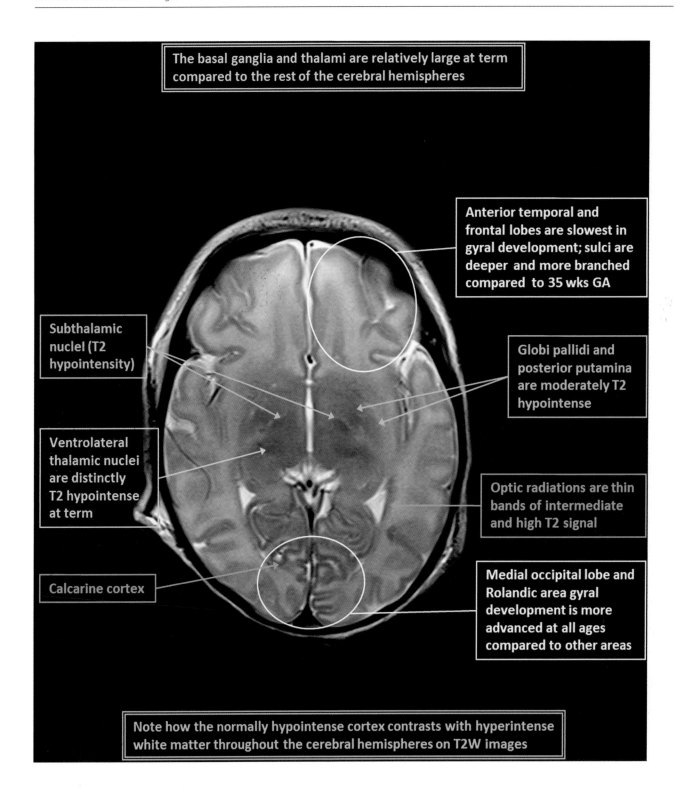

The basal ganglia and thalami are relatively large at term compared to the rest of the cerebral hemispheres

Anterior temporal and frontal lobes are slowest in gyral development; sulci are deeper and more branched compared to 35 wks GA

Subthalamic nuclel (T2 hypointensity)

Globi pallidi and posterior putamina are moderately T2 hypointense

Ventrolateral thalamic nuclei are distinctly T2 hypointense at term

Optic radiations are thin bands of intermediate and high T2 signal

Calcarine cortex

Medial occipital lobe and Rolandic area gyral development is more advanced at all ages compared to other areas

Note how the normally hypointense cortex contrasts with hyperintense white matter throughout the cerebral hemispheres on T2W images

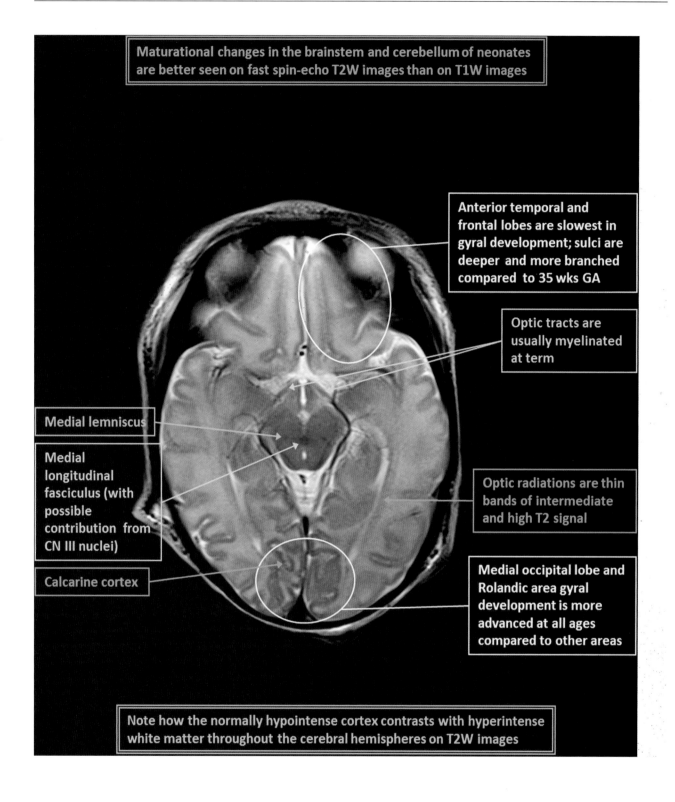

Maturational changes in the brainstem and cerebellum of neonates are better seen on fast spin-echo T2W images than on T1W images

Anterior temporal and frontal lobes are slowest in gyral development; sulci are deeper and more branched compared to 35 wks GA

Optic tracts are usually myelinated at term

Medial lemniscus

Medial longitudinal fasciculus (with possible contribution from CN III nuclei)

Calcarine cortex

Optic radiations are thin bands of intermediate and high T2 signal

Medial occipital lobe and Rolandic area gyral development is more advanced at all ages compared to other areas

Note how the normally hypointense cortex contrasts with hyperintense white matter throughout the cerebral hemispheres on T2W images

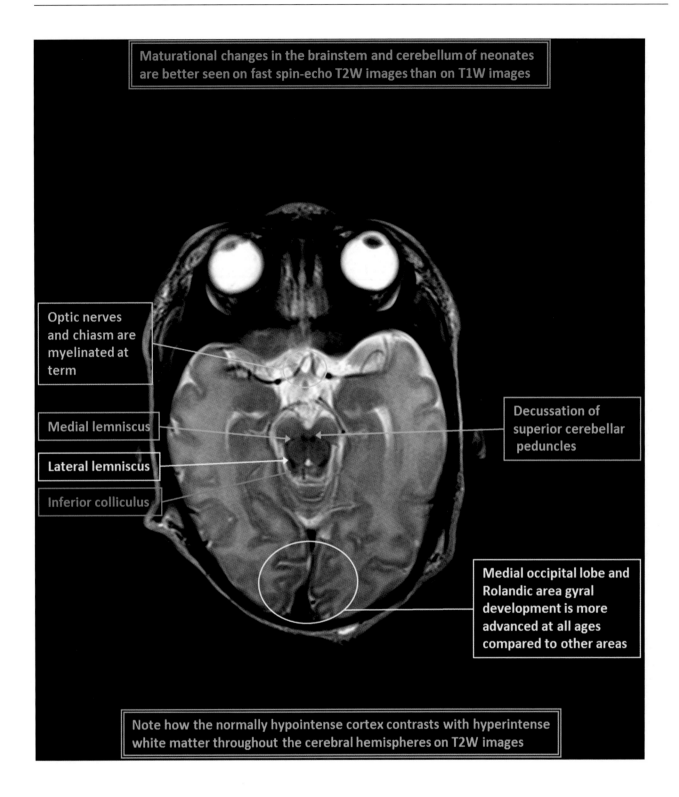

Maturational changes in the brainstem and cerebellum of neonates are better seen on fast spin-echo T2W images than on T1W images

Optic nerves and chiasm are myelinated at term

Medial lemniscus

Lateral lemniscus

Inferior colliculus

Decussation of superior cerebellar peduncles

Medial occipital lobe and Rolandic area gyral development is more advanced at all ages compared to other areas

Note how the normally hypointense cortex contrasts with hyperintense white matter throughout the cerebral hemispheres on T2W images

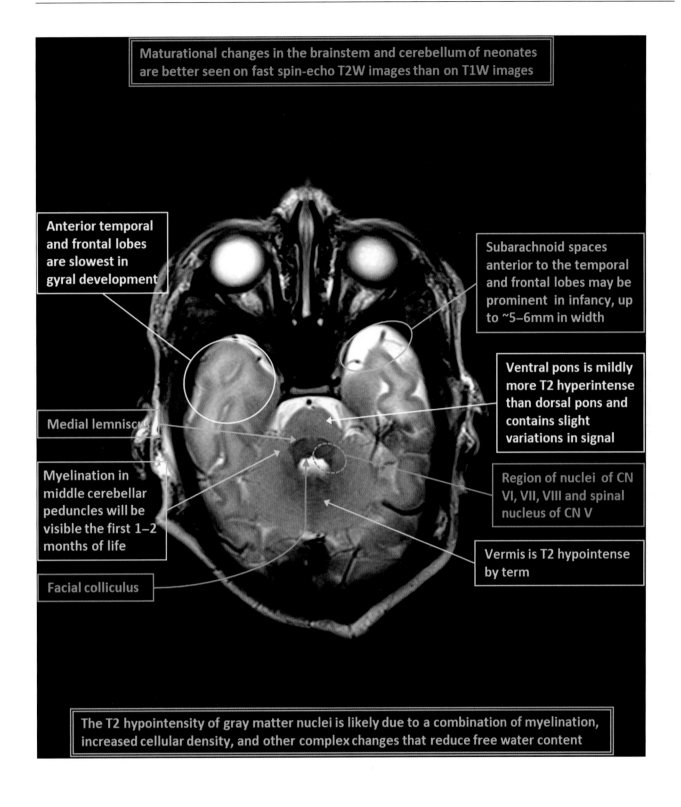

Maturational changes in the brainstem and cerebellum of neonates are better seen on fast spin-echo T2W images than on T1W images

Anterior temporal and frontal lobes are slowest in gyral development

Subarachnoid spaces anterior to the temporal and frontal lobes may be prominent in infancy, up to ~5–6mm in width

Ventral pons is mildly more T2 hyperintense than dorsal pons and contains slight variations in signal

Medial lemniscus

Myelination in middle cerebellar peduncles will be visible the first 1–2 months of life

Region of nuclei of CN VI, VII, VIII and spinal nucleus of CN V

Facial colliculus

Vermis is T2 hypointense by term

The T2 hypointensity of gray matter nuclei is likely due to a combination of myelination, increased cellular density, and other complex changes that reduce free water content

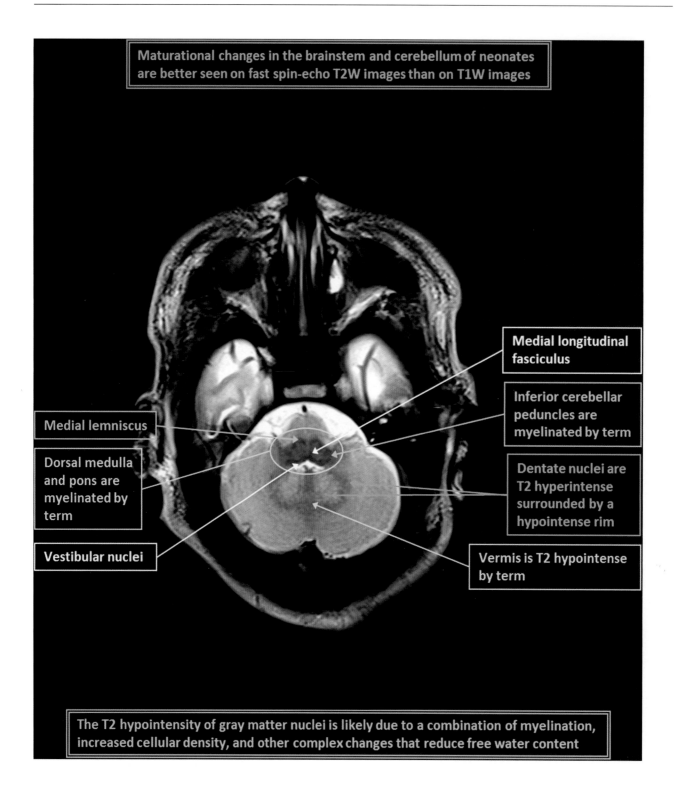

Maturational changes in the brainstem and cerebellum of neonates are better seen on fast spin-echo T2W images than on T1W images

Medial longitudinal fasciculus

Inferior cerebellar peduncles are myelinated by term

Medial lemniscus

Dorsal medulla and pons are myelinated by term

Dentate nuclei are T2 hyperintense surrounded by a hypointense rim

Vestibular nuclei

Vermis is T2 hypointense by term

The T2 hypointensity of gray matter nuclei is likely due to a combination of myelination, increased cellular density, and other complex changes that reduce free water content

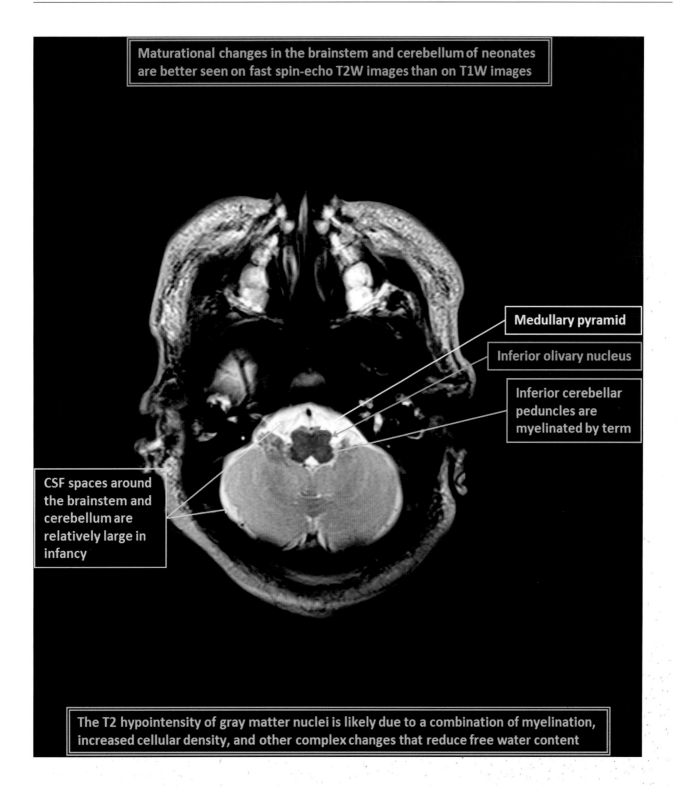

Maturational changes in the brainstem and cerebellum of neonates are better seen on fast spin-echo T2W images than on T1W images

Medullary pyramid

Inferior olivary nucleus

Inferior cerebellar peduncles are myelinated by term

CSF spaces around the brainstem and cerebellum are relatively large in infancy

The T2 hypointensity of gray matter nuclei is likely due to a combination of myelination, increased cellular density, and other complex changes that reduce free water content

40 Weeks, Diffusion Weighted Imaging (DWI) (b=1000 s/mm²)

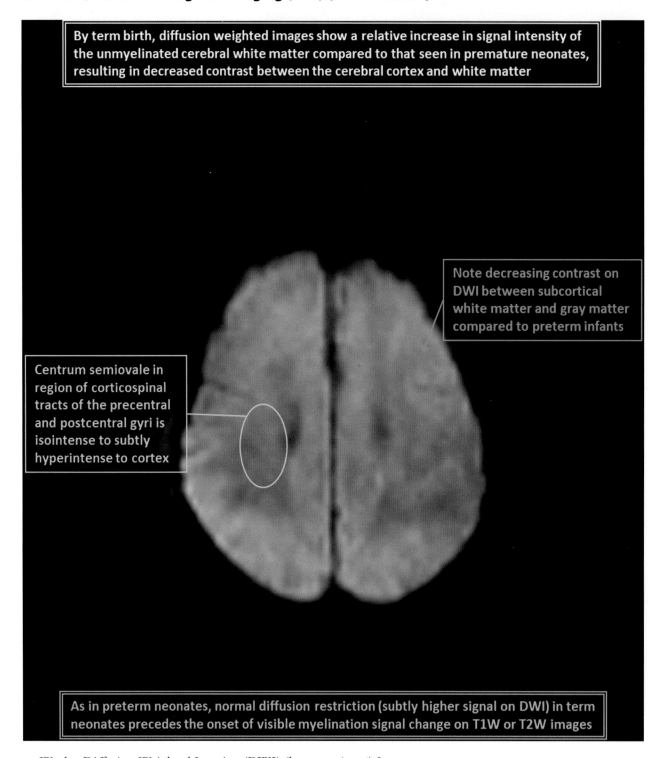

By term birth, diffusion weighted images show a relative increase in signal intensity of the unmyelinated cerebral white matter compared to that seen in premature neonates, resulting in decreased contrast between the cerebral cortex and white matter

Note decreasing contrast on DWI between subcortical white matter and gray matter compared to preterm infants

Centrum semiovale in region of corticospinal tracts of the precentral and postcentral gyri is isointense to subtly hyperintense to cortex

As in preterm neonates, normal diffusion restriction (subtly higher signal on DWI) in term neonates precedes the onset of visible myelination signal change on T1W or T2W images

40 Weeks, Diffusion Weighted Imaging (DWI) (b=1000 s/mm²) Images 1–5

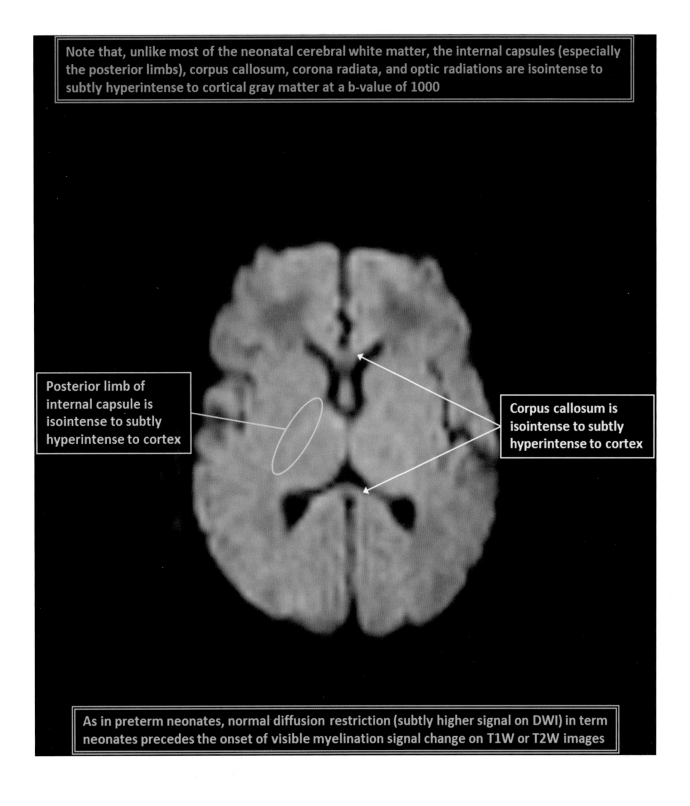

Note that, unlike most of the neonatal cerebral white matter, the internal capsules (especially the posterior limbs), corpus callosum, corona radiata, and optic radiations are isointense to subtly hyperintense to cortical gray matter at a b-value of 1000

Posterior limb of internal capsule is isointense to subtly hyperintense to cortex

Corpus callosum is isointense to subtly hyperintense to cortex

As in preterm neonates, normal diffusion restriction (subtly higher signal on DWI) in term neonates precedes the onset of visible myelination signal change on T1W or T2W images

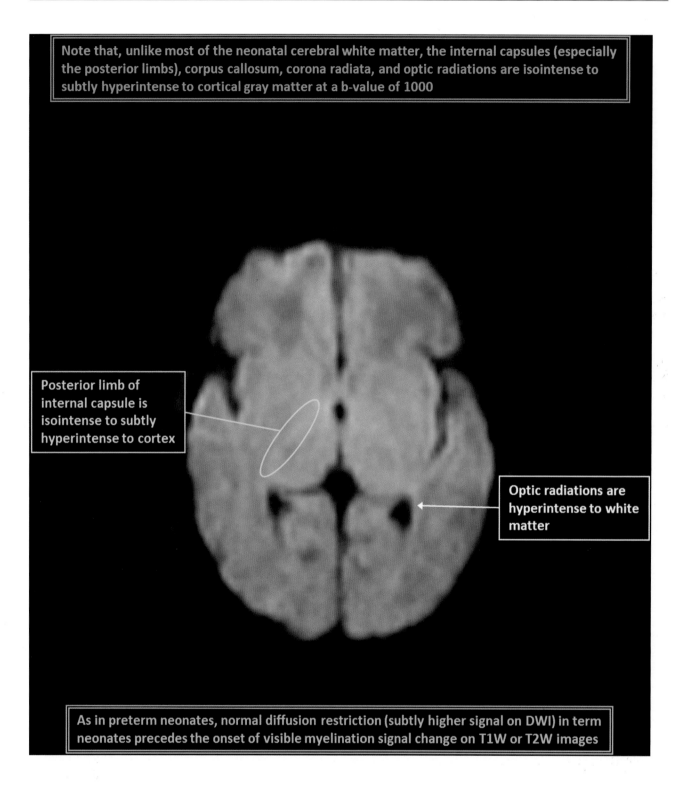

Note that, unlike most of the neonatal cerebral white matter, the internal capsules (especially the posterior limbs), corpus callosum, corona radiata, and optic radiations are isointense to subtly hyperintense to cortical gray matter at a b-value of 1000

Posterior limb of internal capsule is isointense to subtly hyperintense to cortex

Optic radiations are hyperintense to white matter

As in preterm neonates, normal diffusion restriction (subtly higher signal on DWI) in term neonates precedes the onset of visible myelination signal change on T1W or T2W images

For most of the first year of life, the cerebellum as a whole can have a noticeably more hypointense appearance on ADC than the cerebral hemispheres, while on DWI it is isointense to subtly hyperintense to the cerebrum

As in preterm neonates, normal diffusion restriction (subtly higher signal on DWI) in term neonates precedes the onset of visible myelination signal change on T1W or T2W images

For most of the first year of life, the cerebellum as a whole can have a noticeably more hypointense appearance on ADC than the cerebral hemispheres, while on DWI it is isointense to subtly hyperintense to the cerebrum

The central portion of the dentate nuclei and some of the deep cerebellar white matter is hypointense

As in preterm neonates, normal diffusion restriction (subtly higher signal on DWI) in term neonates precedes the onset of visible myelination signal change on T1W or T2W images

40 Weeks, Apparent Diffusion Coefficient (ADC) Map

In term neonates, ADC images continue to have a high contrast appearance due to the higher rate of diffusion in white matter compared to gray matter. Most of the cerebral hemispheric white matter is hyperintense compared to the hypointensity of cerebral cortical gray matter, basal ganglia, and thalami.

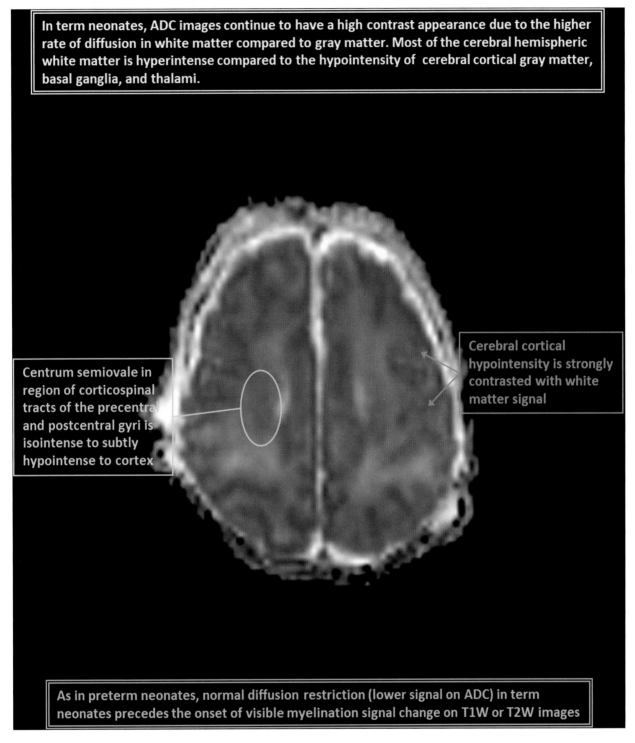

Centrum semiovale in region of corticospinal tracts of the precentral and postcentral gyri is isointense to subtly hypointense to cortex

Cerebral cortical hypointensity is strongly contrasted with white matter signal

As in preterm neonates, normal diffusion restriction (lower signal on ADC) in term neonates precedes the onset of visible myelination signal change on T1W or T2W images

40 Weeks, Apparent Diffusion Coefficient (ADC) Map Images 1–5

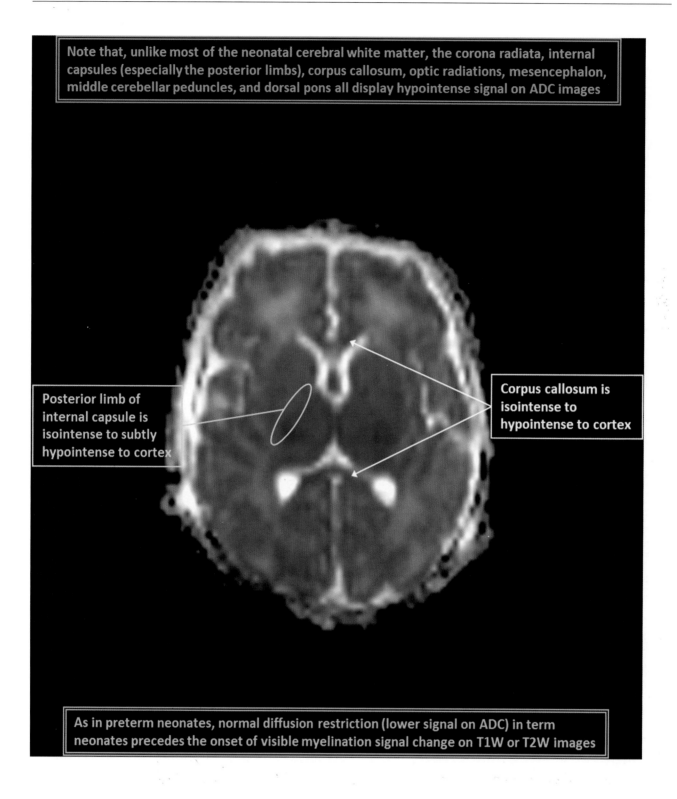

Note that, unlike most of the neonatal cerebral white matter, the corona radiata, internal capsules (especially the posterior limbs), corpus callosum, optic radiations, mesencephalon, middle cerebellar peduncles, and dorsal pons all display hypointense signal on ADC images

Posterior limb of internal capsule is isointense to subtly hypointense to cortex

Corpus callosum is isointense to hypointense to cortex

As in preterm neonates, normal diffusion restriction (lower signal on ADC) in term neonates precedes the onset of visible myelination signal change on T1W or T2W images

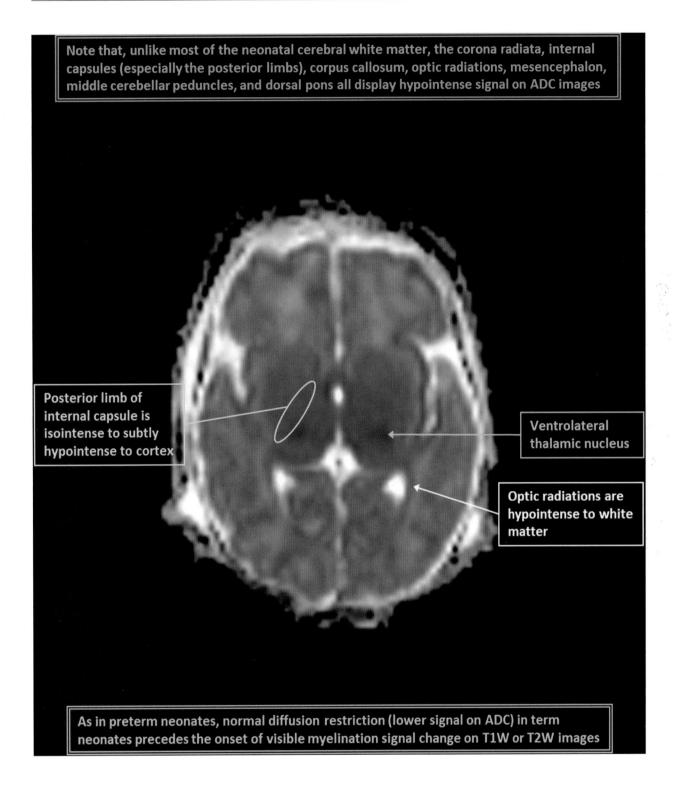

Note that, unlike most of the neonatal cerebral white matter, the corona radiata, internal capsules (especially the posterior limbs), corpus callosum, optic radiations, mesencephalon, middle cerebellar peduncles, and dorsal pons all display hypointense signal on ADC images

Posterior limb of internal capsule is isointense to subtly hypointense to cortex

Ventrolateral thalamic nucleus

Optic radiations are hypointense to white matter

As in preterm neonates, normal diffusion restriction (lower signal on ADC) in term neonates precedes the onset of visible myelination signal change on T1W or T2W images

Note that, unlike most of the neonatal cerebral white matter, the corona radiata, internal capsules (especially the posterior limbs), corpus callosum, optic radiations, mesencephalon, middle cerebellar peduncles, and dorsal pons all display hypointense signal on ADC images

The normal brainstem at term has areas of mildly more hypointense signal on ADC, mainly dorsally and in the central tegmentum of the midbrain

For most of the first year of life, the cerebellum as a whole can have a noticeably more hypointense appearance on ADC than the cerebral hemispheres, while on DWI it is isointense to subtly hyperintense to the cerebrum

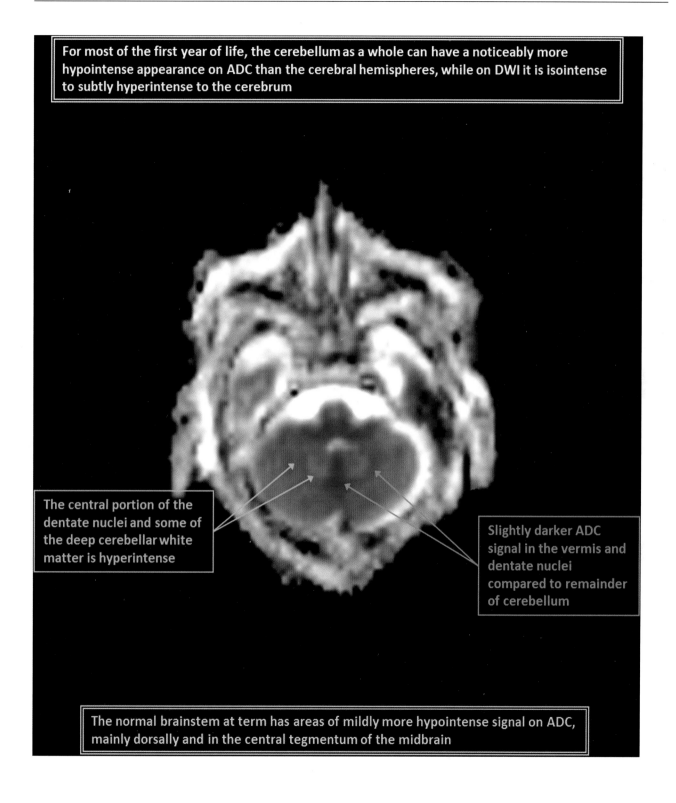

The central portion of the dentate nuclei and some of the deep cerebellar white matter is hyperintense

Slightly darker ADC signal in the vermis and dentate nuclei compared to remainder of cerebellum

The normal brainstem at term has areas of mildly more hypointense signal on ADC, mainly dorsally and in the central tegmentum of the midbrain

40 Weeks, Sagittal T1

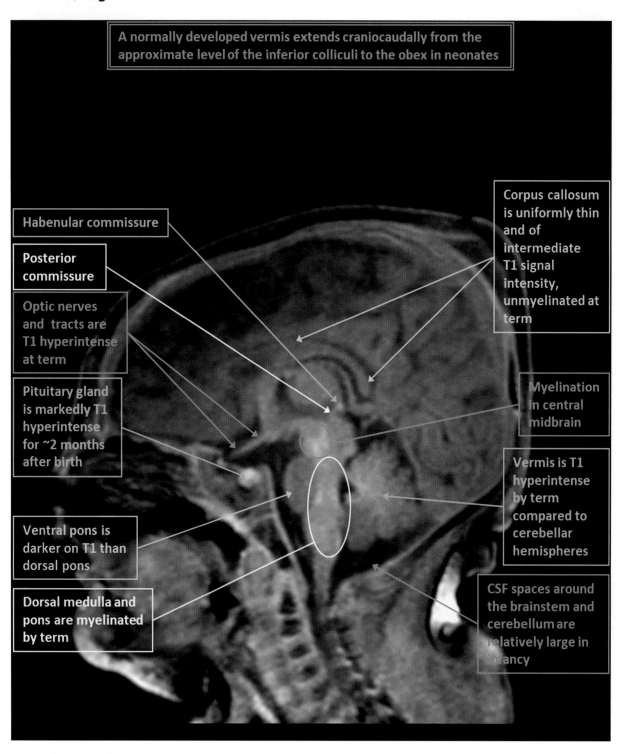

A normally developed vermis extends craniocaudally from the approximate level of the inferior colliculi to the obex in neonates

Habenular commissure

Posterior commissure

Optic nerves and tracts are T1 hyperintense at term

Pituitary gland is markedly T1 hyperintense for ~2 months after birth

Ventral pons is darker on T1 than dorsal pons

Dorsal medulla and pons are myelinated by term

Corpus callosum is uniformly thin and of intermediate T1 signal intensity, unmyelinated at term

Myelination in central midbrain

Vermis is T1 hyperintense by term compared to cerebellar hemispheres

CSF spaces around the brainstem and cerebellum are relatively large in infancy

40 Weeks, Sagittal T1 Images 1–4

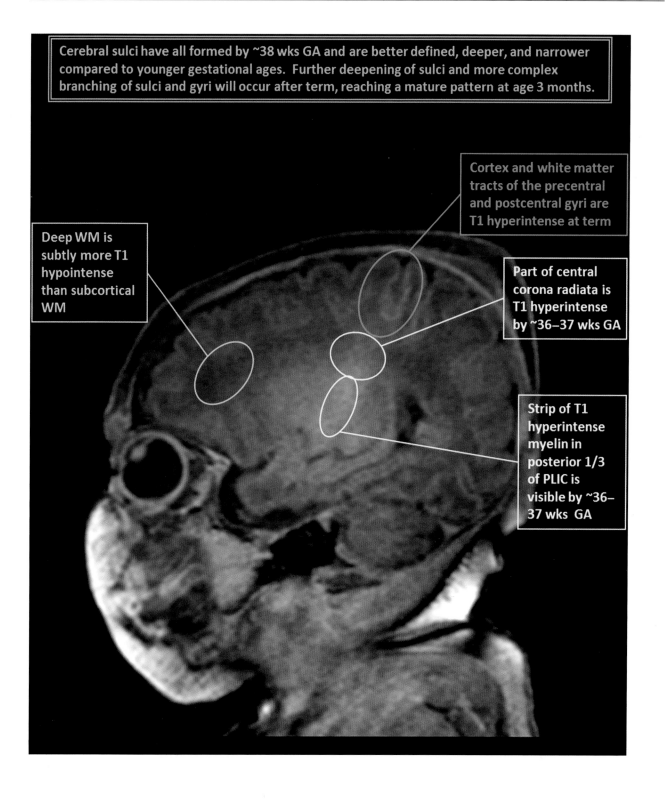

Cerebral sulci have all formed by ~38 wks GA and are better defined, deeper, and narrower compared to younger gestational ages. Further deepening of sulci and more complex branching of sulci and gyri will occur after term, reaching a mature pattern at age 3 months.

Cortex and white matter tracts of the precentral and postcentral gyri are T1 hyperintense at term

Deep WM is subtly more T1 hypointense than subcortical WM

Part of central corona radiata is T1 hyperintense by ~36–37 wks GA

Strip of T1 hyperintense myelin in posterior 1/3 of PLIC is visible by ~36–37 wks GA

40 Weeks, Coronal TSE T2

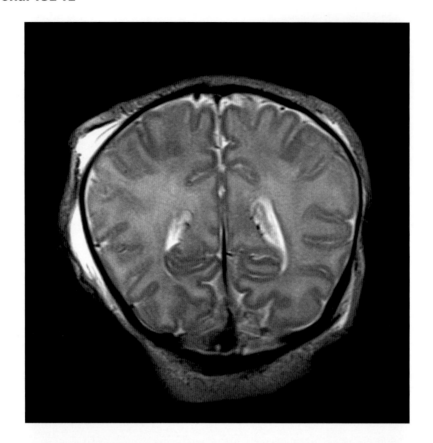

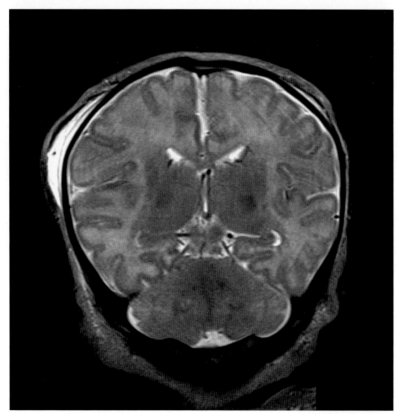

40 Weeks, Coronal TSE T2 Images 1–4

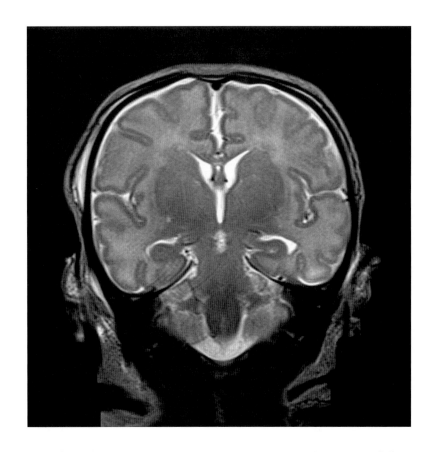

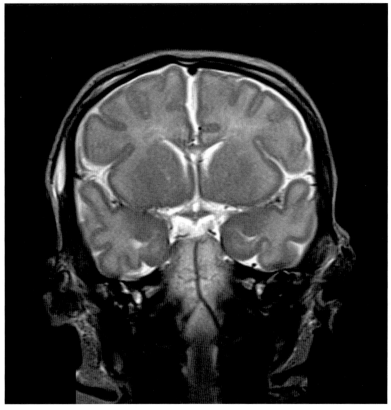

44 Weeks, Axial T1

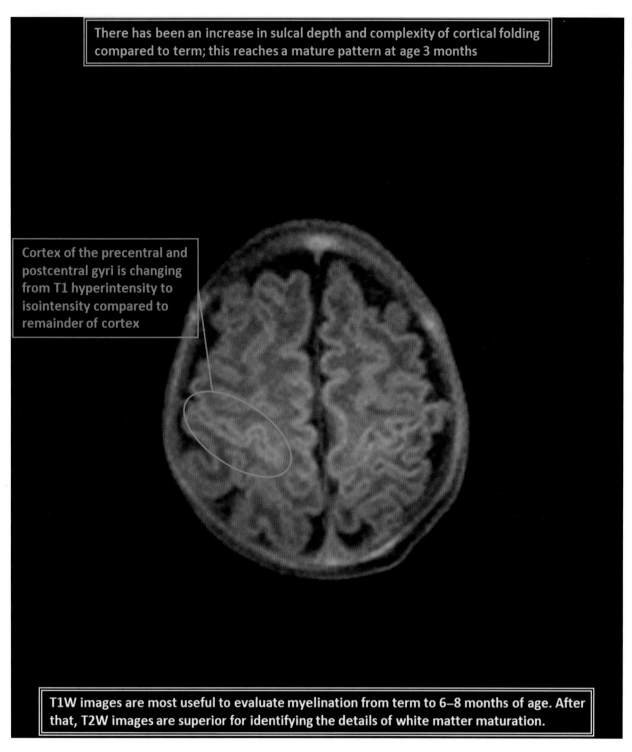

There has been an increase in sulcal depth and complexity of cortical folding compared to term; this reaches a mature pattern at age 3 months

Cortex of the precentral and postcentral gyri is changing from T1 hyperintensity to isointensity compared to remainder of cortex

T1W images are most useful to evaluate myelination from term to 6–8 months of age. After that, T2W images are superior for identifying the details of white matter maturation.

44 Weeks, Axial T1 Images 1–12

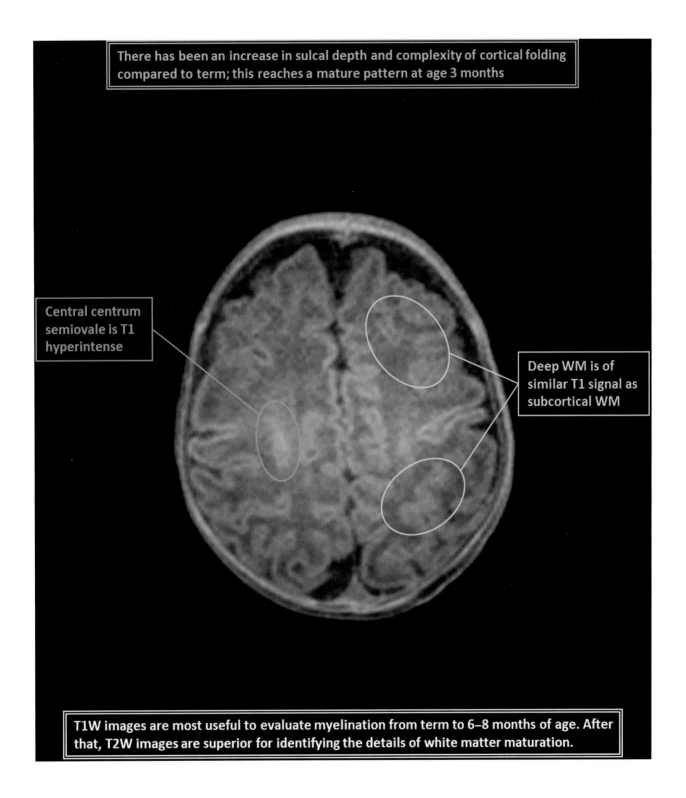

There has been an increase in sulcal depth and complexity of cortical folding compared to term; this reaches a mature pattern at age 3 months

Central centrum semiovale is T1 hyperintense

Deep WM is of similar T1 signal as subcortical WM

T1W images are most useful to evaluate myelination from term to 6–8 months of age. After that, T2W images are superior for identifying the details of white matter maturation.

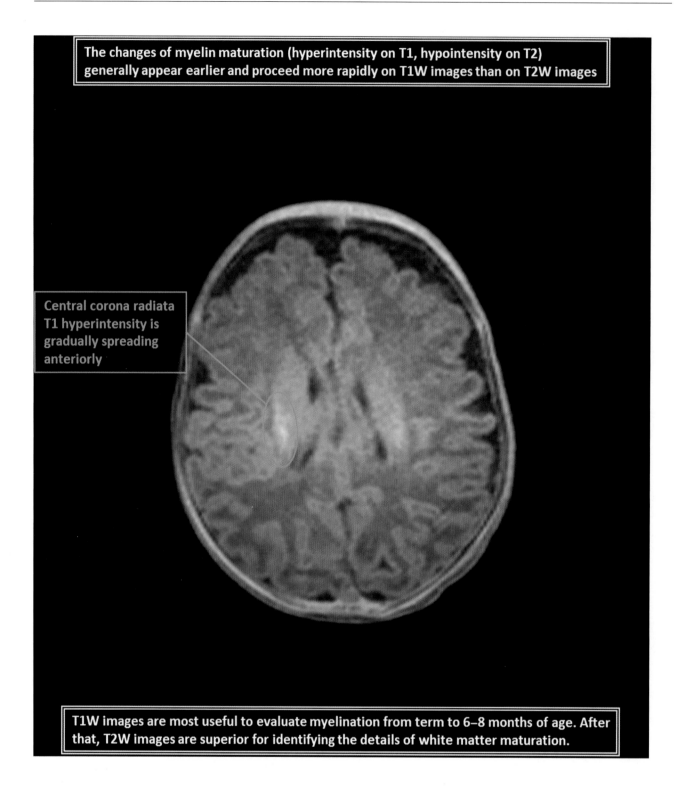

The changes of myelin maturation (hyperintensity on T1, hypointensity on T2) generally appear earlier and proceed more rapidly on T1W images than on T2W images

Central corona radiata T1 hyperintensity is gradually spreading anteriorly

T1W images are most useful to evaluate myelination from term to 6–8 months of age. After that, T2W images are superior for identifying the details of white matter maturation.

The changes of myelin maturation (hyperintensity on T1, hypointensity on T2) generally appear earlier and proceed more rapidly on T1W images than on T2W images

The basal ganglia and thalami are relatively large in young infants compared to the rest of the cerebral hemispheres

Caudate and putamen at mid and superior levels are homogeneous and mildly more T1 hyperintense than posterior thalamus

PLIC myelination on T1 will reach the genu by ~2 months of age

Corpus callosum is thin and of intermediate signal intensity

T1W images are most useful to evaluate myelination from term to 6–8 months of age. After that, T2W images are superior for identifying the details of white matter maturation.

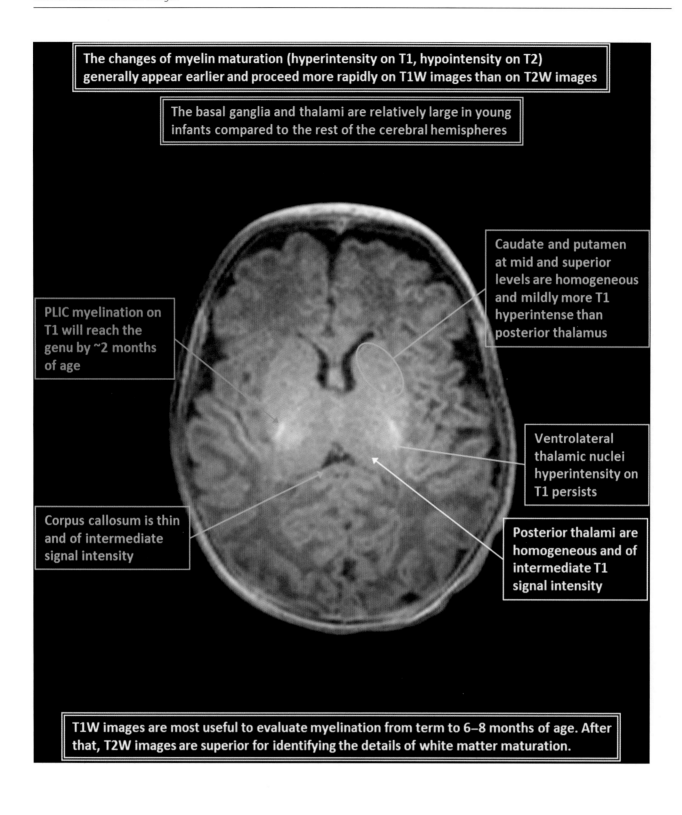

The changes of myelin maturation (hyperintensity on T1, hypointensity on T2) generally appear earlier and proceed more rapidly on T1W images than on T2W images

The basal ganglia and thalami are relatively large in young infants compared to the rest of the cerebral hemispheres

Caudate and putamen at mid and superior levels are homogeneous and mildly more T1 hyperintense than posterior thalamus

PLIC myelination on T1 will reach the genu by ~2 months of age

Ventrolateral thalamic nuclei hyperintensity on T1 persists

Corpus callosum is thin and of intermediate signal intensity

Posterior thalami are homogeneous and of intermediate T1 signal intensity

T1W images are most useful to evaluate myelination from term to 6–8 months of age. After that, T2W images are superior for identifying the details of white matter maturation.

The changes of myelin maturation (hyperintensity on T1, hypointensity on T2) generally appear earlier and proceed more rapidly on T1W images than on T2W images

The basal ganglia and thalami are relatively large in young infants compared to the rest of the cerebral hemispheres

Caudate and putamen at mid and superior levels are homogeneous and mildly more T1 hyperintense than posterior thalamus

PLIC myelination on T1 will reach the genu by ~2 months of age

Ventrolateral thalamic nuclei hyperintensity on T1 persists

Posterior thalami are homogeneous and of intermediate T1 signal intensity

T1W images are most useful to evaluate myelination from term to 6–8 months of age. After that, T2W images are superior for identifying the details of white matter maturation.

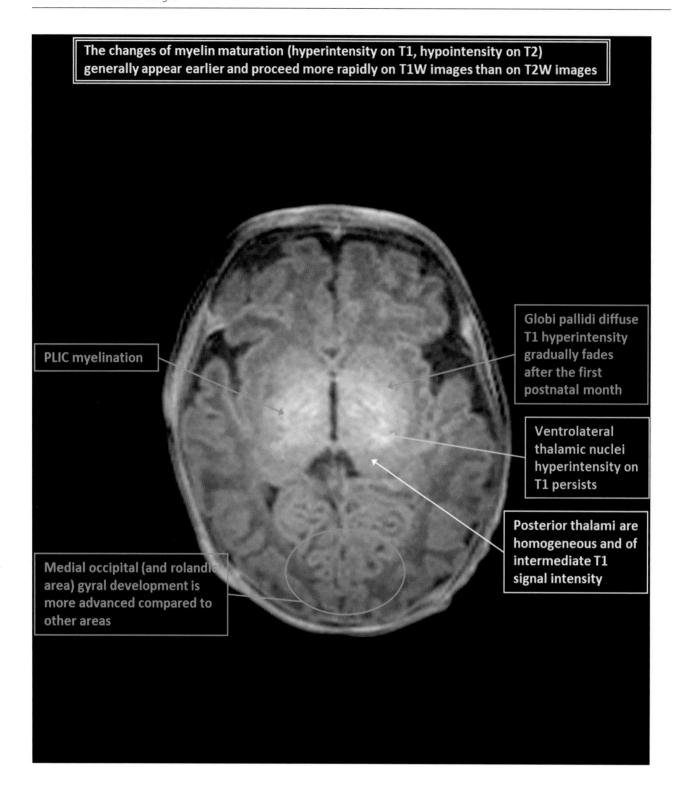

The changes of myelin maturation (hyperintensity on T1, hypointensity on T2) generally appear earlier and proceed more rapidly on T1W images than on T2W images

PLIC myelination

Globi pallidi diffuse T1 hyperintensity gradually fades after the first postnatal month

Ventrolateral thalamic nuclei hyperintensity on T1 persists

Posterior thalami are homogeneous and of intermediate T1 signal intensity

Medial occipital (and rolandic area) gyral development is more advanced compared to other areas

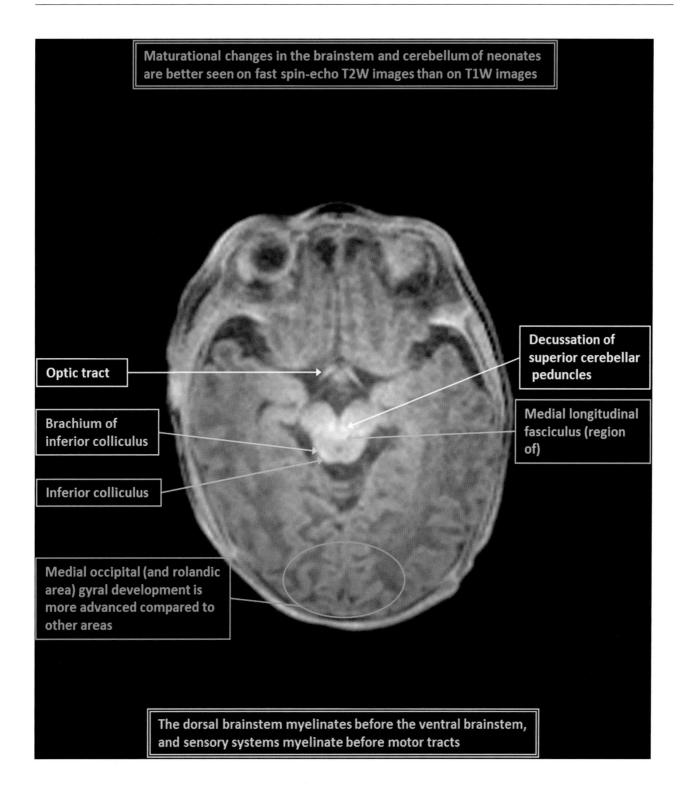

Maturational changes in the brainstem and cerebellum of neonates are better seen on fast spin-echo T2W images than on T1W images

Optic tract

Brachium of inferior colliculus

Inferior colliculus

Medial occipital (and rolandic area) gyral development is more advanced compared to other areas

Decussation of superior cerebellar peduncles

Medial longitudinal fasciculus (region of)

The dorsal brainstem myelinates before the ventral brainstem, and sensory systems myelinate before motor tracts

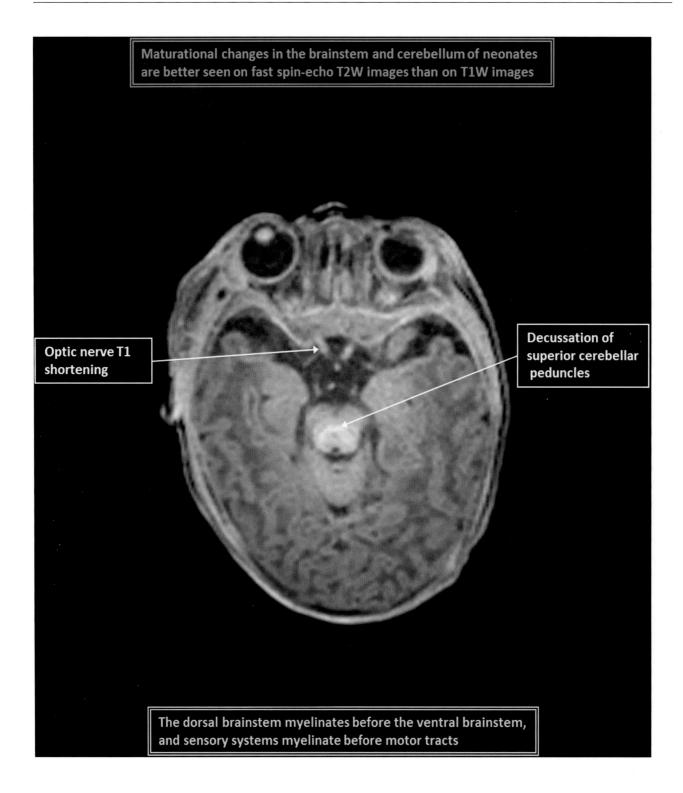

Maturational changes in the brainstem and cerebellum of neonates are better seen on fast spin-echo T2W images than on T1W images

Optic nerve T1 shortening

Decussation of superior cerebellar peduncles

The dorsal brainstem myelinates before the ventral brainstem, and sensory systems myelinate before motor tracts

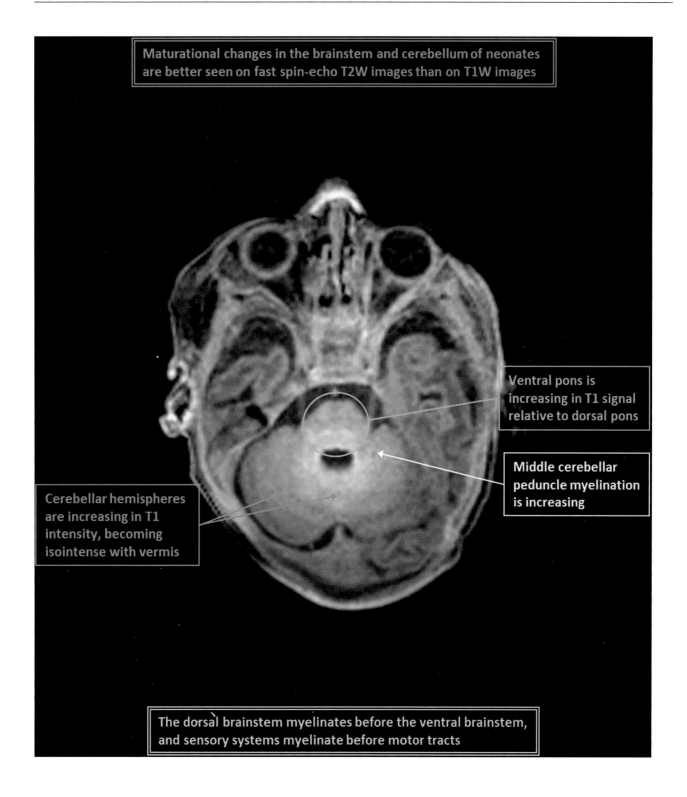

Maturational changes in the brainstem and cerebellum of neonates are better seen on fast spin-echo T2W images than on T1W images

Ventral pons is increasing in T1 signal relative to dorsal pons

Middle cerebellar peduncle myelination is increasing

Cerebellar hemispheres are increasing in T1 intensity, becoming isointense with vermis

The dorsal brainstem myelinates before the ventral brainstem, and sensory systems myelinate before motor tracts

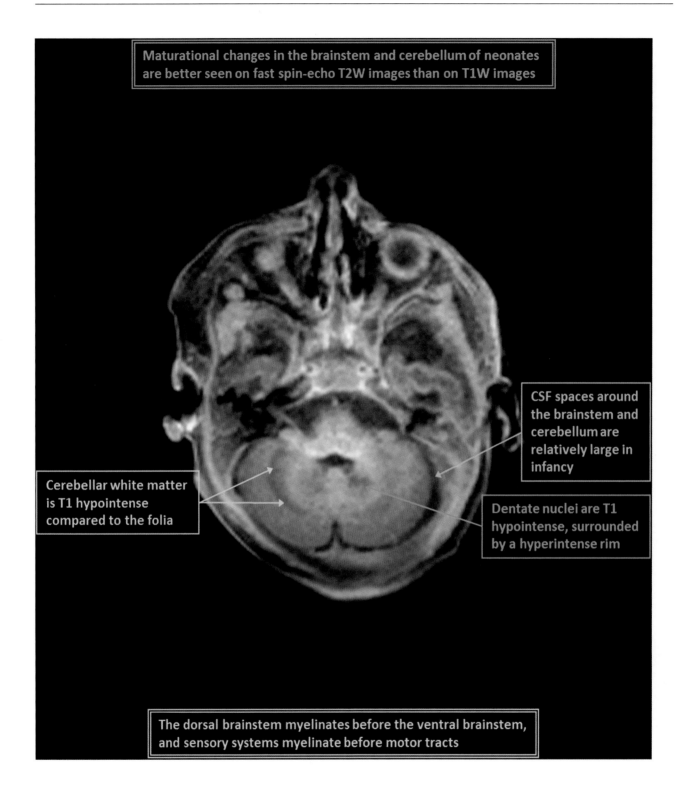

Maturational changes in the brainstem and cerebellum of neonates are better seen on fast spin-echo T2W images than on T1W images

CSF spaces around the brainstem and cerebellum are relatively large in infancy

Cerebellar white matter is T1 hypointense compared to the folia

Dentate nuclei are T1 hypointense, surrounded by a hyperintense rim

The dorsal brainstem myelinates before the ventral brainstem, and sensory systems myelinate before motor tracts

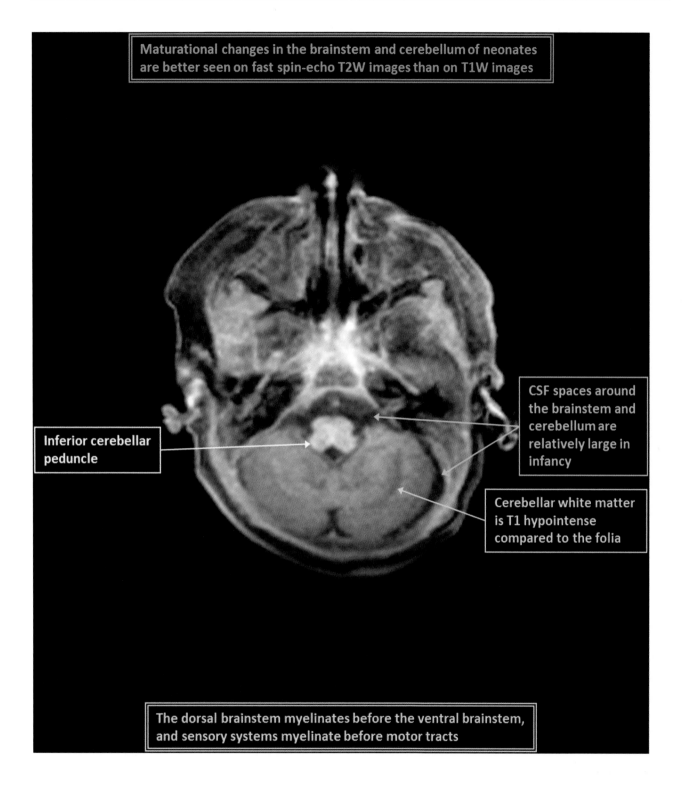

Maturational changes in the brainstem and cerebellum of neonates are better seen on fast spin-echo T2W images than on T1W images

Inferior cerebellar peduncle

CSF spaces around the brainstem and cerebellum are relatively large in infancy

Cerebellar white matter is T1 hypointense compared to the folia

The dorsal brainstem myelinates before the ventral brainstem, and sensory systems myelinate before motor tracts

44 Weeks, Axial TSE T2

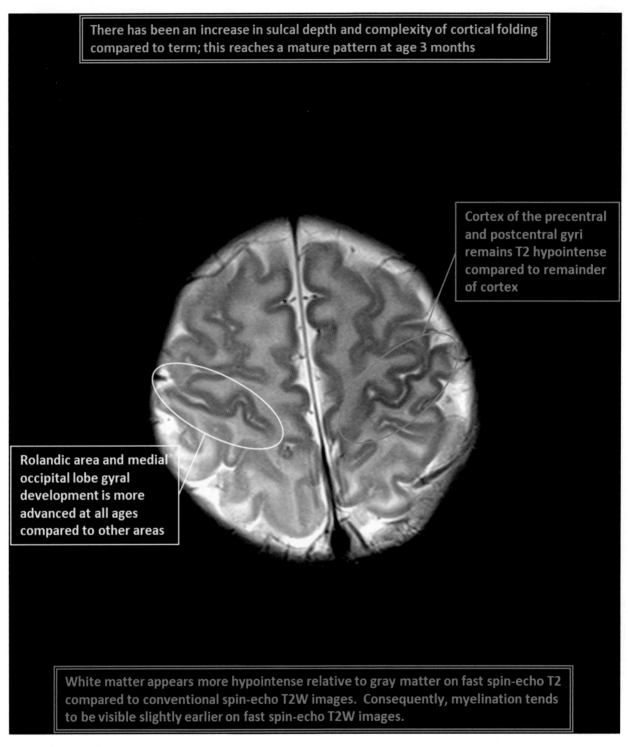

There has been an increase in sulcal depth and complexity of cortical folding compared to term; this reaches a mature pattern at age 3 months

Cortex of the precentral and postcentral gyri remains T2 hypointense compared to remainder of cortex

Rolandic area and medial occipital lobe gyral development is more advanced at all ages compared to other areas

White matter appears more hypointense relative to gray matter on fast spin-echo T2 compared to conventional spin-echo T2W images. Consequently, myelination tends to be visible slightly earlier on fast spin-echo T2W images.

44 Weeks, Axial TSE T2 Images 1–12

There has been an increase in sulcal depth and complexity of cortical folding compared to term; this reaches a mature pattern at age 3 months

Subarachnoid spaces over the cerebral convexities and in the interhemispheric fissure are ~0–3 mm wide in infancy

Small portion of central centrum semiovale is T2 hypointense

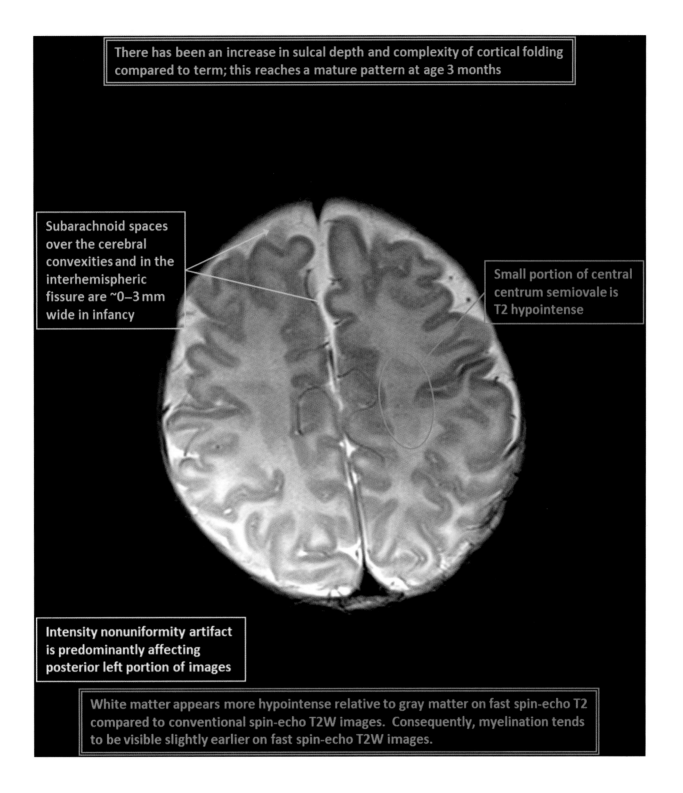

Intensity nonuniformity artifact is predominantly affecting posterior left portion of images

White matter appears more hypointense relative to gray matter on fast spin-echo T2 compared to conventional spin-echo T2W images. Consequently, myelination tends to be visible slightly earlier on fast spin-echo T2W images.

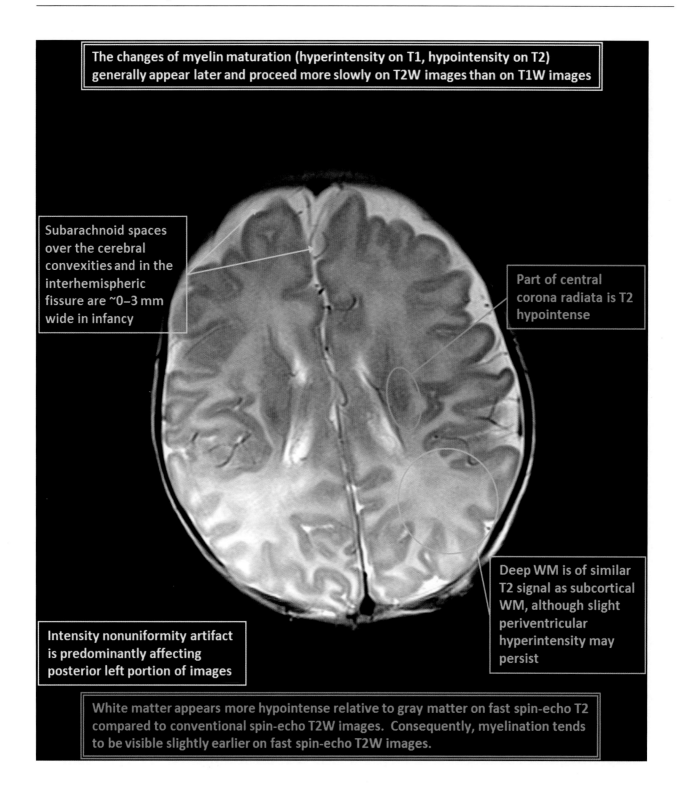

The changes of myelin maturation (hyperintensity on T1, hypointensity on T2) generally appear later and proceed more slowly on T2W images than on T1W images

Subarachnoid spaces over the cerebral convexities and in the interhemispheric fissure are ~0–3 mm wide in infancy

Part of central corona radiata is T2 hypointense

Intensity nonuniformity artifact is predominantly affecting posterior left portion of images

Deep WM is of similar T2 signal as subcortical WM, although slight periventricular hyperintensity may persist

White matter appears more hypointense relative to gray matter on fast spin-echo T2 compared to conventional spin-echo T2W images. Consequently, myelination tends to be visible slightly earlier on fast spin-echo T2W images.

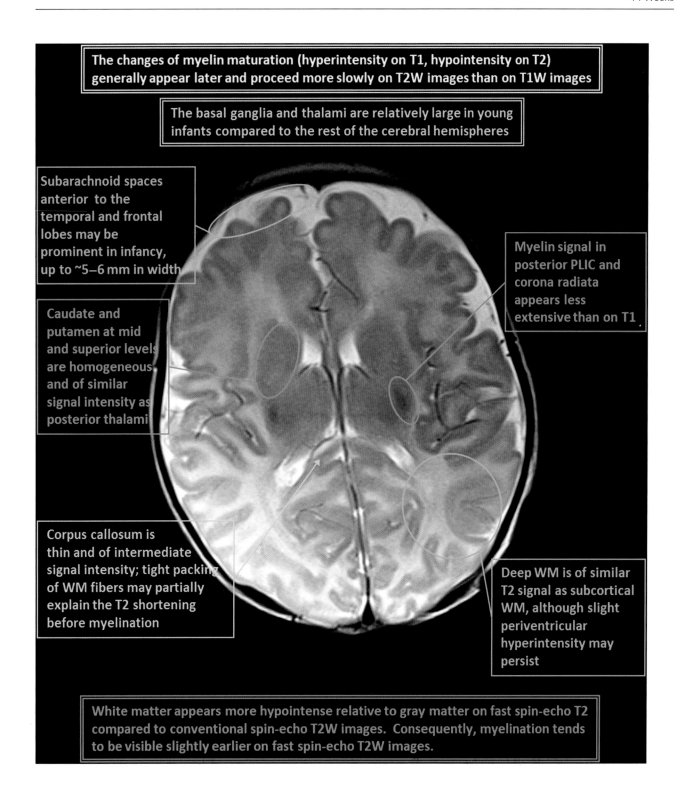

The changes of myelin maturation (hyperintensity on T1, hypointensity on T2) generally appear later and proceed more slowly on T2W images than on T1W images

The basal ganglia and thalami are relatively large in young infants compared to the rest of the cerebral hemispheres

Subarachnoid spaces anterior to the temporal and frontal lobes may be prominent in infancy, up to ~5–6 mm in width

Caudate and putamen at mid and superior levels are homogeneous, and of similar signal intensity as posterior thalami

Myelin signal in posterior PLIC and corona radiata appears less extensive than on T1

Corpus callosum is thin and of intermediate signal intensity; tight packing of WM fibers may partially explain the T2 shortening before myelination

Deep WM is of similar T2 signal as subcortical WM, although slight periventricular hyperintensity may persist

White matter appears more hypointense relative to gray matter on fast spin-echo T2 compared to conventional spin-echo T2W images. Consequently, myelination tends to be visible slightly earlier on fast spin-echo T2W images.

The changes of myelin maturation (hyperintensity on T1, hypointensity on T2) generally appear later and proceed more slowly on T2W images than on T1W images

The basal ganglia and thalami are relatively large in young infants compared to the rest of the cerebral hemispheres

Subarachnoid spaces anterior to the temporal and frontal lobes may be prominent in infancy up to ~5–6 mm in width

Globi pallidi may be very slightly T2 hyperintense superiorly

Short strip of T2 hypointense myelin in posterior 1/3 of PLIC is not significantly changed from term. Note how this progresses more slowly on T2 compared to T1W images.

Caudate and putamen at mid and superior levels are homogeneous, and of similar signal intensity as posterior thalami

Ventrolateral thalamic nuclei marked T2 hypointensity persists

Medial occipital (and rolandic area) gyral development is more advanced compared to other areas

Posterior thalami are homogeneous and of intermediate T2 signal intensity

Intensity nonuniformity artifact is predominantly affecting posterior left portion of images

Note how the normally hypointense cortex contrasts with hyperintense white matter throughout the cerebral hemispheres on T2W images

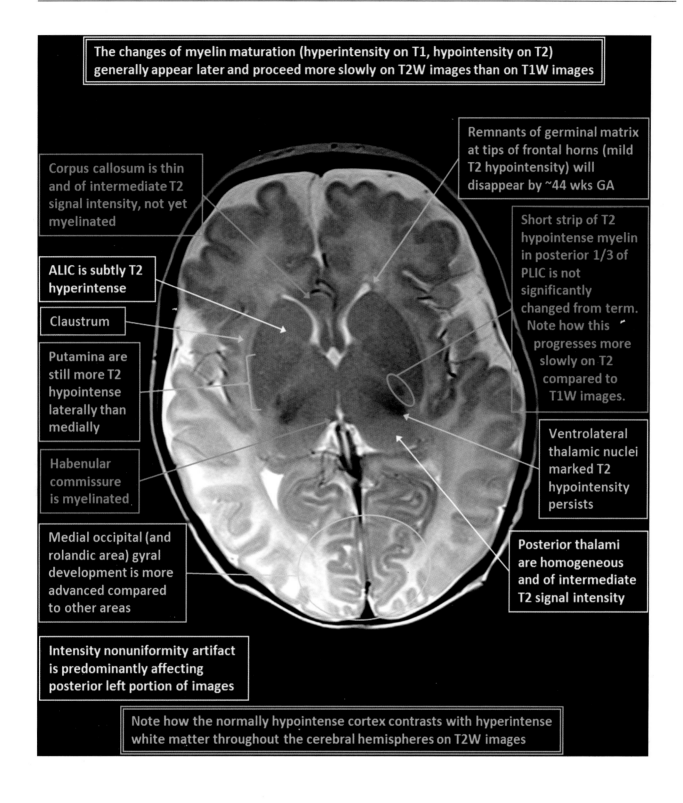

The changes of myelin maturation (hyperintensity on T1, hypointensity on T2) generally appear later and proceed more slowly on T2W images than on T1W images

Remnants of germinal matrix at tips of frontal horns (mild T2 hypointensity) will disappear by ~44 wks GA

Corpus callosum is thin and of intermediate T2 signal intensity, not yet myelinated

Short strip of T2 hypointense myelin in posterior 1/3 of PLIC is not significantly changed from term. Note how this progresses more slowly on T2 compared to T1W images.

ALIC is subtly T2 hyperintense

Claustrum

Putamina are still more T2 hypointense laterally than medially

Ventrolateral thalamic nuclei marked T2 hypointensity persists

Habenular commissure is myelinated

Medial occipital (and rolandic area) gyral development is more advanced compared to other areas

Posterior thalami are homogeneous and of intermediate T2 signal intensity

Intensity nonuniformity artifact is predominantly affecting posterior left portion of images

Note how the normally hypointense cortex contrasts with hyperintense white matter throughout the cerebral hemispheres on T2W images

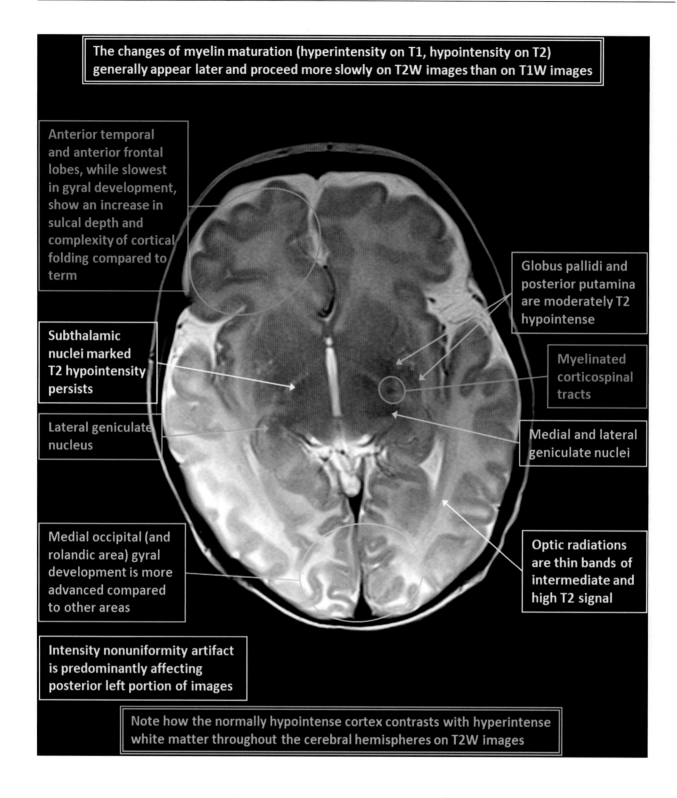

The changes of myelin maturation (hyperintensity on T1, hypointensity on T2) generally appear later and proceed more slowly on T2W images than on T1W images

Anterior temporal and anterior frontal lobes, while slowest in gyral development, show an increase in sulcal depth and complexity of cortical folding compared to term

Globus pallidi and posterior putamina are moderately T2 hypointense

Subthalamic nuclei marked T2 hypointensity persists

Myelinated corticospinal tracts

Lateral geniculate nucleus

Medial and lateral geniculate nuclei

Medial occipital (and rolandic area) gyral development is more advanced compared to other areas

Optic radiations are thin bands of intermediate and high T2 signal

Intensity nonuniformity artifact is predominantly affecting posterior left portion of images

Note how the normally hypointense cortex contrasts with hyperintense white matter throughout the cerebral hemispheres on T2W images

The changes of myelin maturation (hyperintensity on T1, hypointensity on T2) generally appear later and proceed more slowly on T2W images than on T1W images

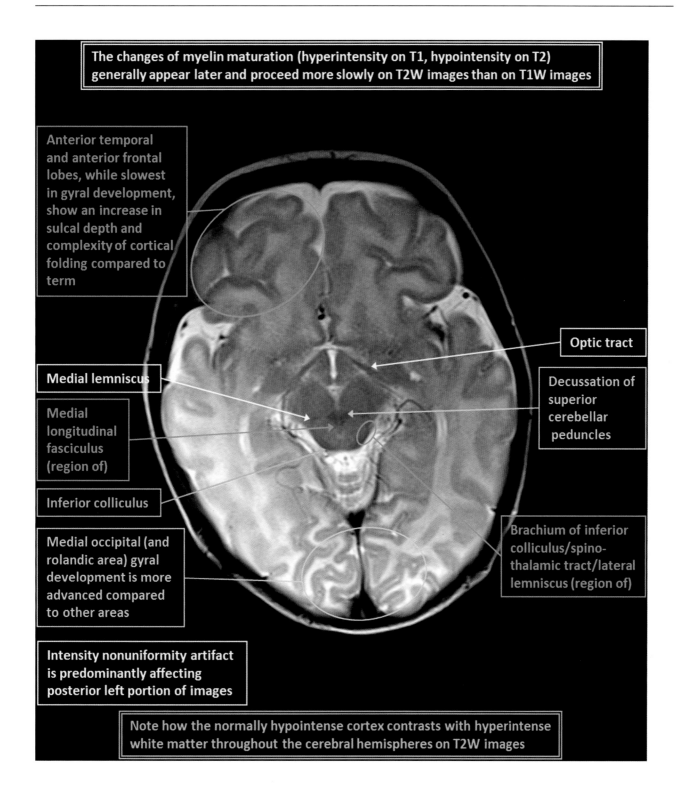

Anterior temporal and anterior frontal lobes, while slowest in gyral development, show an increase in sulcal depth and complexity of cortical folding compared to term

Optic tract

Medial lemniscus

Decussation of superior cerebellar peduncles

Medial longitudinal fasciculus (region of)

Inferior colliculus

Medial occipital (and rolandic area) gyral development is more advanced compared to other areas

Brachium of inferior colliculus/spino-thalamic tract/lateral lemniscus (region of)

Intensity nonuniformity artifact is predominantly affecting posterior left portion of images

Note how the normally hypointense cortex contrasts with hyperintense white matter throughout the cerebral hemispheres on T2W images

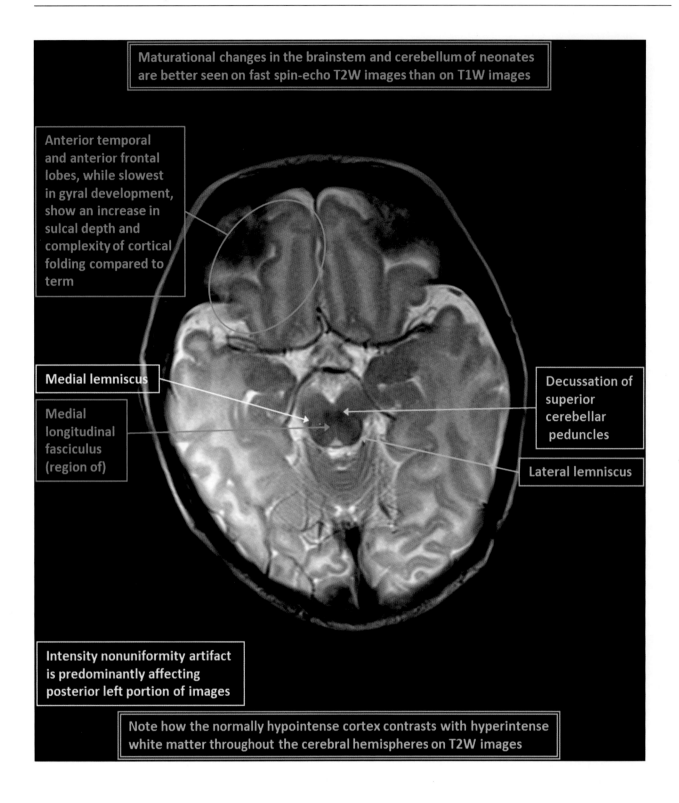

Maturational changes in the brainstem and cerebellum of neonates are better seen on fast spin-echo T2W images than on T1W images

Anterior temporal and anterior frontal lobes, while slowest in gyral development, show an increase in sulcal depth and complexity of cortical folding compared to term

Medial lemniscus

Medial longitudinal fasciculus (region of)

Decussation of superior cerebellar peduncles

Lateral lemniscus

Intensity nonuniformity artifact is predominantly affecting posterior left portion of images

Note how the normally hypointense cortex contrasts with hyperintense white matter throughout the cerebral hemispheres on T2W images

Maturational changes in the brainstem and cerebellum of neonates are better seen on fast spin-echo T2W images than on T1W images

Anterior temporal and anterior frontal lobes are slowest in gyral development

Subarachnoid spaces anterior to the temporal and frontal lobes may be prominent in infancy, up to ~5-6mm in width

Ventral pons is mildly more T2 hyperintense than dorsal pons

Medial lemniscus

Central tegmental tract (region of)

Middle cerebellar peduncle myelination becomes visible in the first 1-2 months of life

Superior cerebellar peduncle

Region of nuclei of CN VI, VII, VIII and spinal nucleus of CN V

Dentate nuclei are T2 hyperintense, surrounded by a hypointense rim

Vermian T2 hypointensity is less conspicuous as cerebellar hemisphere myelination increases

Facial colliculus

The T2 hypointensity of gray matter nuclei is likely due to a combination of myelination, increased cellular density, and other complex changes that reduce free water content

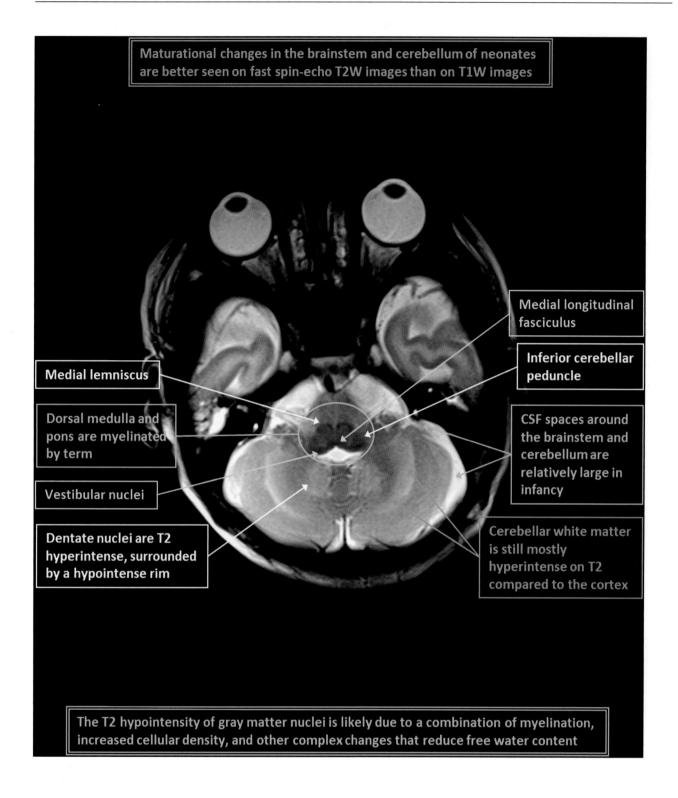

Maturational changes in the brainstem and cerebellum of neonates are better seen on fast spin-echo T2W images than on T1W images

Medial longitudinal fasciculus

Inferior cerebellar peduncle

Medial lemniscus

Dorsal medulla and pons are myelinated by term

Vestibular nuclei

Dentate nuclei are T2 hyperintense, surrounded by a hypointense rim

CSF spaces around the brainstem and cerebellum are relatively large in infancy

Cerebellar white matter is still mostly hyperintense on T2 compared to the cortex

The T2 hypointensity of gray matter nuclei is likely due to a combination of myelination, increased cellular density, and other complex changes that reduce free water content

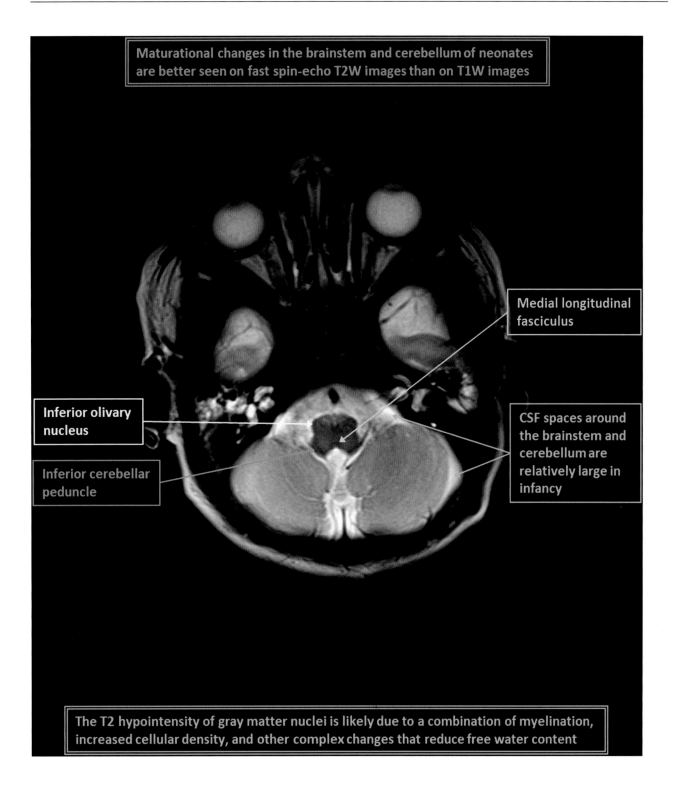

Maturational changes in the brainstem and cerebellum of neonates are better seen on fast spin-echo T2W images than on T1W images

Medial longitudinal fasciculus

Inferior olivary nucleus

Inferior cerebellar peduncle

CSF spaces around the brainstem and cerebellum are relatively large in infancy

The T2 hypointensity of gray matter nuclei is likely due to a combination of myelination, increased cellular density, and other complex changes that reduce free water content

44 Weeks, Sagittal T1

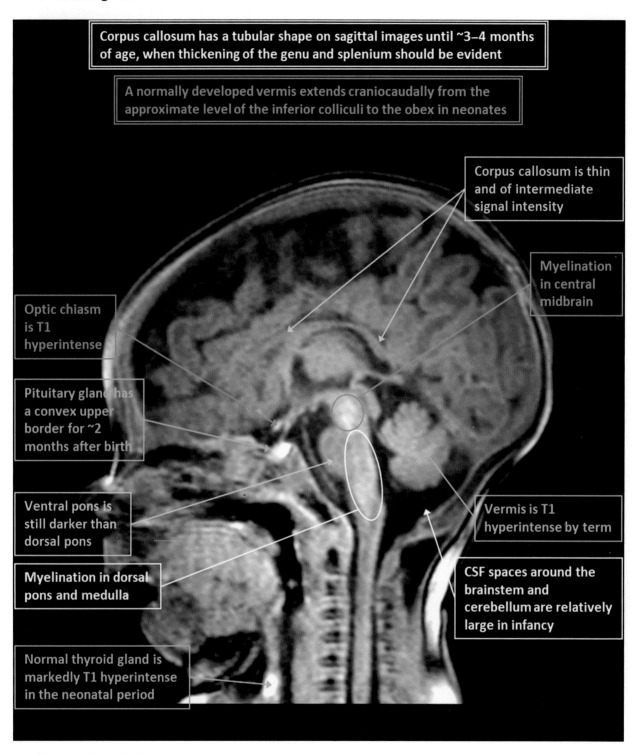

Corpus callosum has a tubular shape on sagittal images until ~3–4 months of age, when thickening of the genu and splenium should be evident

A normally developed vermis extends craniocaudally from the approximate level of the inferior colliculi to the obex in neonates

Corpus callosum is thin and of intermediate signal intensity

Myelination in central midbrain

Optic chiasm is T1 hyperintense

Pituitary gland has a convex upper border for ~2 months after birth

Ventral pons is still darker than dorsal pons

Myelination in dorsal pons and medulla

Vermis is T1 hyperintense by term

CSF spaces around the brainstem and cerebellum are relatively large in infancy

Normal thyroid gland is markedly T1 hyperintense in the neonatal period

44 Weeks, Sagittal T1 Images 1–4

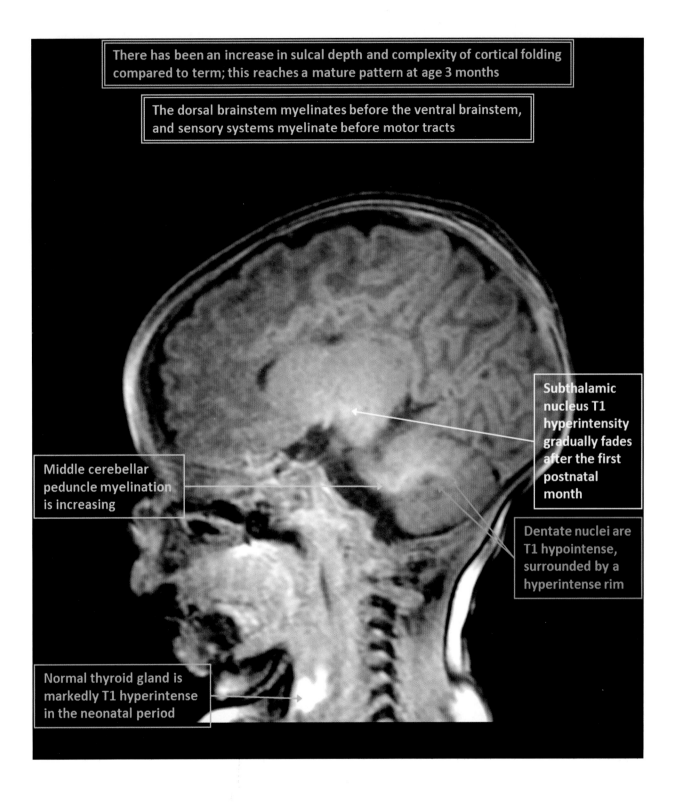

There has been an increase in sulcal depth and complexity of cortical folding compared to term; this reaches a mature pattern at age 3 months

The dorsal brainstem myelinates before the ventral brainstem, and sensory systems myelinate before motor tracts

Subthalamic nucleus T1 hyperintensity gradually fades after the first postnatal month

Middle cerebellar peduncle myelination is increasing

Dentate nuclei are T1 hypointense, surrounded by a hyperintense rim

Normal thyroid gland is markedly T1 hyperintense in the neonatal period

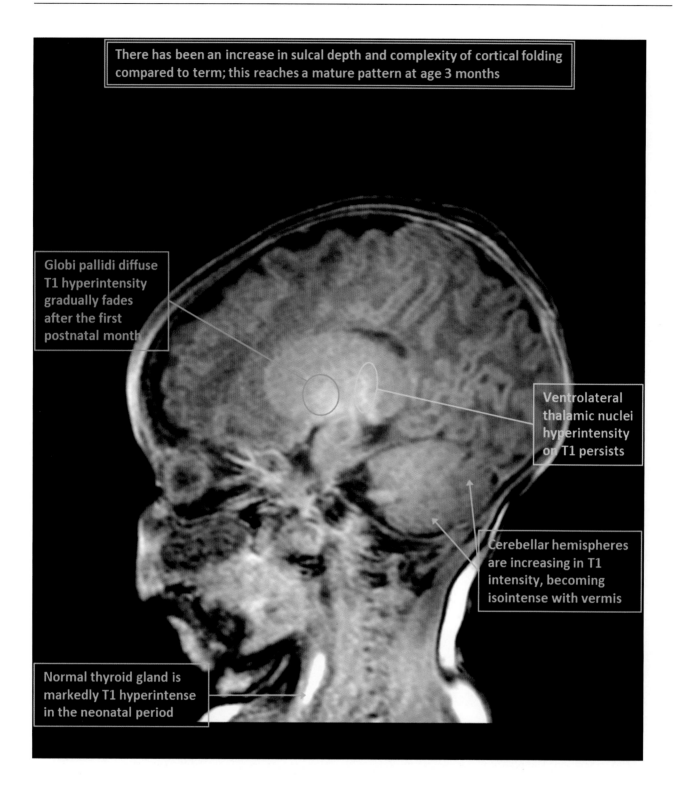

There has been an increase in sulcal depth and complexity of cortical folding compared to term; this reaches a mature pattern at age 3 months

Globi pallidi diffuse T1 hyperintensity gradually fades after the first postnatal month

Ventrolateral thalamic nuclei hyperintensity on T1 persists

Cerebellar hemispheres are increasing in T1 intensity, becoming isointense with vermis

Normal thyroid gland is markedly T1 hyperintense in the neonatal period

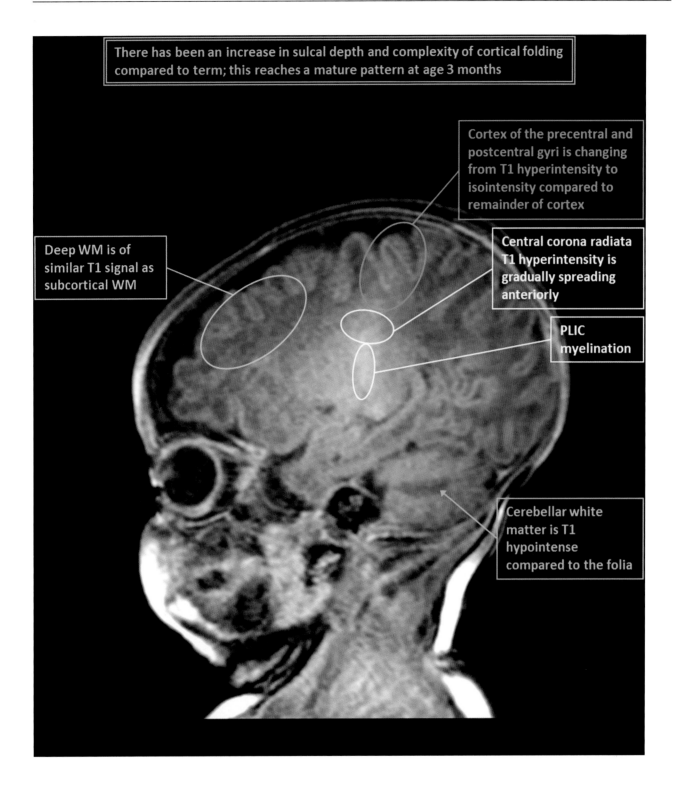

There has been an increase in sulcal depth and complexity of cortical folding compared to term; this reaches a mature pattern at age 3 months

Cortex of the precentral and postcentral gyri is changing from T1 hyperintensity to isointensity compared to remainder of cortex

Central corona radiata T1 hyperintensity is gradually spreading anteriorly

Deep WM is of similar T1 signal as subcortical WM

PLIC myelination

Cerebellar white matter is T1 hypointense compared to the folia

44 Weeks, Coronal TSE T2

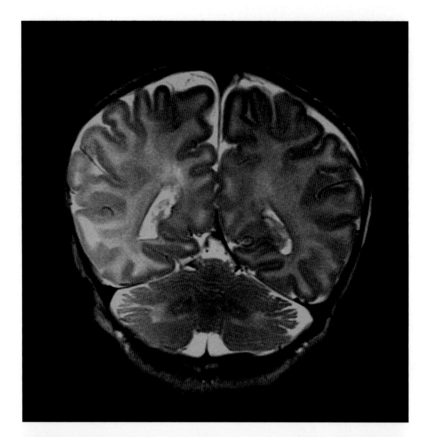

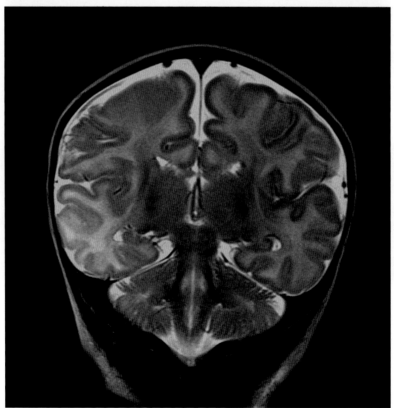

44 Weeks, Coronal TSE T2 Images 1–4

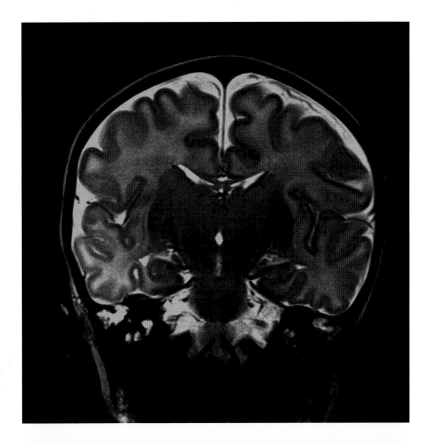

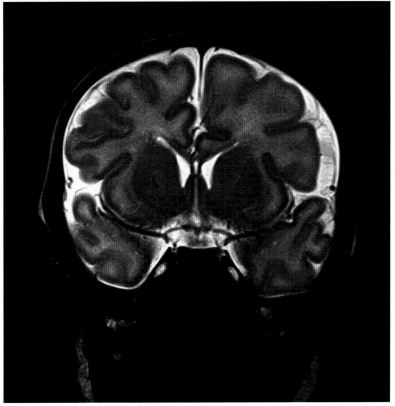

3 Months, Axial T1

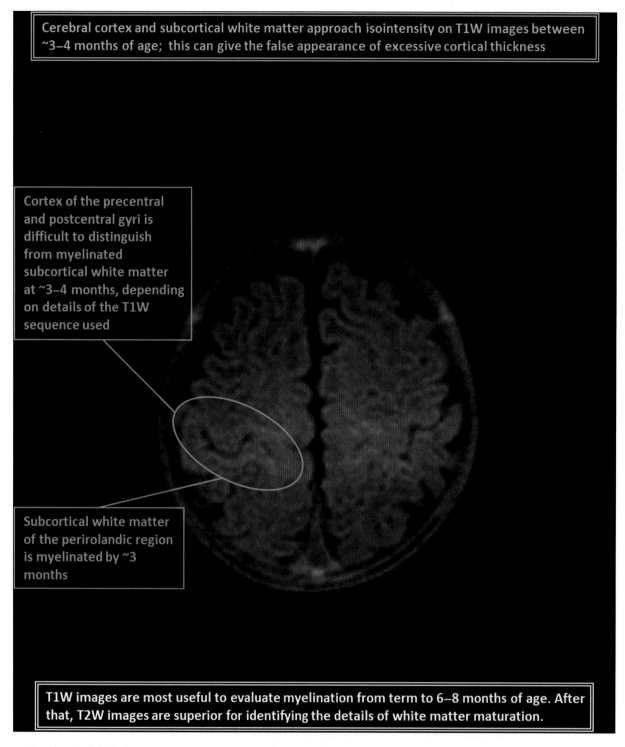

Cerebral cortex and subcortical white matter approach isointensity on T1W images between ~3–4 months of age; this can give the false appearance of excessive cortical thickness

Cortex of the precentral and postcentral gyri is difficult to distinguish from myelinated subcortical white matter at ~3–4 months, depending on details of the T1W sequence used

Subcortical white matter of the perirolandic region is myelinated by ~3 months

T1W images are most useful to evaluate myelination from term to 6–8 months of age. After that, T2W images are superior for identifying the details of white matter maturation.

3 Months, Axial T1 Images 1–12

Cerebral cortex and subcortical white matter approach isointensity on T1W images between ~3–4 months of age; this can give the false appearance of excessive cortical thickness

Centrum semiovale myelination is increased (frontal more than parietal) compared to age 1 month

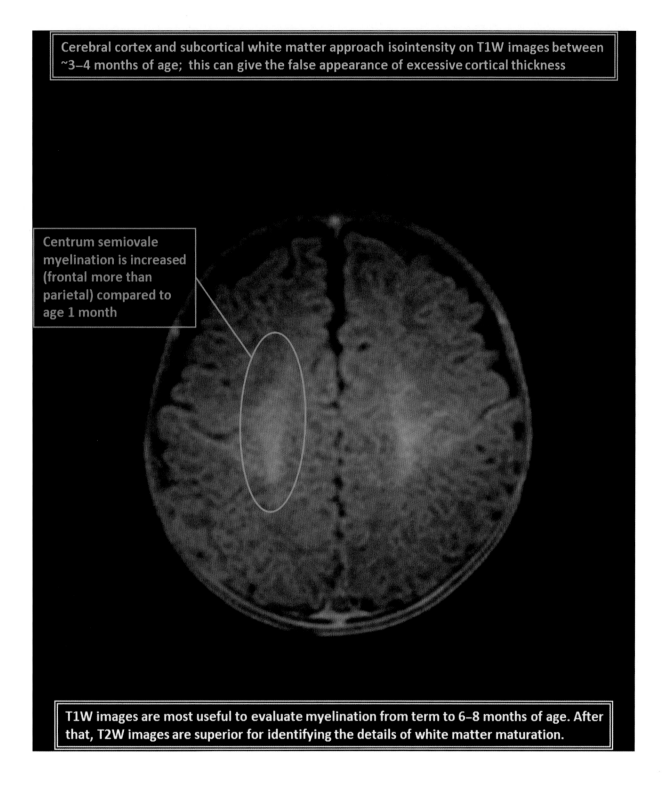

T1W images are most useful to evaluate myelination from term to 6–8 months of age. After that, T2W images are superior for identifying the details of white matter maturation.

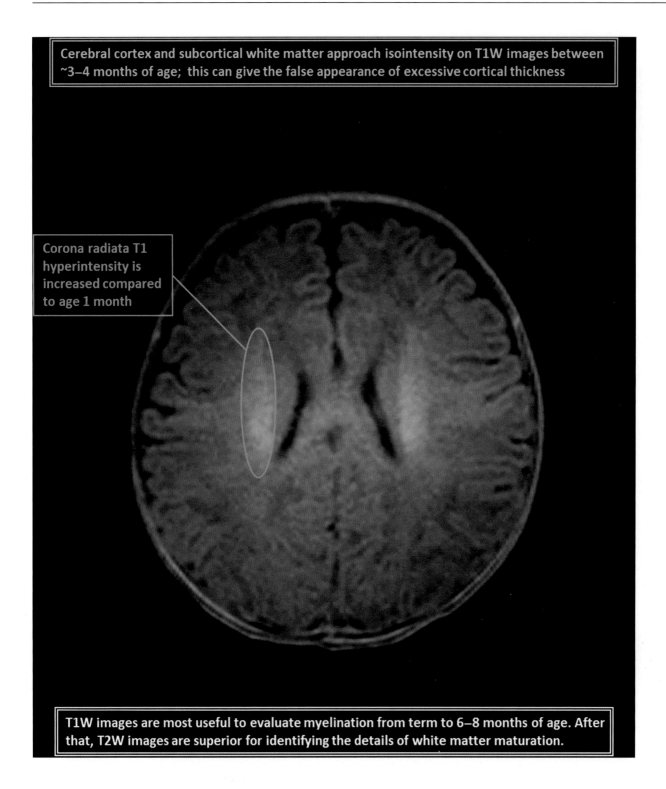

Cerebral cortex and subcortical white matter approach isointensity on T1W images between ~3–4 months of age; this can give the false appearance of excessive cortical thickness

Corona radiata T1 hyperintensity is increased compared to age 1 month

T1W images are most useful to evaluate myelination from term to 6–8 months of age. After that, T2W images are superior for identifying the details of white matter maturation.

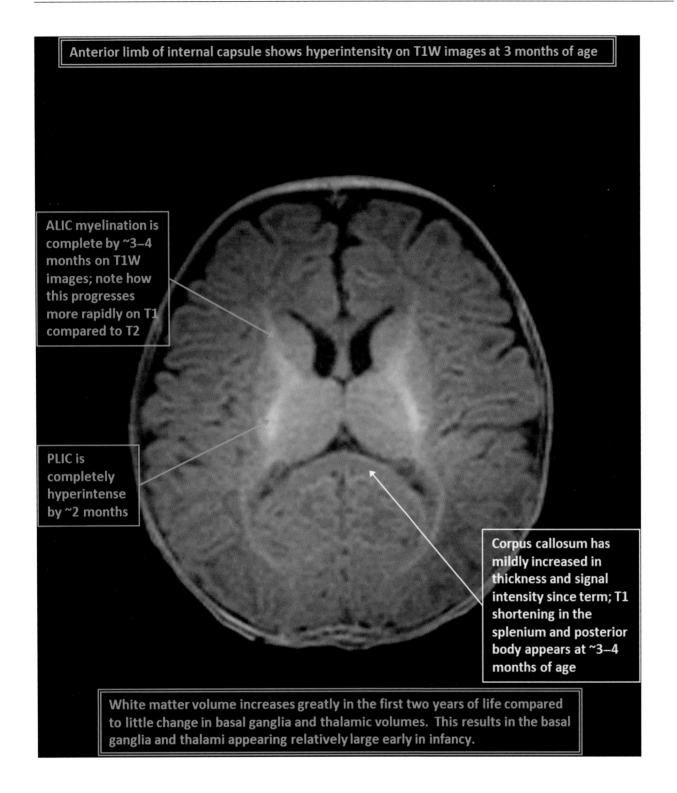

Anterior limb of internal capsule shows hyperintensity on T1W images at 3 months of age

ALIC myelination is complete by ~3–4 months on T1W images; note how this progresses more rapidly on T1 compared to T2

PLIC is completely hyperintense by ~2 months

Corpus callosum has mildly increased in thickness and signal intensity since term; T1 shortening in the splenium and posterior body appears at ~3–4 months of age

White matter volume increases greatly in the first two years of life compared to little change in basal ganglia and thalamic volumes. This results in the basal ganglia and thalami appearing relatively large early in infancy.

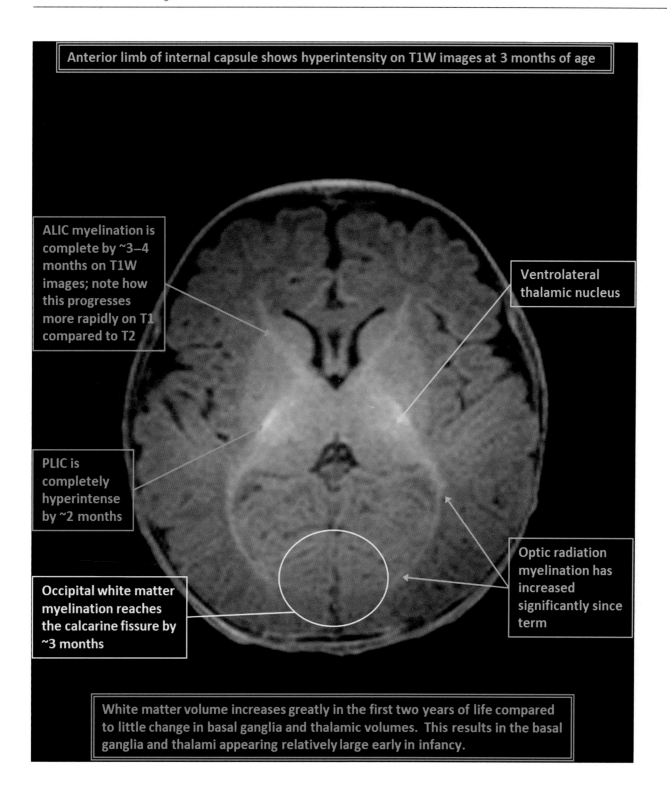

Anterior limb of internal capsule shows hyperintensity on T1W images at 3 months of age

ALIC myelination is complete by ~3–4 months on T1W images; note how this progresses more rapidly on T1 compared to T2

Ventrolateral thalamic nucleus

PLIC is completely hyperintense by ~2 months

Occipital white matter myelination reaches the calcarine fissure by ~3 months

Optic radiation myelination has increased significantly since term

White matter volume increases greatly in the first two years of life compared to little change in basal ganglia and thalamic volumes. This results in the basal ganglia and thalami appearing relatively large early in infancy.

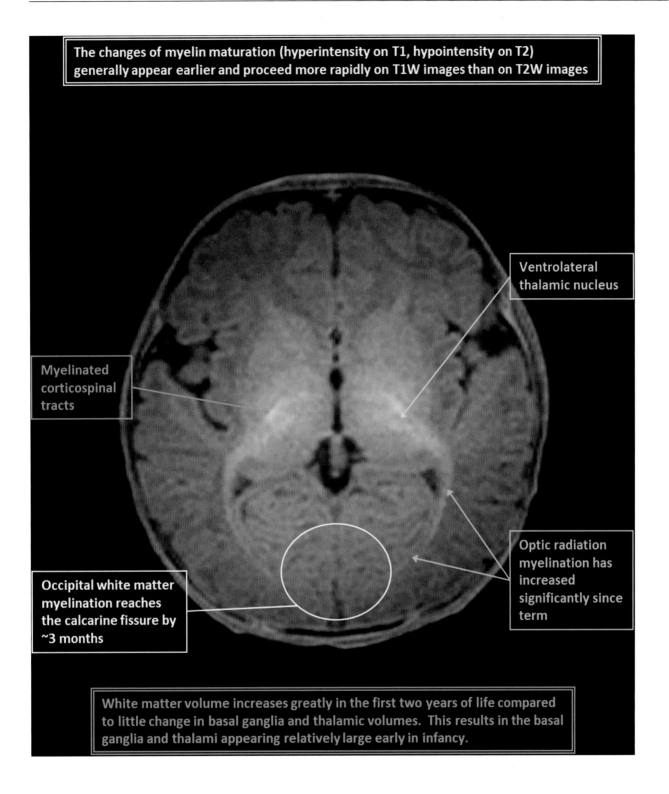

The changes of myelin maturation (hyperintensity on T1, hypointensity on T2) generally appear earlier and proceed more rapidly on T1W images than on T2W images

Ventrolateral thalamic nucleus

Myelinated corticospinal tracts

Optic radiation myelination has increased significantly since term

Occipital white matter myelination reaches the calcarine fissure by ~3 months

White matter volume increases greatly in the first two years of life compared to little change in basal ganglia and thalamic volumes. This results in the basal ganglia and thalami appearing relatively large early in infancy.

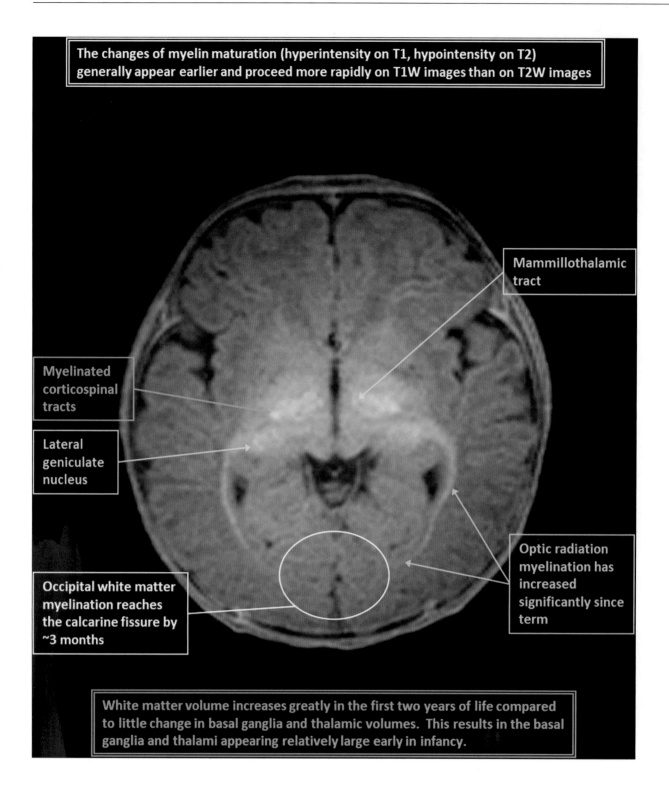

The changes of myelin maturation (hyperintensity on T1, hypointensity on T2) generally appear earlier and proceed more rapidly on T1W images than on T2W images

Mammillothalamic tract

Myelinated corticospinal tracts

Lateral geniculate nucleus

Optic radiation myelination has increased significantly since term

Occipital white matter myelination reaches the calcarine fissure by ~3 months

White matter volume increases greatly in the first two years of life compared to little change in basal ganglia and thalamic volumes. This results in the basal ganglia and thalami appearing relatively large early in infancy.

The changes of myelin maturation (hyperintensity on T1, hypointensity on T2) generally appear earlier and proceed more rapidly on T1W images than on T2W images

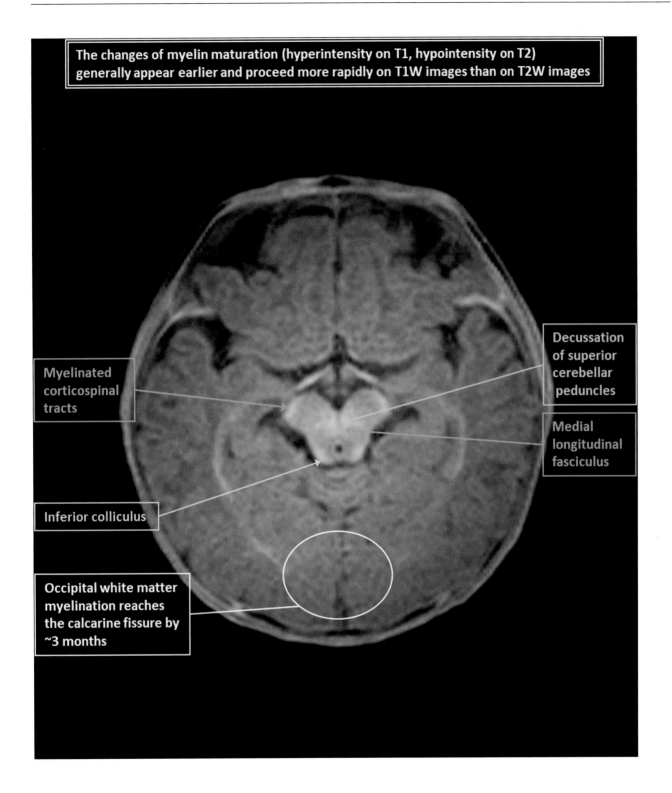

Myelinated corticospinal tracts

Decussation of superior cerebellar peduncles

Medial longitudinal fasciculus

Inferior colliculus

Occipital white matter myelination reaches the calcarine fissure by ~3 months

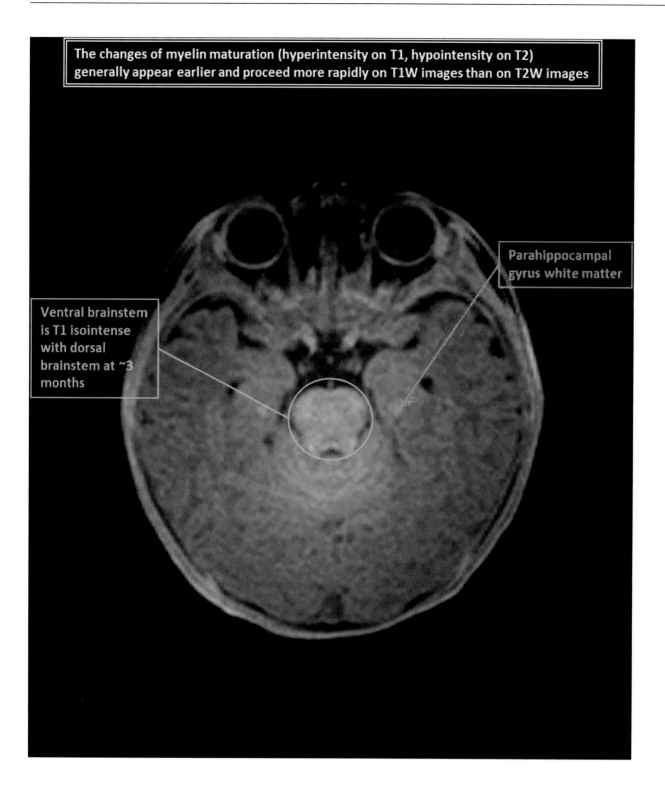

The changes of myelin maturation (hyperintensity on T1, hypointensity on T2) generally appear earlier and proceed more rapidly on T1W images than on T2W images

Parahippocampal gyrus white matter

Ventral brainstem is T1 isointense with dorsal brainstem at ~3 months

The changes of myelin maturation (hyperintensity on T1, hypointensity on T2) generally appear earlier and proceed more rapidly on T1W images than on T2W images

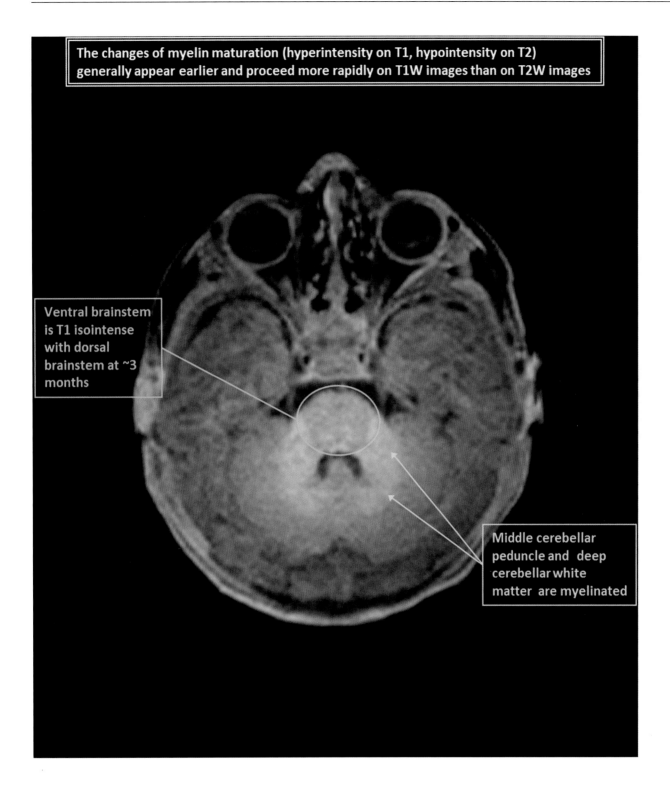

Ventral brainstem is T1 isointense with dorsal brainstem at ~3 months

Middle cerebellar peduncle and deep cerebellar white matter are myelinated

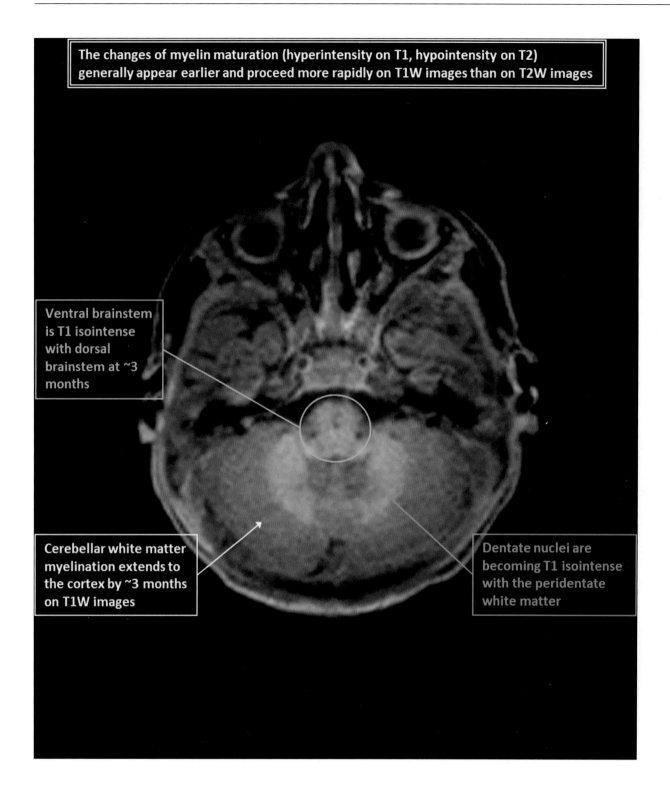

The changes of myelin maturation (hyperintensity on T1, hypointensity on T2) generally appear earlier and proceed more rapidly on T1W images than on T2W images

Ventral brainstem is T1 isointense with dorsal brainstem at ~3 months

Cerebellar white matter myelination extends to the cortex by ~3 months on T1W images

Dentate nuclei are becoming T1 isointense with the peridentate white matter

The changes of myelin maturation (hyperintensity on T1, hypointensity on T2) generally appear earlier and proceed more rapidly on T1W images than on T2W images

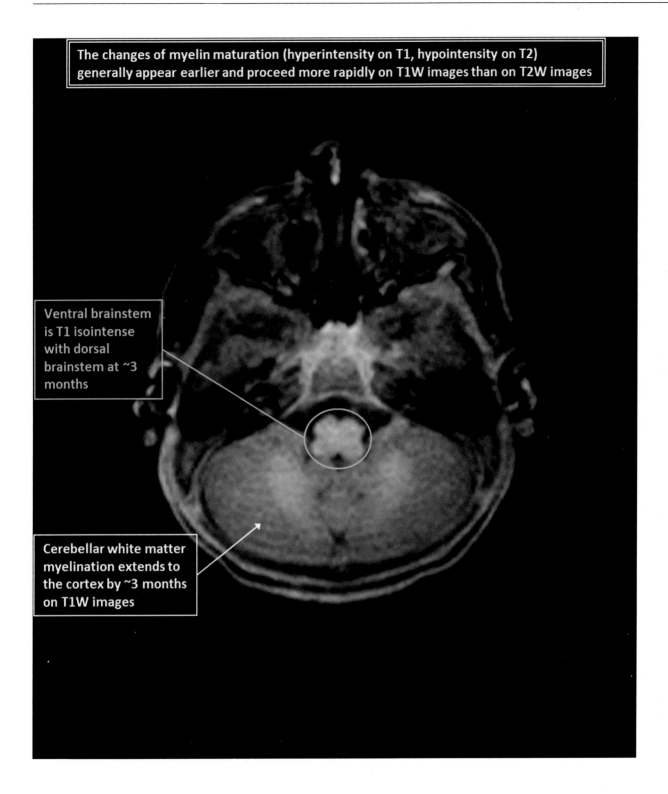

Ventral brainstem is T1 isointense with dorsal brainstem at ~3 months

Cerebellar white matter myelination extends to the cortex by ~3 months on T1W images

3 Months, Axial TSE T2

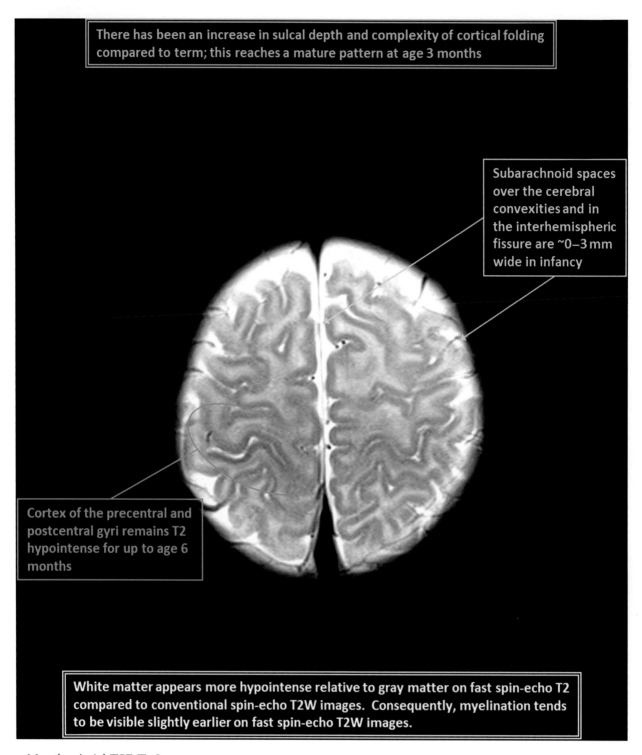

There has been an increase in sulcal depth and complexity of cortical folding compared to term; this reaches a mature pattern at age 3 months

Subarachnoid spaces over the cerebral convexities and in the interhemispheric fissure are ~0–3 mm wide in infancy

Cortex of the precentral and postcentral gyri remains T2 hypointense for up to age 6 months

White matter appears more hypointense relative to gray matter on fast spin-echo T2 compared to conventional spin-echo T2W images. Consequently, myelination tends to be visible slightly earlier on fast spin-echo T2W images.

3 Months, Axial TSE T2 Images 1–12

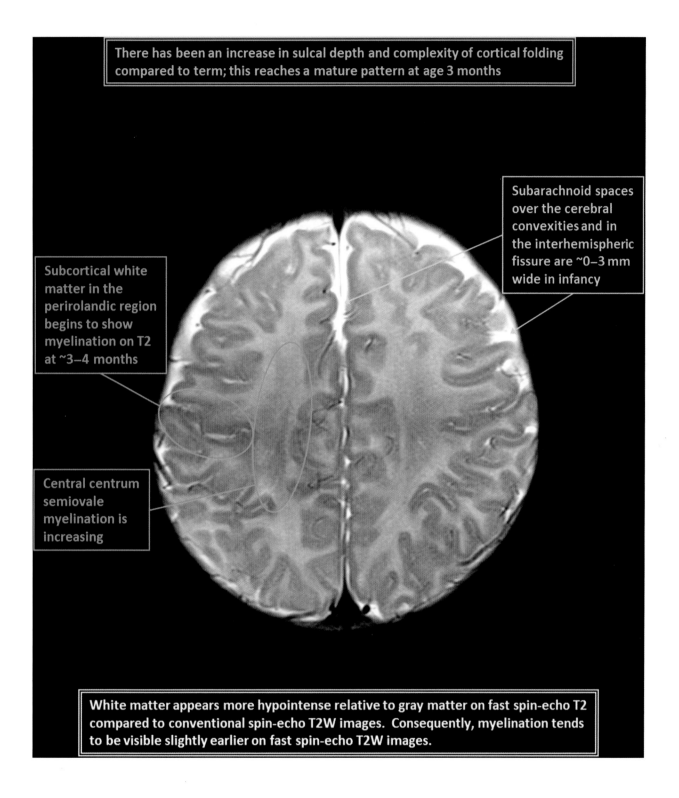

There has been an increase in sulcal depth and complexity of cortical folding compared to term; this reaches a mature pattern at age 3 months

Subarachnoid spaces over the cerebral convexities and in the interhemispheric fissure are ~0–3 mm wide in infancy

Subcortical white matter in the perirolandic region begins to show myelination on T2 at ~3–4 months

Central centrum semiovale myelination is increasing

White matter appears more hypointense relative to gray matter on fast spin-echo T2 compared to conventional spin-echo T2W images. Consequently, myelination tends to be visible slightly earlier on fast spin-echo T2W images.

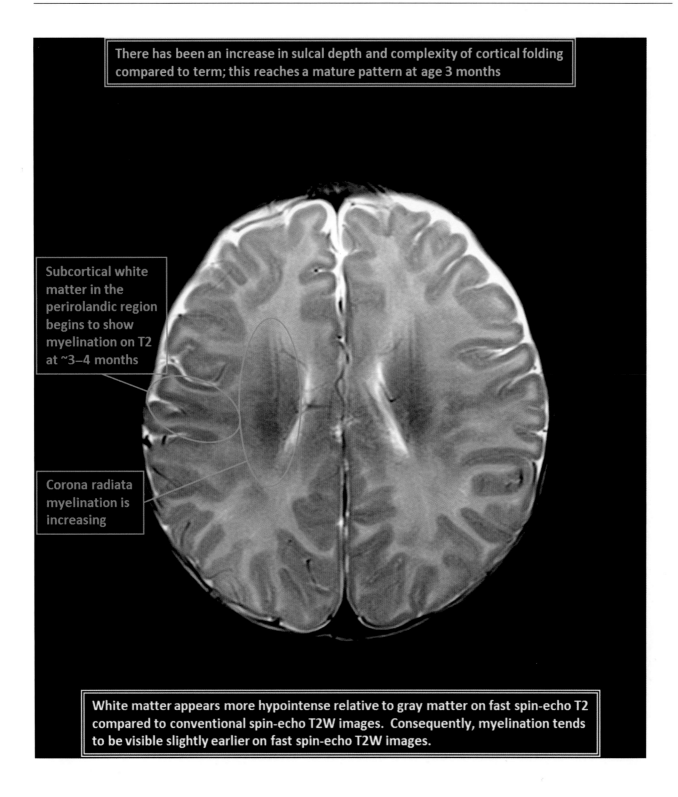

There has been an increase in sulcal depth and complexity of cortical folding compared to term; this reaches a mature pattern at age 3 months

Subcortical white matter in the perirolandic region begins to show myelination on T2 at ~3–4 months

Corona radiata myelination is increasing

White matter appears more hypointense relative to gray matter on fast spin-echo T2 compared to conventional spin-echo T2W images. Consequently, myelination tends to be visible slightly earlier on fast spin-echo T2W images.

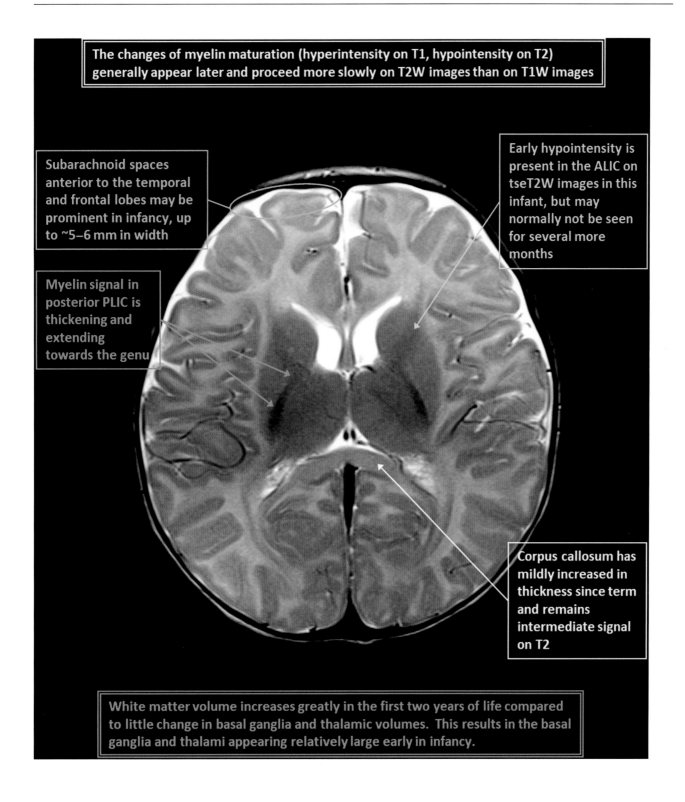

The changes of myelin maturation (hyperintensity on T1, hypointensity on T2) generally appear later and proceed more slowly on T2W images than on T1W images

Subarachnoid spaces anterior to the temporal and frontal lobes may be prominent in infancy, up to ~5–6 mm in width

Early hypointensity is present in the ALIC on tseT2W images in this infant, but may normally not be seen for several more months

Myelin signal in posterior PLIC is thickening and extending towards the genu

Corpus callosum has mildly increased in thickness since term and remains intermediate signal on T2

White matter volume increases greatly in the first two years of life compared to little change in basal ganglia and thalamic volumes. This results in the basal ganglia and thalami appearing relatively large early in infancy.

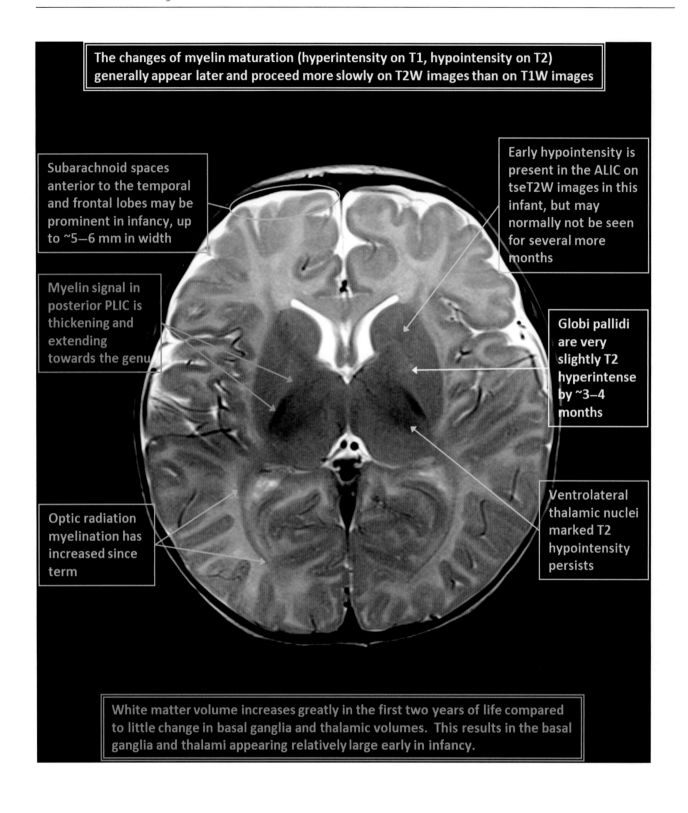

The changes of myelin maturation (hyperintensity on T1, hypointensity on T2) generally appear later and proceed more slowly on T2W images than on T1W images

Subarachnoid spaces anterior to the temporal and frontal lobes may be prominent in infancy, up to ~5–6 mm in width

Early hypointensity is present in the ALIC on tseT2W images in this infant, but may normally not be seen for several more months

Myelin signal in posterior PLIC is thickening and extending towards the genu

Globi pallidi are very slightly T2 hyperintense by ~3–4 months

Optic radiation myelination has increased since term

Ventrolateral thalamic nuclei marked T2 hypointensity persists

White matter volume increases greatly in the first two years of life compared to little change in basal ganglia and thalamic volumes. This results in the basal ganglia and thalami appearing relatively large early in infancy.

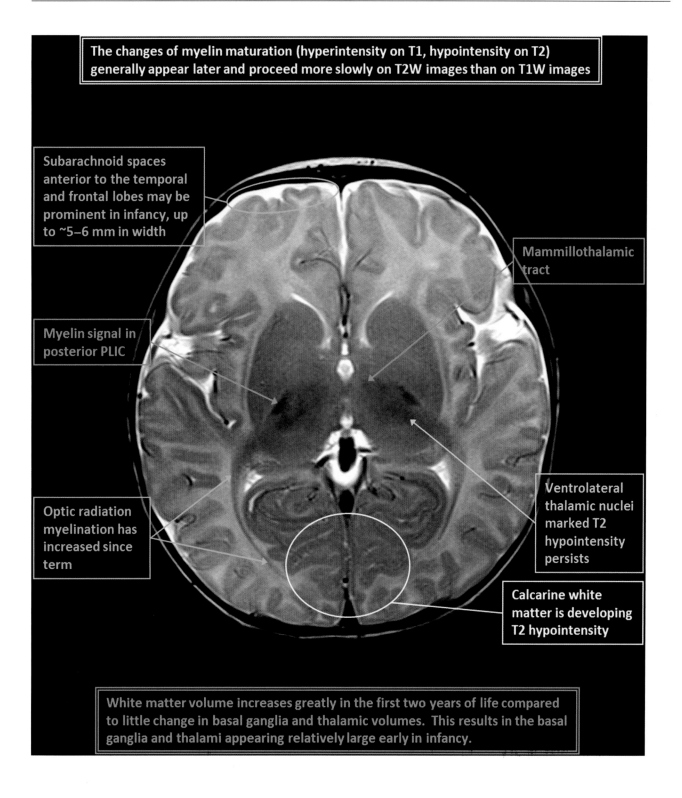

The changes of myelin maturation (hyperintensity on T1, hypointensity on T2) generally appear later and proceed more slowly on T2W images than on T1W images

Subarachnoid spaces anterior to the temporal and frontal lobes may be prominent in infancy, up to ~5–6 mm in width

Mammillothalamic tract

Myelin signal in posterior PLIC

Optic radiation myelination has increased since term

Ventrolateral thalamic nuclei marked T2 hypointensity persists

Calcarine white matter is developing T2 hypointensity

White matter volume increases greatly in the first two years of life compared to little change in basal ganglia and thalamic volumes. This results in the basal ganglia and thalami appearing relatively large early in infancy.

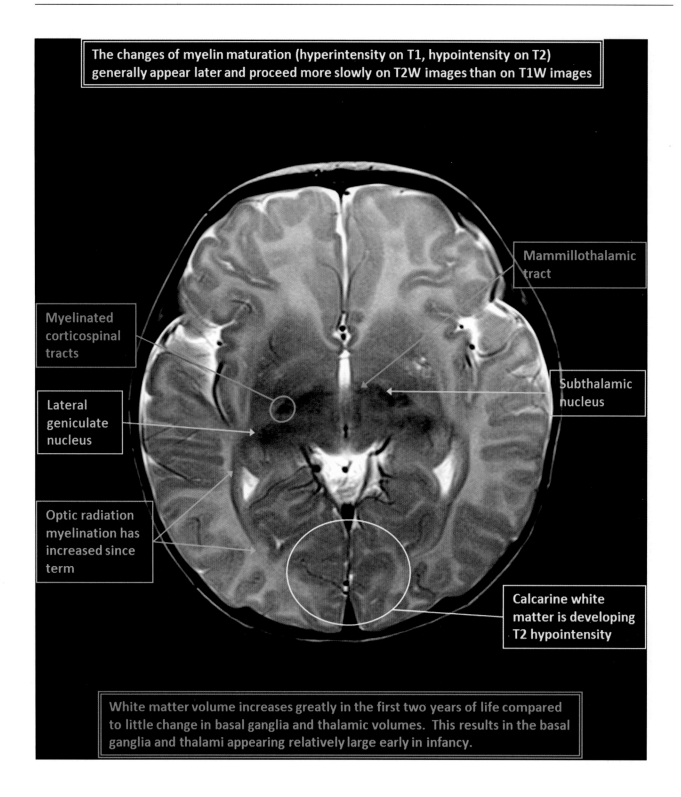

The changes of myelin maturation (hyperintensity on T1, hypointensity on T2) generally appear later and proceed more slowly on T2W images than on T1W images

Mammillothalamic tract

Myelinated corticospinal tracts

Lateral geniculate nucleus

Subthalamic nucleus

Optic radiation myelination has increased since term

Calcarine white matter is developing T2 hypointensity

White matter volume increases greatly in the first two years of life compared to little change in basal ganglia and thalamic volumes. This results in the basal ganglia and thalami appearing relatively large early in infancy.

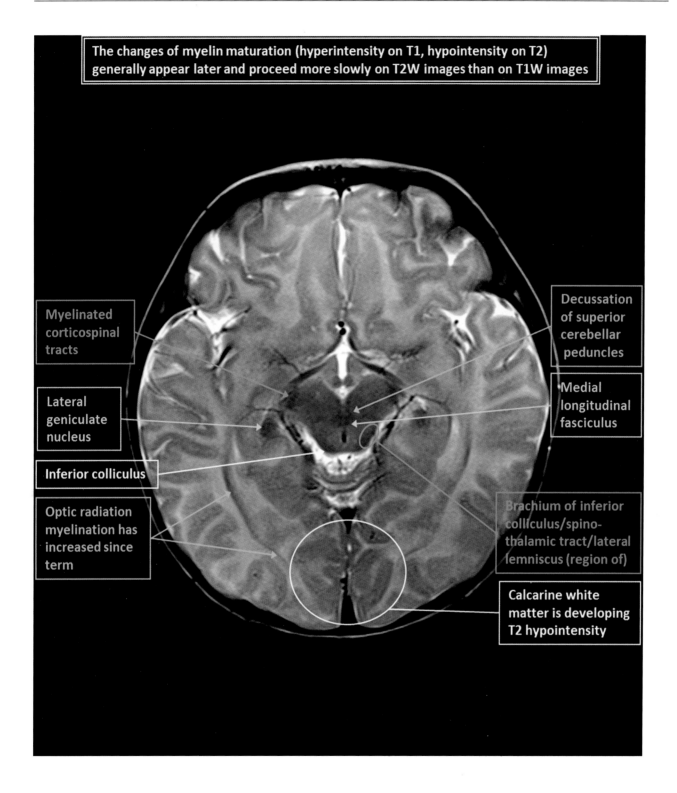

The changes of myelin maturation (hyperintensity on T1, hypointensity on T2) generally appear later and proceed more slowly on T2W images than on T1W images

Myelinated corticospinal tracts

Lateral geniculate nucleus

Inferior colliculus

Optic radiation myelination has increased since term

Decussation of superior cerebellar peduncles

Medial longitudinal fasciculus

Brachium of inferior colliculus/spino-thalamic tract/lateral lemniscus (region of)

Calcarine white matter is developing T2 hypointensity

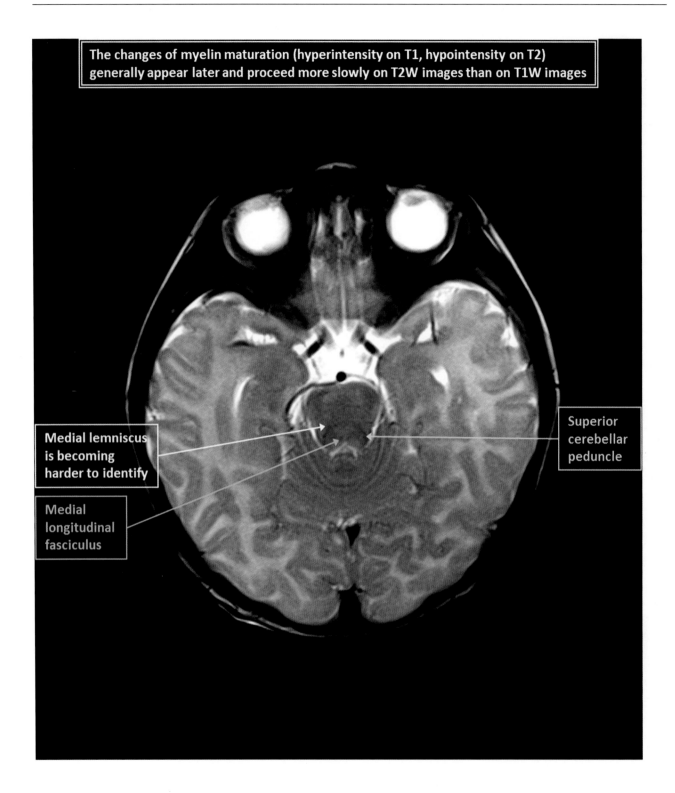

The changes of myelin maturation (hyperintensity on T1, hypointensity on T2) generally appear later and proceed more slowly on T2W images than on T1W images

Medial lemniscus is becoming harder to identify

Medial longitudinal fasciculus

Superior cerebellar peduncle

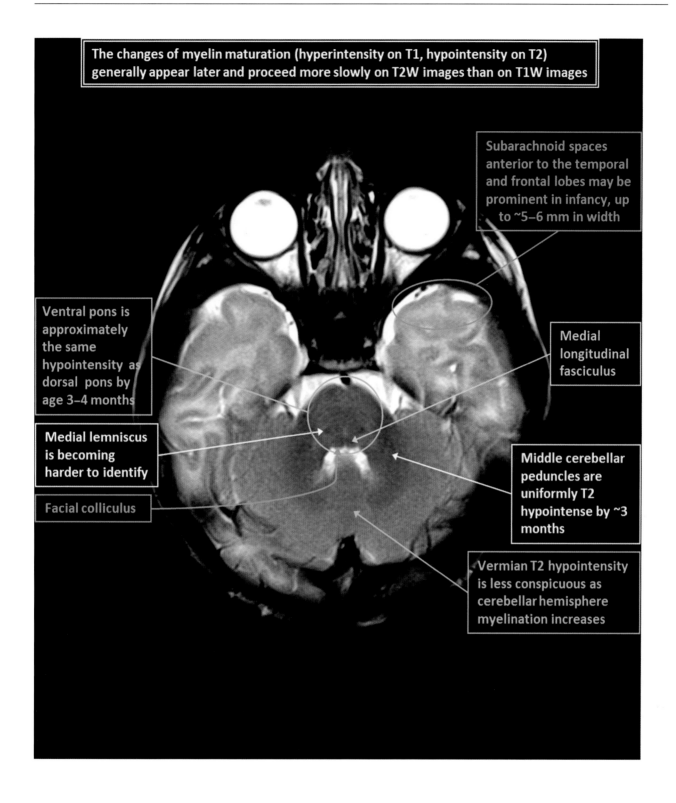

The changes of myelin maturation (hyperintensity on T1, hypointensity on T2) generally appear later and proceed more slowly on T2W images than on T1W images

Subarachnoid spaces anterior to the temporal and frontal lobes may be prominent in infancy, up to ~5–6 mm in width

Ventral pons is approximately the same hypointensity as dorsal pons by age 3–4 months

Medial longitudinal fasciculus

Medial lemniscus is becoming harder to identify

Facial colliculus

Middle cerebellar peduncles are uniformly T2 hypointense by ~3 months

Vermian T2 hypointensity is less conspicuous as cerebellar hemisphere myelination increases

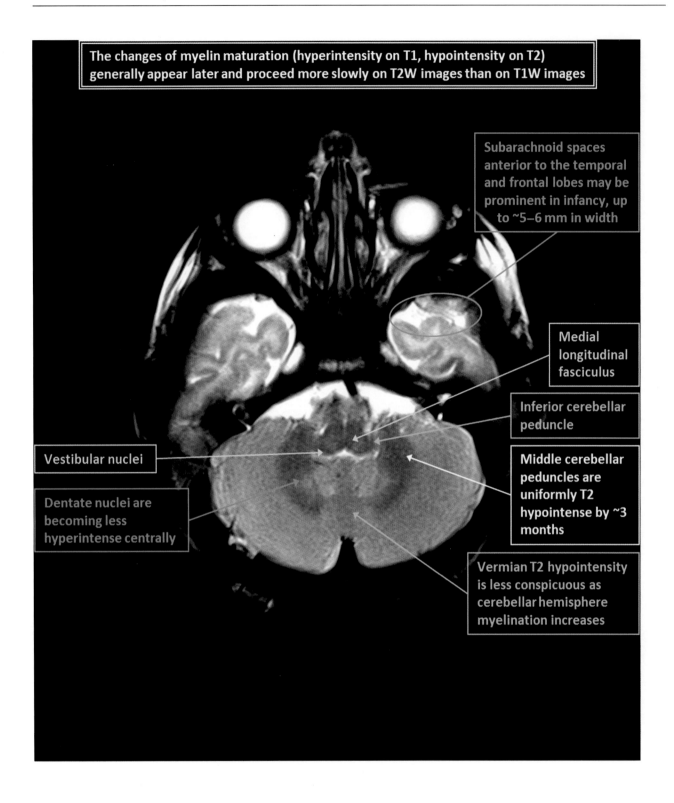

The changes of myelin maturation (hyperintensity on T1, hypointensity on T2) generally appear later and proceed more slowly on T2W images than on T1W images

Subarachnoid spaces anterior to the temporal and frontal lobes may be prominent in infancy, up to ~5–6 mm in width

Medial longitudinal fasciculus

Inferior cerebellar peduncle

Vestibular nuclei

Middle cerebellar peduncles are uniformly T2 hypointense by ~3 months

Dentate nuclei are becoming less hyperintense centrally

Vermian T2 hypointensity is less conspicuous as cerebellar hemisphere myelination increases

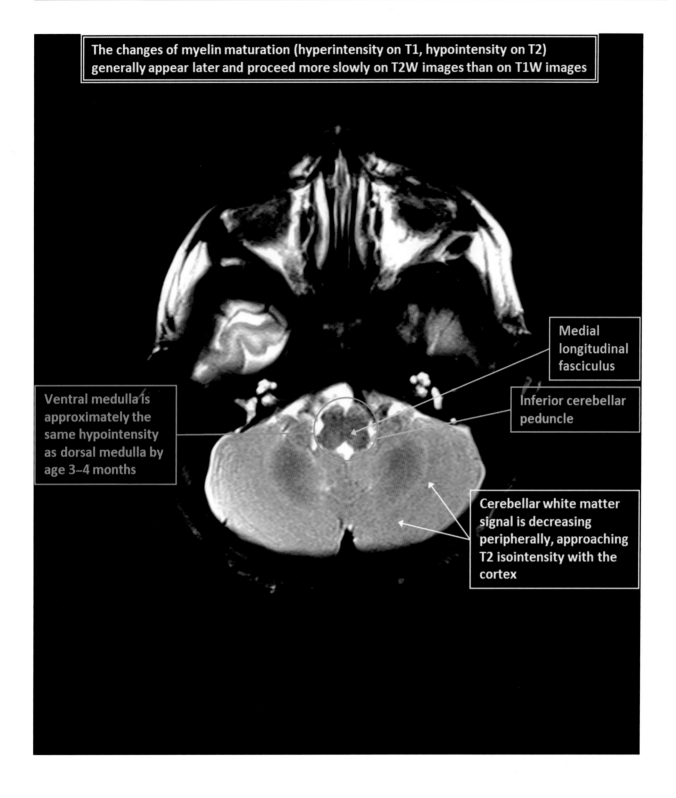

The changes of myelin maturation (hyperintensity on T1, hypointensity on T2) generally appear later and proceed more slowly on T2W images than on T1W images

Medial longitudinal fasciculus

Inferior cerebellar peduncle

Ventral medulla is approximately the same hypointensity as dorsal medulla by age 3–4 months

Cerebellar white matter signal is decreasing peripherally, approaching T2 isointensity with the cortex

3 Months, Diffusion Weighted Imaging (DWI) (b=1000 s/mm²)

Diffusion restriction increases during white matter maturation, which results in a gradual increase in WM signal intensity and thus a reduction in GM-WM contrast on diffusion weighted images from the neonatal period up to ~5 months of age

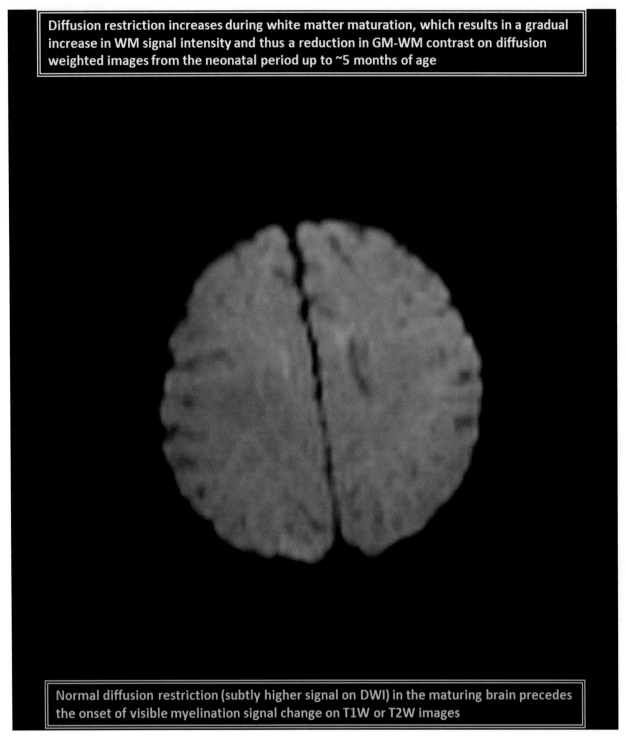

Normal diffusion restriction (subtly higher signal on DWI) in the maturing brain precedes the onset of visible myelination signal change on T1W or T2W images

3 Months, Diffusion Weighted Imaging (DWI) (b=1000 s/mm²) Images 1–5

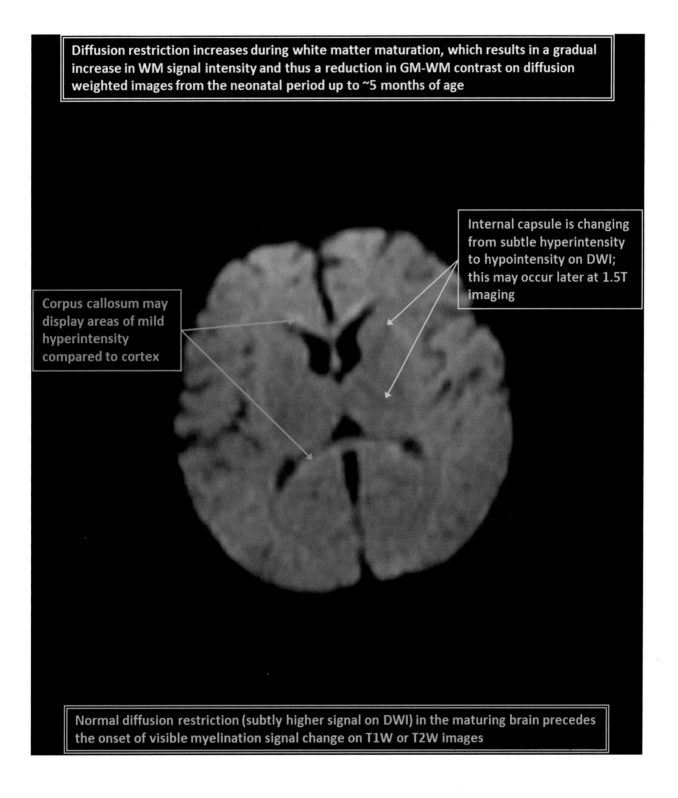

Diffusion restriction increases during white matter maturation, which results in a gradual increase in WM signal intensity and thus a reduction in GM-WM contrast on diffusion weighted images from the neonatal period up to ~5 months of age

Internal capsule is changing from subtle hyperintensity to hypointensity on DWI; this may occur later at 1.5T imaging

Corpus callosum may display areas of mild hyperintensity compared to cortex

Normal diffusion restriction (subtly higher signal on DWI) in the maturing brain precedes the onset of visible myelination signal change on T1W or T2W images

Diffusion restriction increases during white matter maturation, which results in a gradual increase in WM signal intensity and thus a reduction in GM-WM contrast on diffusion weighted images from the neonatal period up to ~5 months of age

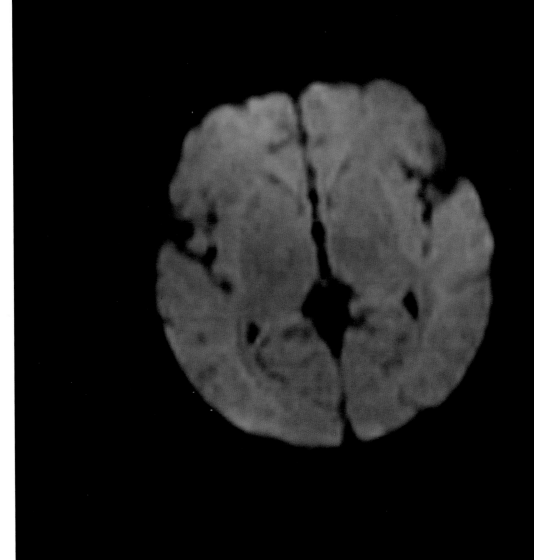

Normal diffusion restriction (subtly higher signal on DWI) in the maturing brain precedes the onset of visible myelination signal change on T1W or T2W images

For most of the first year of life, the cerebellum as a whole can have a noticeably more hypointense appearance on ADC than the cerebral hemispheres, while on DWI it is isointense to subtly hyperintense to the cerebrum

Normal diffusion restriction (subtly higher signal on DWI) in the maturing brain precedes the onset of visible myelination signal change on T1W or T2W images

For most of the first year of life, the cerebellum as a whole can have a noticeably more hypointense appearance on ADC than the cerebral hemispheres, while on DWI it is isointense to subtly hyperintense to the cerebrum

Cerebellar white matter hypointensity is increasingly obvious

Normal diffusion restriction (subtly higher signal on DWI) in the maturing brain precedes the onset of visible myelination signal change on T1W or T2W images

3 Months, Apparent Diffusion Coefficient (ADC) Map

The high contrast appearance between white matter and gray matter found on ADC images in neonates has diminished, reflecting the rapid decrease in ADC values of WM during the first five months of life

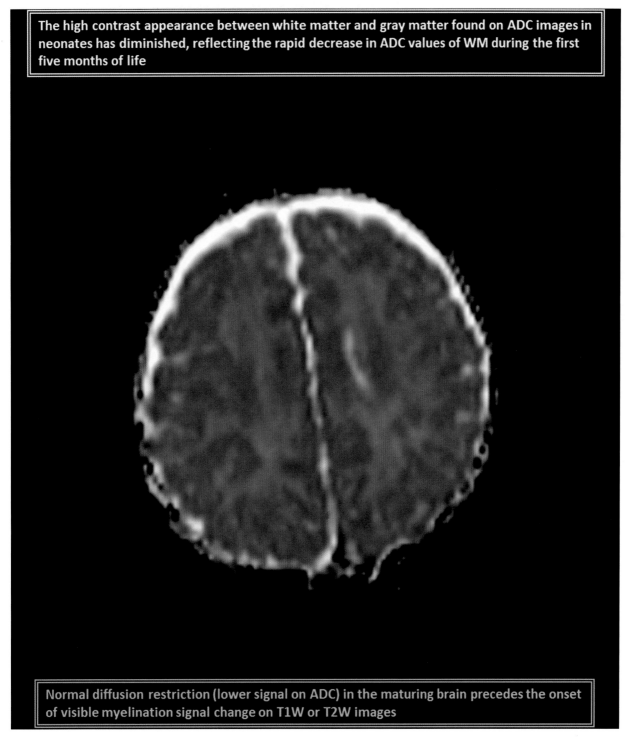

Normal diffusion restriction (lower signal on ADC) in the maturing brain precedes the onset of visible myelination signal change on T1W or T2W images

3 Months, Apparent Diffusion Coefficient (ADC) Map Images 1–5

The high contrast appearance between white matter and gray matter found on ADC images in neonates has diminished, reflecting the rapid decrease in ADC values of WM during the first five months of life

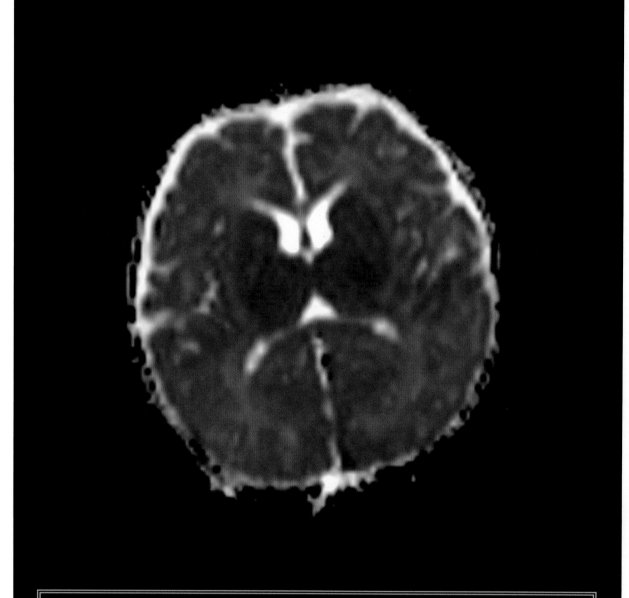

Normal diffusion restriction (lower signal on ADC) in the maturing brain precedes the onset of visible myelination signal change on T1W or T2W images

The high contrast appearance between white matter and gray matter found on ADC images in neonates has diminished, reflecting the rapid decrease in ADC values of WM during the first five months of life

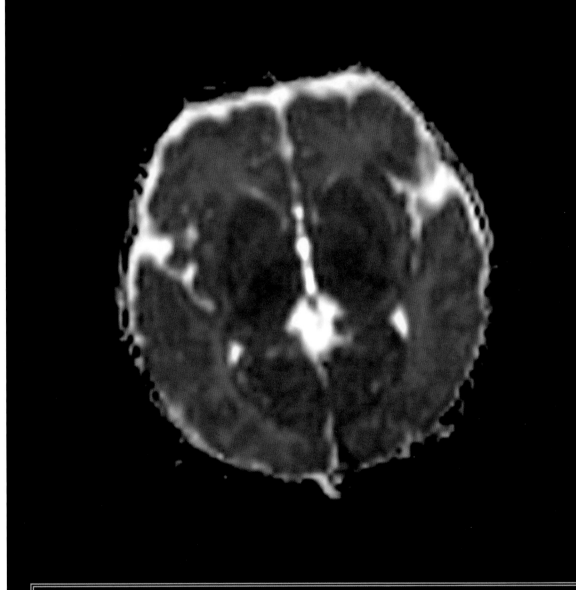

Normal diffusion restriction (lower signal on ADC) in the maturing brain precedes the onset of visible myelination signal change on T1W or T2W images

For most of the first year of life, the cerebellum as a whole can have a noticeably more hypointense appearance on ADC than the cerebral hemispheres, while on DWI it is isointense to subtly hyperintense to the cerebrum

Normal diffusion restriction (lower signal on ADC) in the maturing brain precedes the onset of visible myelination signal change on T1W or T2W images

For most of the first year of life, the cerebellum as a whole can have a noticeably more hypointense appearance on ADC than the cerebral hemispheres, while on DWI it is isointense to subtly hyperintense to the cerebrum

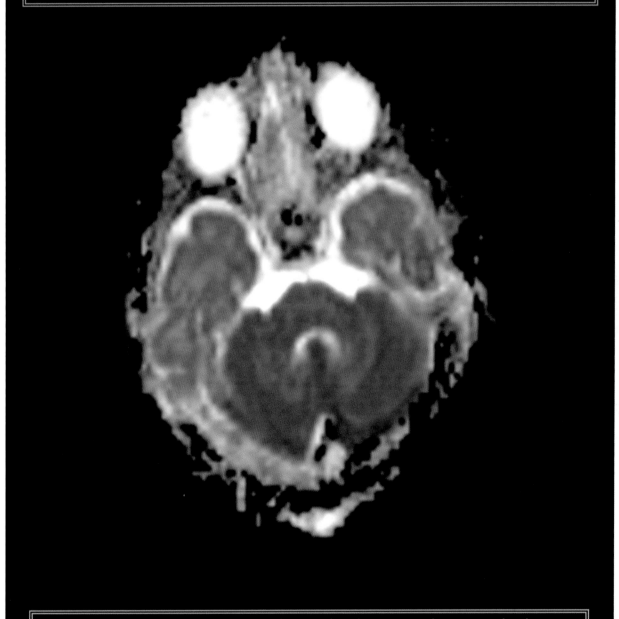

Normal diffusion restriction (lower signal on ADC) in the maturing brain precedes the onset of visible myelination signal change on T1W or T2W images

3 Months, Sagittal T1

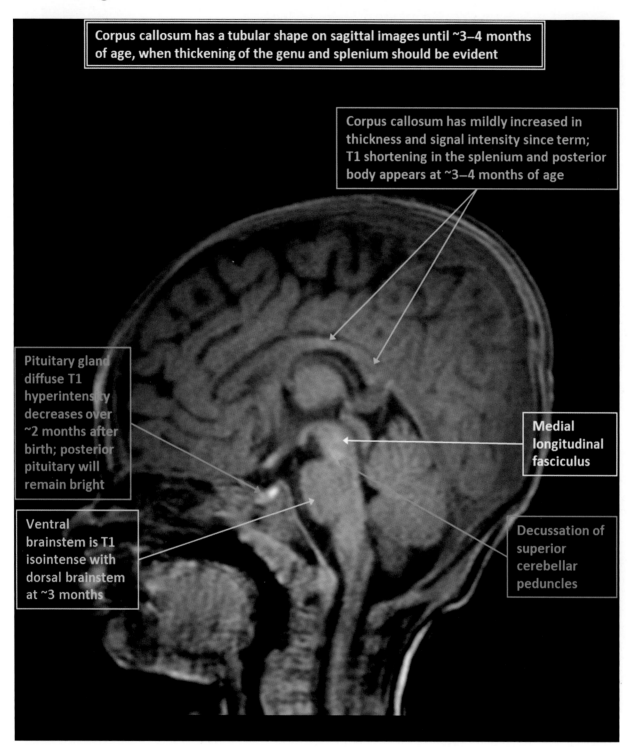

Corpus callosum has a tubular shape on sagittal images until ~3–4 months of age, when thickening of the genu and splenium should be evident

Corpus callosum has mildly increased in thickness and signal intensity since term; T1 shortening in the splenium and posterior body appears at ~3–4 months of age

Pituitary gland diffuse T1 hyperintensity decreases over ~2 months after birth; posterior pituitary will remain bright

Medial longitudinal fasciculus

Ventral brainstem is T1 isointense with dorsal brainstem at ~3 months

Decussation of superior cerebellar peduncles

3 Months, Sagittal T1 Images 1–4

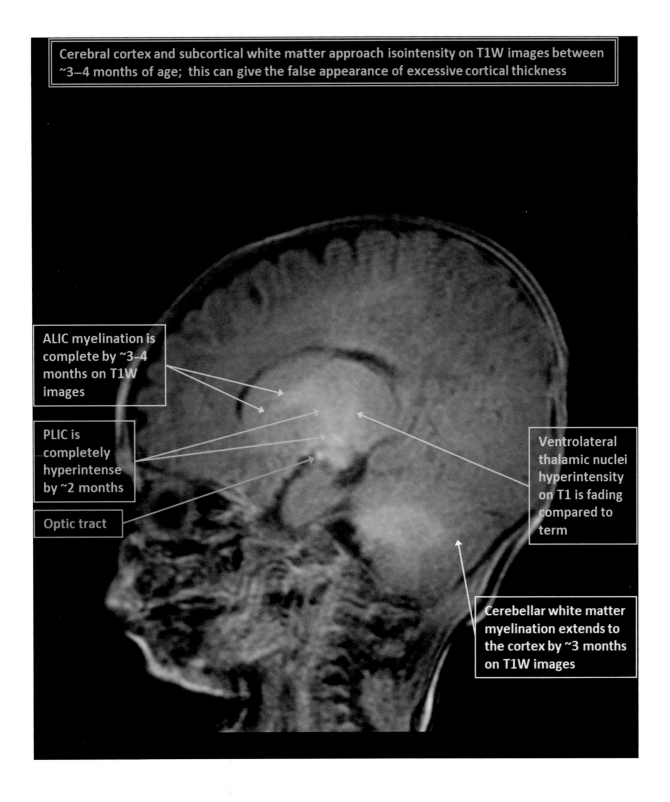

Cerebral cortex and subcortical white matter approach isointensity on T1W images between ~3–4 months of age; this can give the false appearance of excessive cortical thickness

ALIC myelination is complete by ~3–4 months on T1W images

PLIC is completely hyperintense by ~2 months

Optic tract

Ventrolateral thalamic nuclei hyperintensity on T1 is fading compared to term

Cerebellar white matter myelination extends to the cortex by ~3 months on T1W images

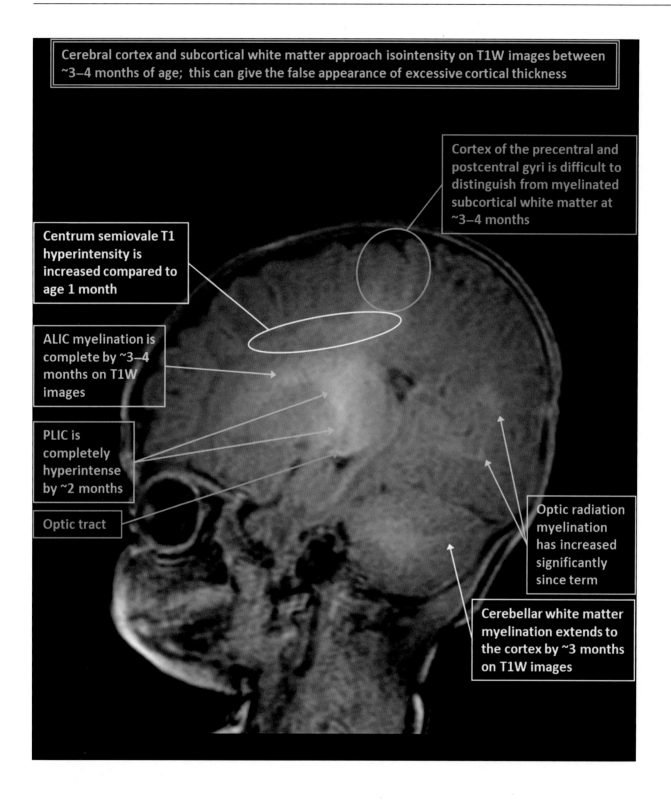

Cerebral cortex and subcortical white matter approach isointensity on T1W images between ~3–4 months of age; this can give the false appearance of excessive cortical thickness

Cortex of the precentral and postcentral gyri is difficult to distinguish from myelinated subcortical white matter at ~3–4 months

Centrum semiovale T1 hyperintensity is increased compared to age 1 month

ALIC myelination is complete by ~3–4 months on T1W images

PLIC is completely hyperintense by ~2 months

Optic tract

Optic radiation myelination has increased significantly since term

Cerebellar white matter myelination extends to the cortex by ~3 months on T1W images

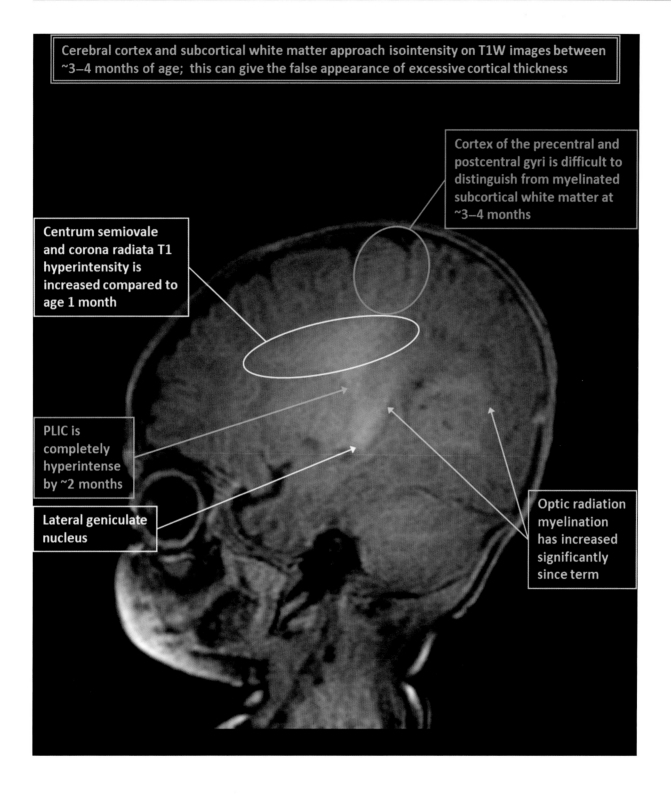

Cerebral cortex and subcortical white matter approach isointensity on T1W images between ~3–4 months of age; this can give the false appearance of excessive cortical thickness

Cortex of the precentral and postcentral gyri is difficult to distinguish from myelinated subcortical white matter at ~3–4 months

Centrum semiovale and corona radiata T1 hyperintensity is increased compared to age 1 month

PLIC is completely hyperintense by ~2 months

Lateral geniculate nucleus

Optic radiation myelination has increased significantly since term

3 Months, Coronal TSE T2

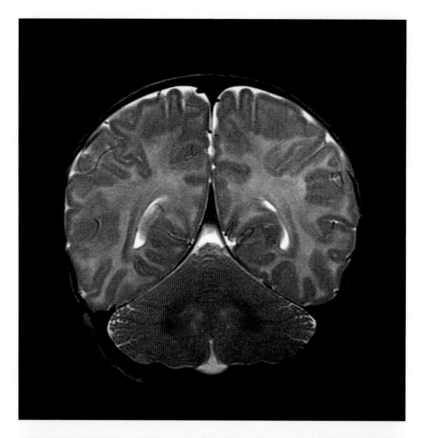

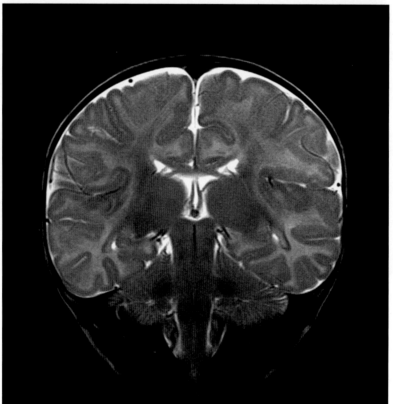

3 Months, Coronal TSE T2 Images 1–4

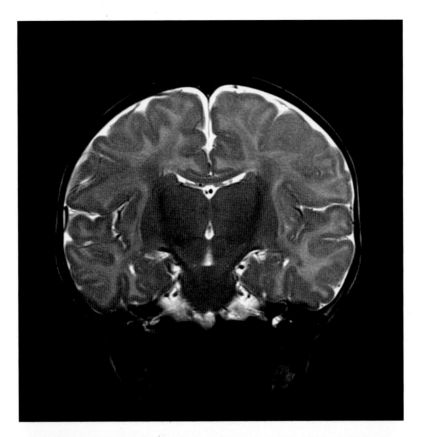

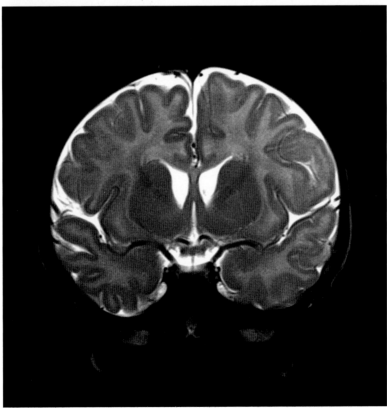

6 Months, Axial T1

As subcortical white matter in different regions pass through a period of isointensity with cortex on T1W images, it can give the false appearance of excessive cortical thickness. This phenomenon occurs predominantly between ~4–8 months of age.

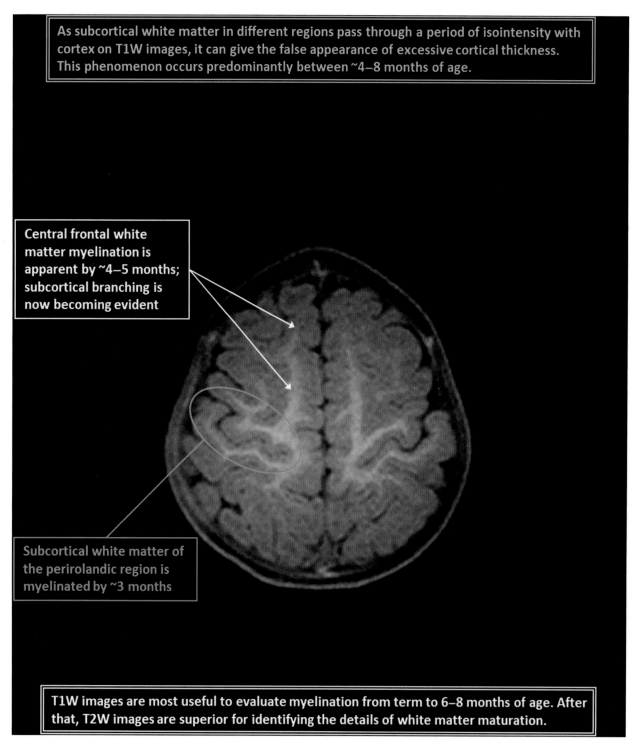

Central frontal white matter myelination is apparent by ~4–5 months; subcortical branching is now becoming evident

Subcortical white matter of the perirolandic region is myelinated by ~3 months

T1W images are most useful to evaluate myelination from term to 6–8 months of age. After that, T2W images are superior for identifying the details of white matter maturation.

6 Months, Axial T1 Images 1–12

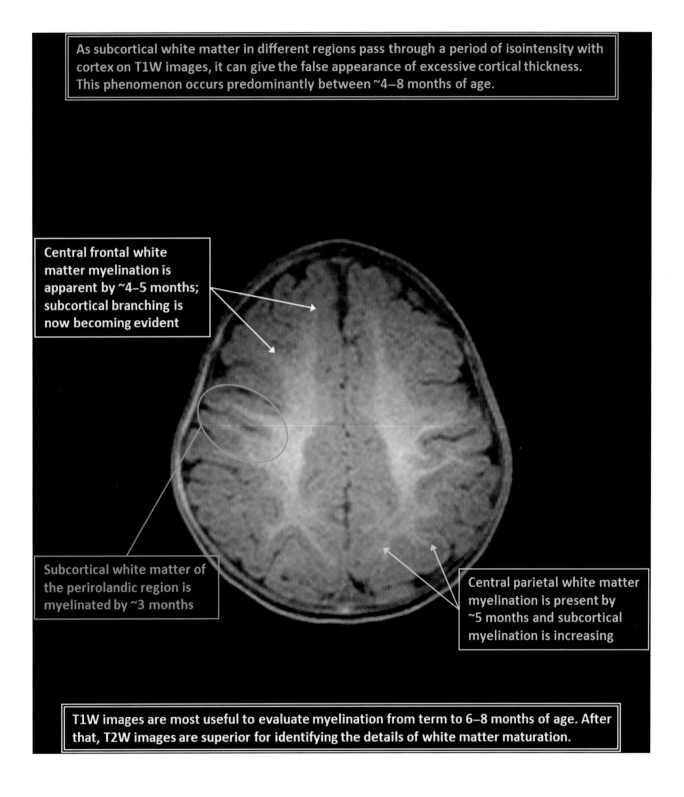

As subcortical white matter in different regions pass through a period of isointensity with cortex on T1W images, it can give the false appearance of excessive cortical thickness. This phenomenon occurs predominantly between ~4–8 months of age.

Central frontal white matter myelination is apparent by ~4–5 months; subcortical branching is now becoming evident

Subcortical white matter of the perirolandic region is myelinated by ~3 months

Central parietal white matter myelination is present by ~5 months and subcortical myelination is increasing

T1W images are most useful to evaluate myelination from term to 6–8 months of age. After that, T2W images are superior for identifying the details of white matter maturation.

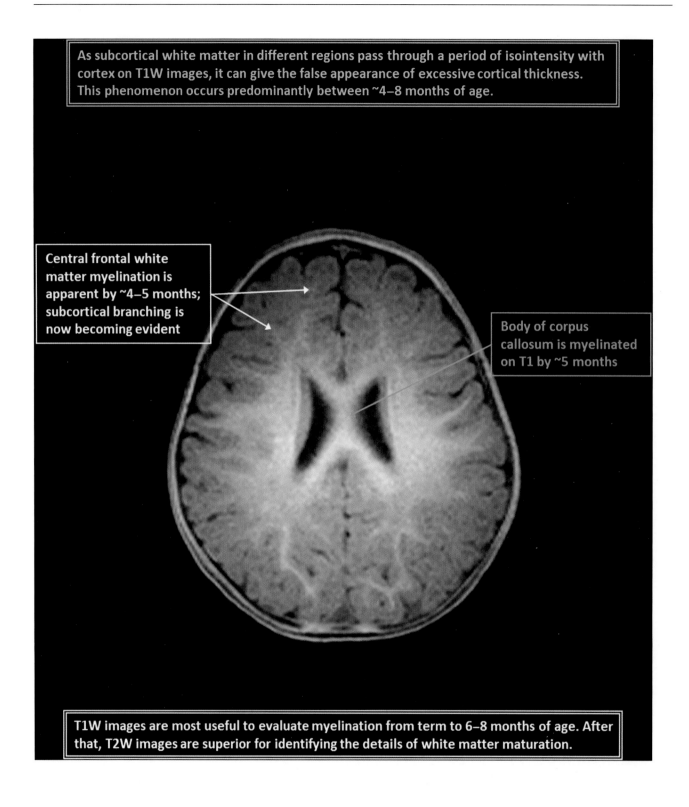

As subcortical white matter in different regions pass through a period of isointensity with cortex on T1W images, it can give the false appearance of excessive cortical thickness. This phenomenon occurs predominantly between ~4–8 months of age.

Central frontal white matter myelination is apparent by ~4–5 months; subcortical branching is now becoming evident

Body of corpus callosum is myelinated on T1 by ~5 months

T1W images are most useful to evaluate myelination from term to 6–8 months of age. After that, T2W images are superior for identifying the details of white matter maturation.

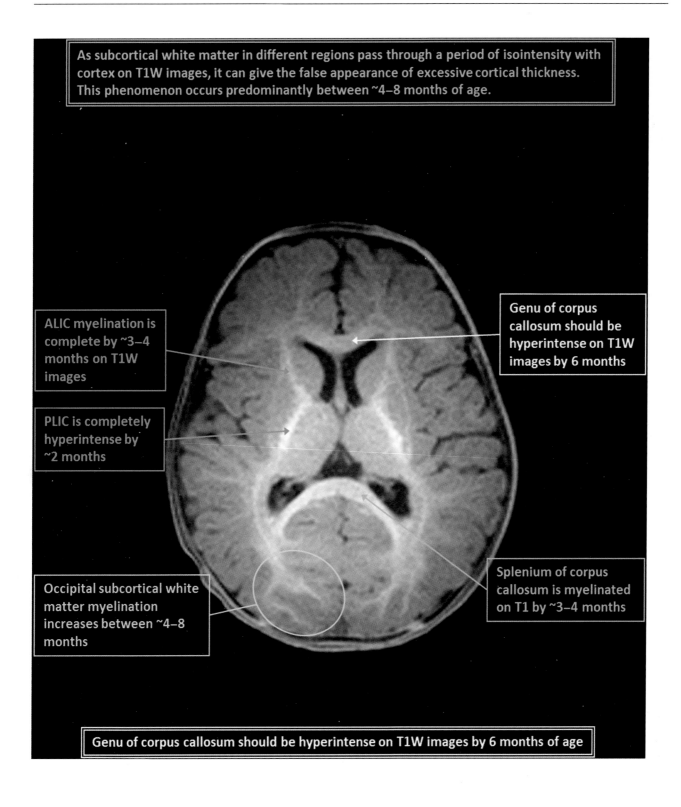

As subcortical white matter in different regions pass through a period of isointensity with cortex on T1W images, it can give the false appearance of excessive cortical thickness. This phenomenon occurs predominantly between ~4–8 months of age.

Genu of corpus callosum should be hyperintense on T1W images by 6 months

ALIC myelination is complete by ~3–4 months on T1W images

PLIC is completely hyperintense by ~2 months

Occipital subcortical white matter myelination increases between ~4–8 months

Splenium of corpus callosum is myelinated on T1 by ~3–4 months

Genu of corpus callosum should be hyperintense on T1W images by 6 months of age

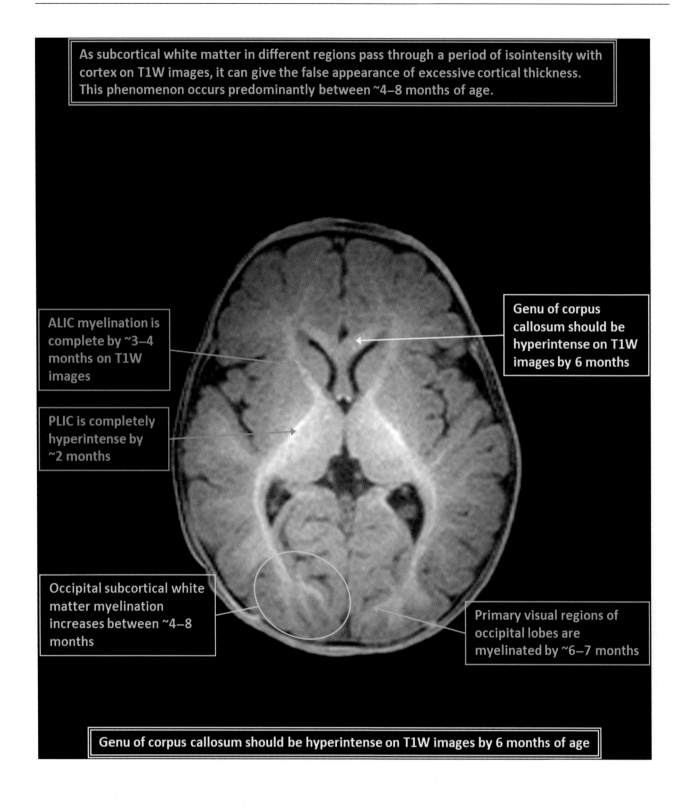

As subcortical white matter in different regions pass through a period of isointensity with cortex on T1W images, it can give the false appearance of excessive cortical thickness. This phenomenon occurs predominantly between ~4–8 months of age.

Genu of corpus callosum should be hyperintense on T1W images by 6 months

ALIC myelination is complete by ~3–4 months on T1W images

PLIC is completely hyperintense by ~2 months

Occipital subcortical white matter myelination increases between ~4–8 months

Primary visual regions of occipital lobes are myelinated by ~6–7 months

Genu of corpus callosum should be hyperintense on T1W images by 6 months of age

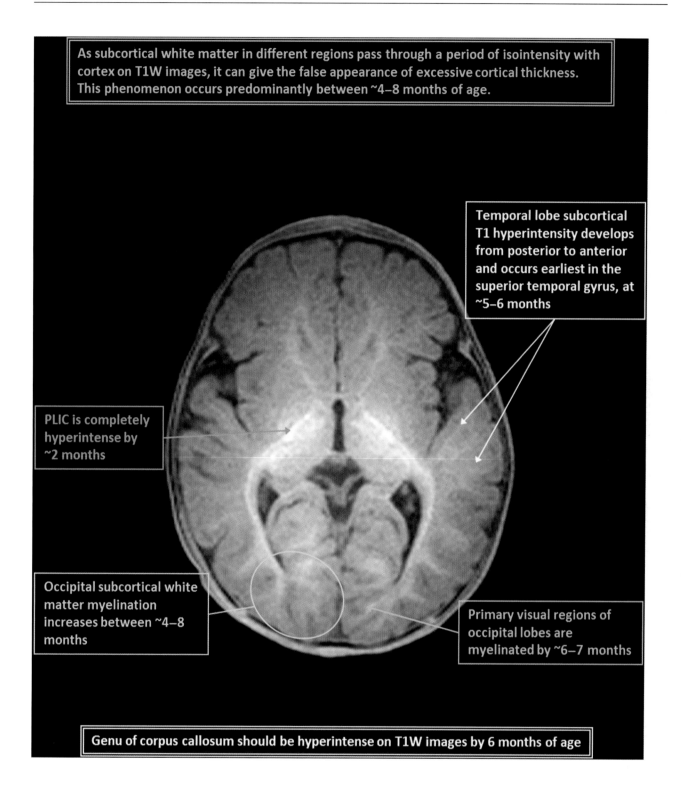

As subcortical white matter in different regions pass through a period of isointensity with cortex on T1W images, it can give the false appearance of excessive cortical thickness. This phenomenon occurs predominantly between ~4–8 months of age.

Temporal lobe subcortical T1 hyperintensity develops from posterior to anterior and occurs earliest in the superior temporal gyrus, at ~5–6 months

PLIC is completely hyperintense by ~2 months

Occipital subcortical white matter myelination increases between ~4–8 months

Primary visual regions of occipital lobes are myelinated by ~6–7 months

Genu of corpus callosum should be hyperintense on T1W images by 6 months of age

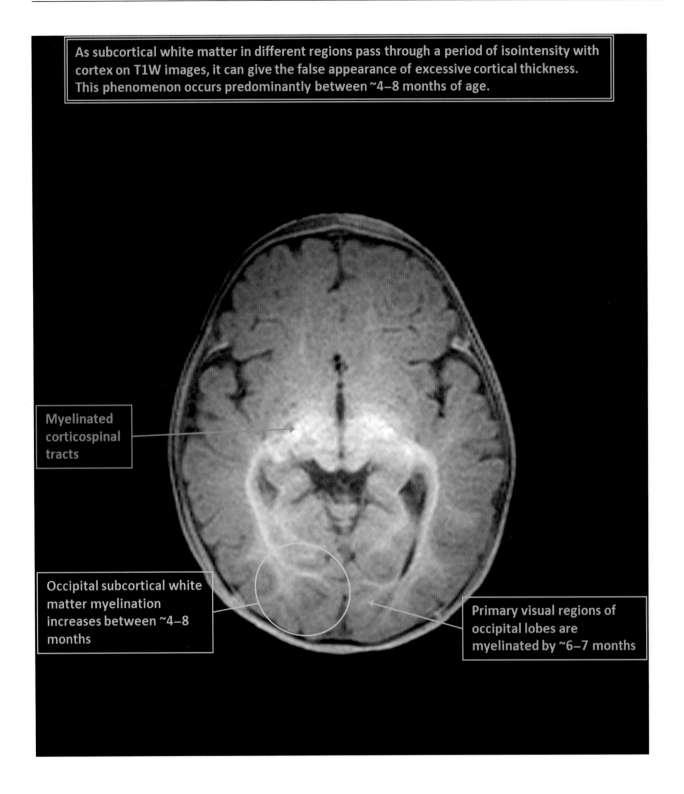

As subcortical white matter in different regions pass through a period of isointensity with cortex on T1W images, it can give the false appearance of excessive cortical thickness. This phenomenon occurs predominantly between ~4–8 months of age.

Myelinated corticospinal tracts

Occipital subcortical white matter myelination increases between ~4–8 months

Primary visual regions of occipital lobes are myelinated by ~6–7 months

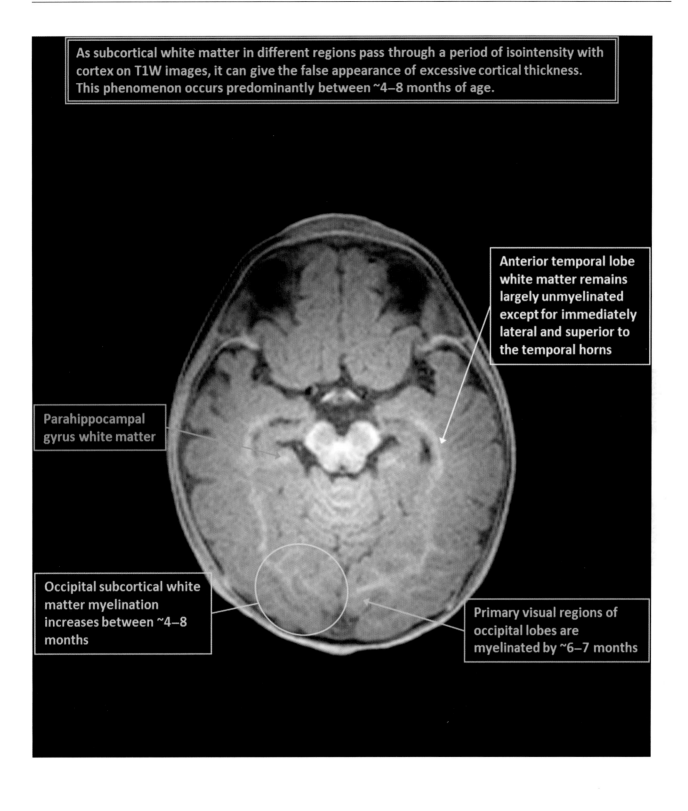

As subcortical white matter in different regions pass through a period of isointensity with cortex on T1W images, it can give the false appearance of excessive cortical thickness. This phenomenon occurs predominantly between ~4–8 months of age.

Anterior temporal lobe white matter remains largely unmyelinated except for immediately lateral and superior to the temporal horns

Parahippocampal gyrus white matter

Occipital subcortical white matter myelination increases between ~4–8 months

Primary visual regions of occipital lobes are myelinated by ~6–7 months

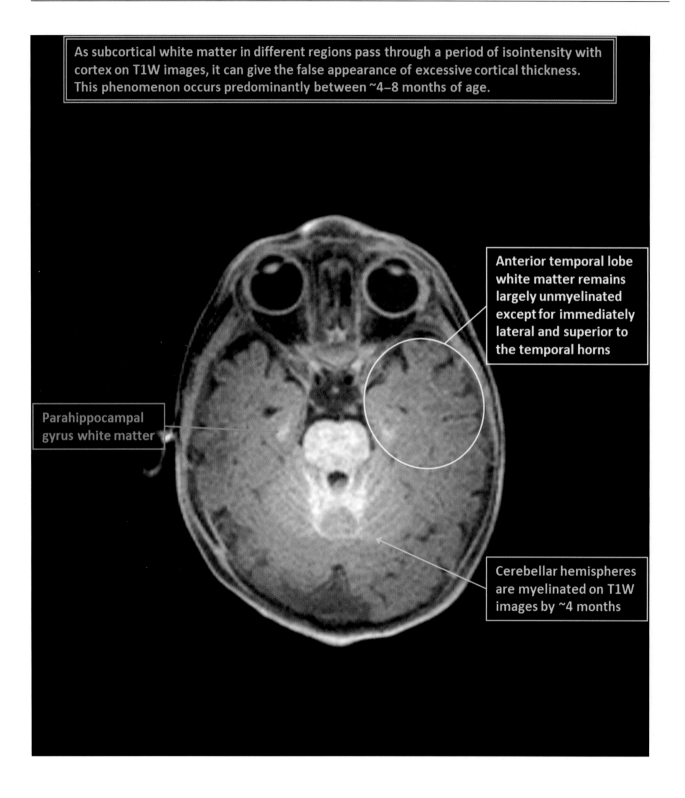

As subcortical white matter in different regions pass through a period of isointensity with cortex on T1W images, it can give the false appearance of excessive cortical thickness. This phenomenon occurs predominantly between ~4–8 months of age.

Anterior temporal lobe white matter remains largely unmyelinated except for immediately lateral and superior to the temporal horns

Parahippocampal gyrus white matter

Cerebellar hemispheres are myelinated on T1W images by ~4 months

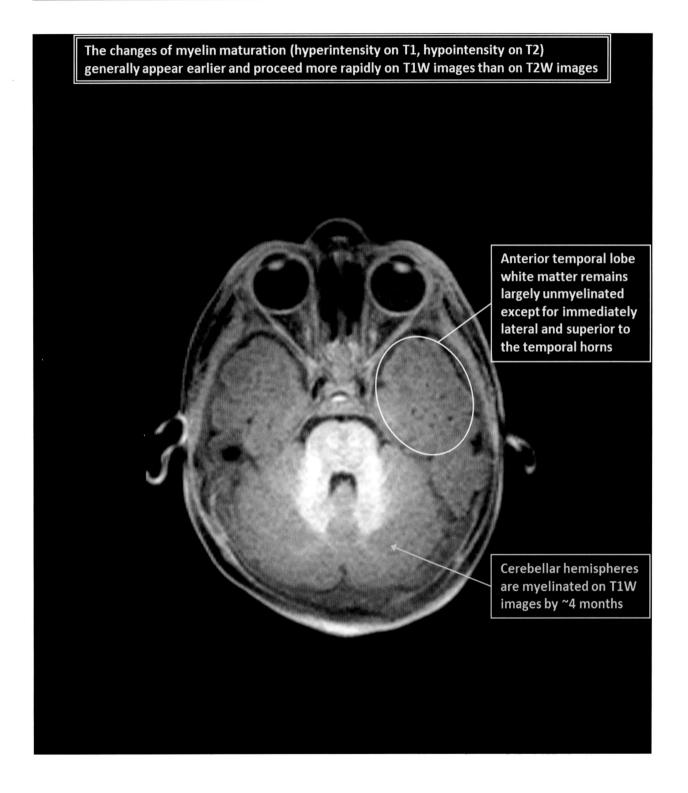

The changes of myelin maturation (hyperintensity on T1, hypointensity on T2) generally appear earlier and proceed more rapidly on T1W images than on T2W images

Anterior temporal lobe white matter remains largely unmyelinated except for immediately lateral and superior to the temporal horns

Cerebellar hemispheres are myelinated on T1W images by ~4 months

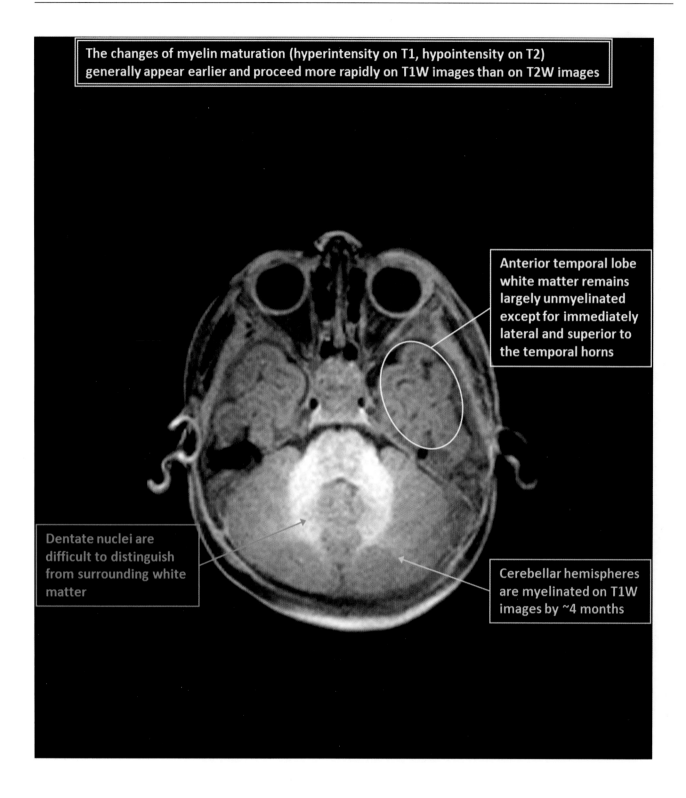

The changes of myelin maturation (hyperintensity on T1, hypointensity on T2) generally appear earlier and proceed more rapidly on T1W images than on T2W images

Anterior temporal lobe white matter remains largely unmyelinated except for immediately lateral and superior to the temporal horns

Dentate nuclei are difficult to distinguish from surrounding white matter

Cerebellar hemispheres are myelinated on T1W images by ~4 months

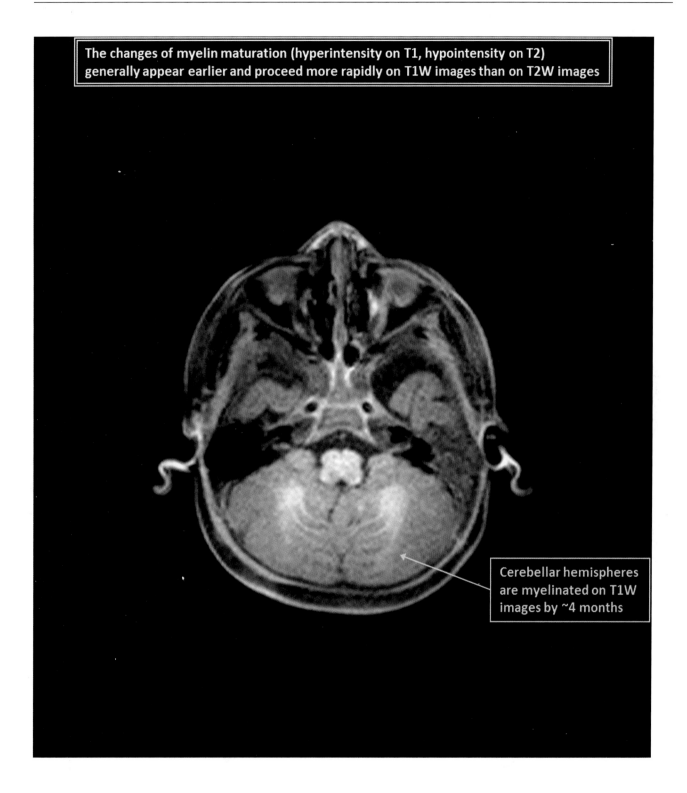

The changes of myelin maturation (hyperintensity on T1, hypointensity on T2) generally appear earlier and proceed more rapidly on T1W images than on T2W images

Cerebellar hemispheres are myelinated on T1W images by ~4 months

6 Months, Axial TSE T2

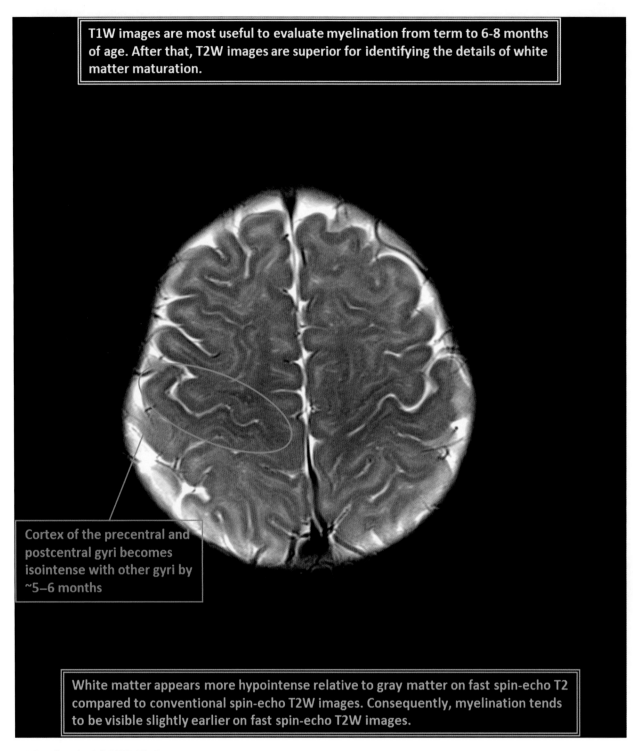

T1W images are most useful to evaluate myelination from term to 6-8 months of age. After that, T2W images are superior for identifying the details of white matter maturation.

Cortex of the precentral and postcentral gyri becomes isointense with other gyri by ~5–6 months

White matter appears more hypointense relative to gray matter on fast spin-echo T2 compared to conventional spin-echo T2W images. Consequently, myelination tends to be visible slightly earlier on fast spin-echo T2W images.

6 Months, Axial TSE T2 Images 1-12

T1W images are most useful to evaluate myelination from term to 6–8 months of age. After that, T2W images are superior for identifying the details of white matter maturation.

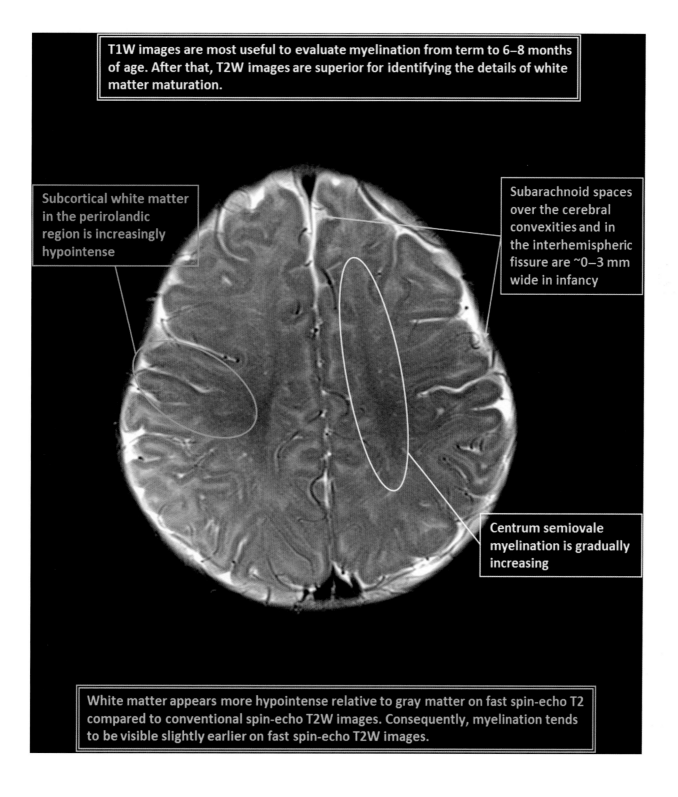

Subcortical white matter in the perirolandic region is increasingly hypointense

Subarachnoid spaces over the cerebral convexities and in the interhemispheric fissure are ~0–3 mm wide in infancy

Centrum semiovale myelination is gradually increasing

White matter appears more hypointense relative to gray matter on fast spin-echo T2 compared to conventional spin-echo T2W images. Consequently, myelination tends to be visible slightly earlier on fast spin-echo T2W images.

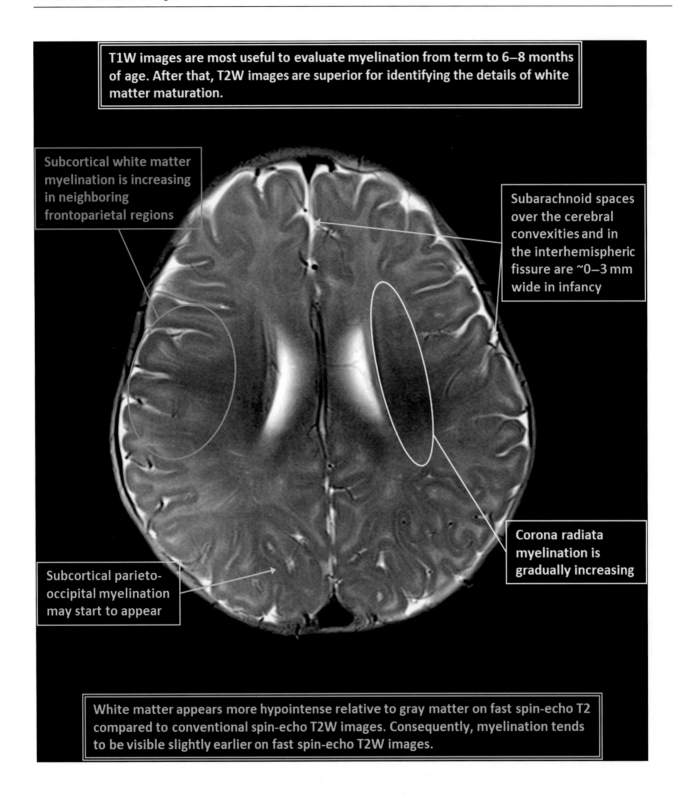

T1W images are most useful to evaluate myelination from term to 6–8 months of age. After that, T2W images are superior for identifying the details of white matter maturation.

Subcortical white matter myelination is increasing in neighboring frontoparietal regions

Subarachnoid spaces over the cerebral convexities and in the interhemispheric fissure are ~0–3 mm wide in infancy

Subcortical parieto-occipital myelination may start to appear

Corona radiata myelination is gradually increasing

White matter appears more hypointense relative to gray matter on fast spin-echo T2 compared to conventional spin-echo T2W images. Consequently, myelination tends to be visible slightly earlier on fast spin-echo T2W images.

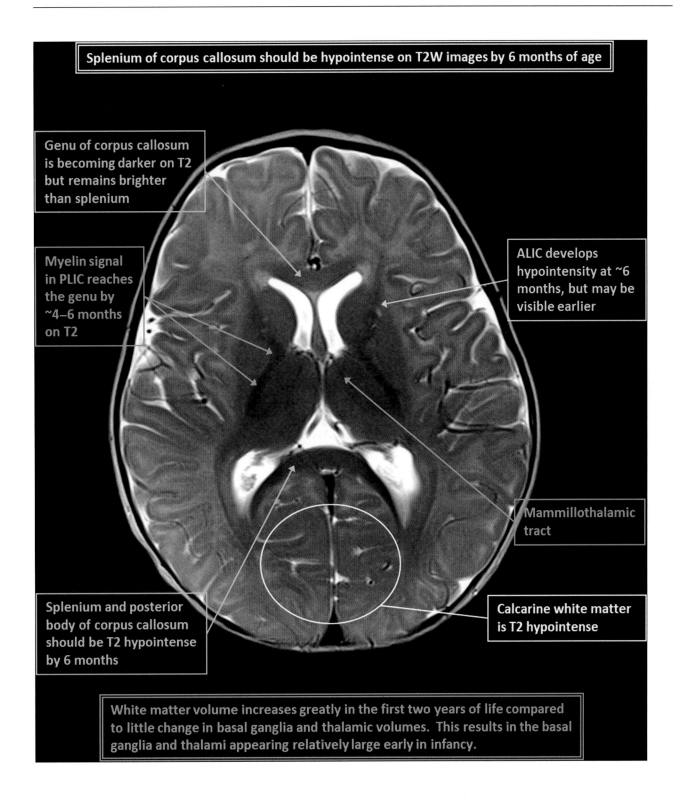

Splenium of corpus callosum should be hypointense on T2W images by 6 months of age

Genu of corpus callosum is becoming darker on T2 but remains brighter than splenium

Myelin signal in PLIC reaches the genu by ~4–6 months on T2

ALIC develops hypointensity at ~6 months, but may be visible earlier

Mammillothalamic tract

Splenium and posterior body of corpus callosum should be T2 hypointense by 6 months

Calcarine white matter is T2 hypointense

White matter volume increases greatly in the first two years of life compared to little change in basal ganglia and thalamic volumes. This results in the basal ganglia and thalami appearing relatively large early in infancy.

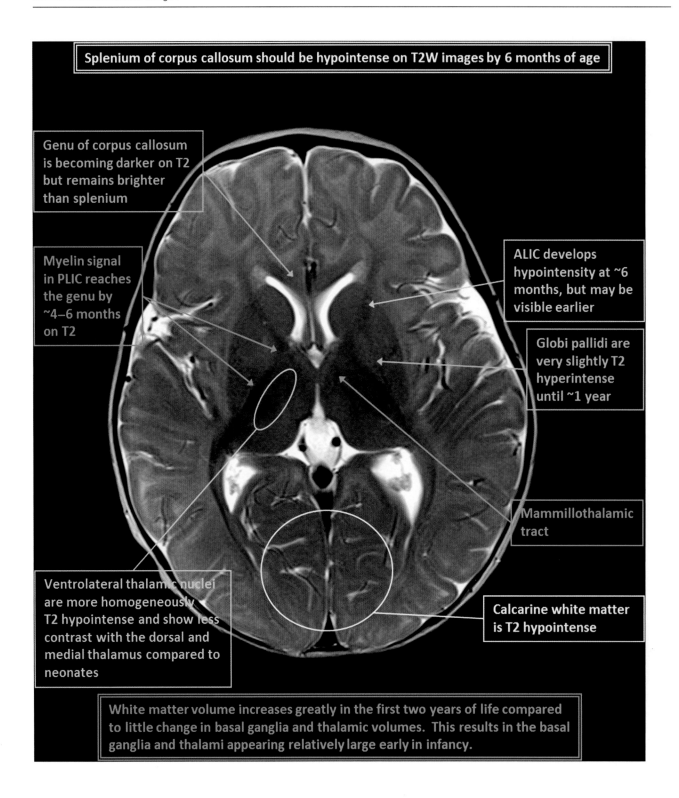

Splenium of corpus callosum should be hypointense on T2W images by 6 months of age

Genu of corpus callosum is becoming darker on T2 but remains brighter than splenium

Myelin signal in PLIC reaches the genu by ~4–6 months on T2

ALIC develops hypointensity at ~6 months, but may be visible earlier

Globi pallidi are very slightly T2 hyperintense until ~1 year

Mammillothalamic tract

Ventrolateral thalamic nuclei are more homogeneously T2 hypointense and show less contrast with the dorsal and medial thalamus compared to neonates

Calcarine white matter is T2 hypointense

White matter volume increases greatly in the first two years of life compared to little change in basal ganglia and thalamic volumes. This results in the basal ganglia and thalami appearing relatively large early in infancy.

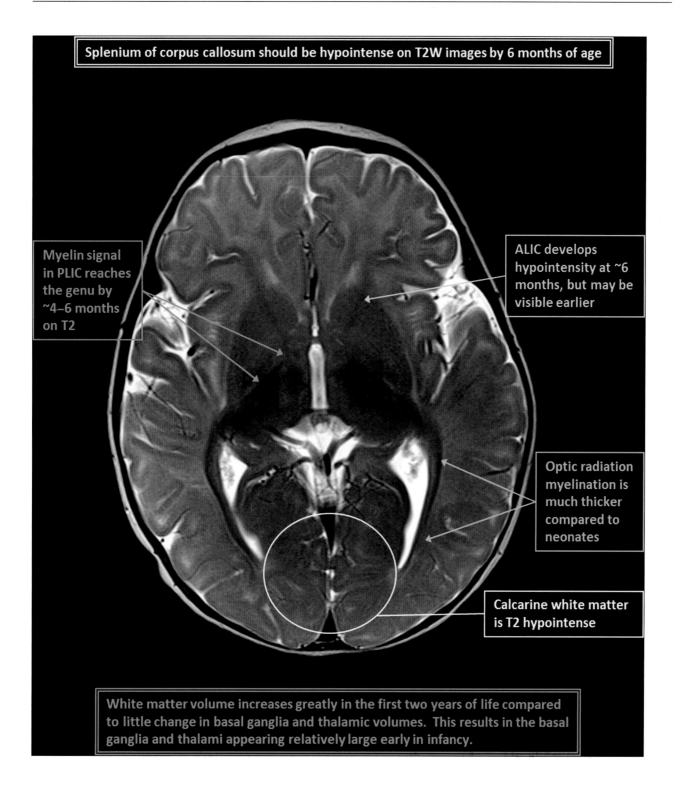

Splenium of corpus callosum should be hypointense on T2W images by 6 months of age

Myelin signal in PLIC reaches the genu by ~4–6 months on T2

ALIC develops hypointensity at ~6 months, but may be visible earlier

Optic radiation myelination is much thicker compared to neonates

Calcarine white matter is T2 hypointense

White matter volume increases greatly in the first two years of life compared to little change in basal ganglia and thalamic volumes. This results in the basal ganglia and thalami appearing relatively large early in infancy.

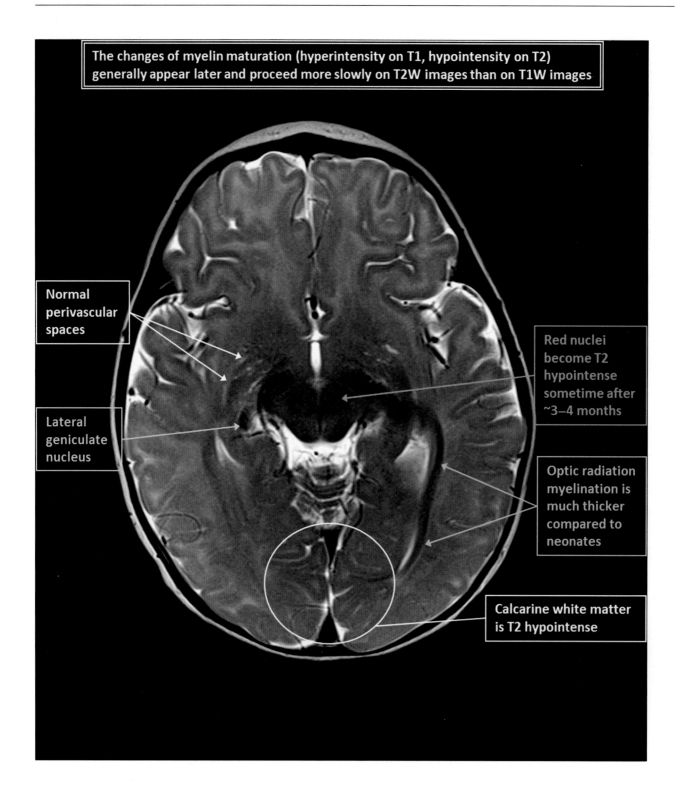

The changes of myelin maturation (hyperintensity on T1, hypointensity on T2) generally appear later and proceed more slowly on T2W images than on T1W images

Normal perivascular spaces

Lateral geniculate nucleus

Red nuclei become T2 hypointense sometime after ~3–4 months

Optic radiation myelination is much thicker compared to neonates

Calcarine white matter is T2 hypointense

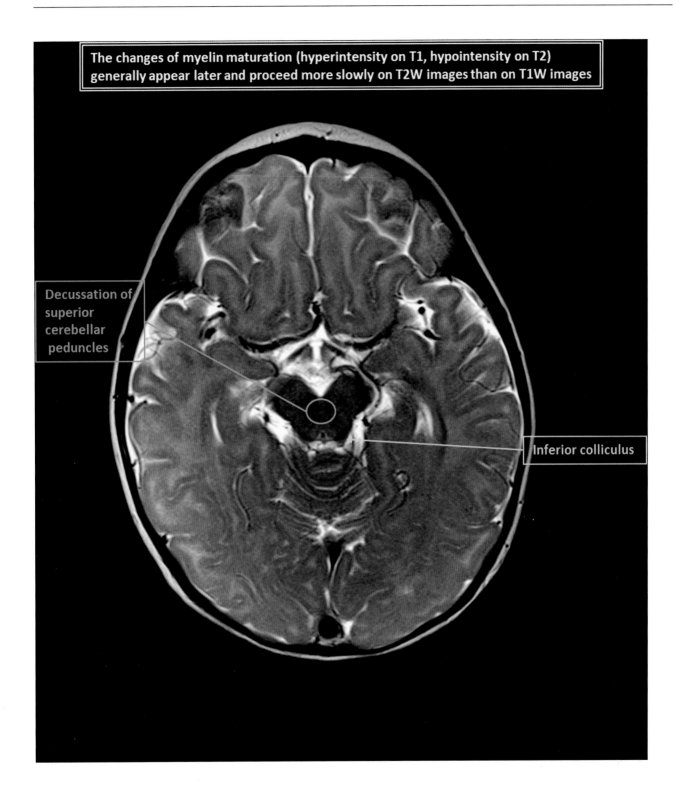

The changes of myelin maturation (hyperintensity on T1, hypointensity on T2) generally appear later and proceed more slowly on T2W images than on T1W images

Decussation of superior cerebellar peduncles

Inferior colliculus

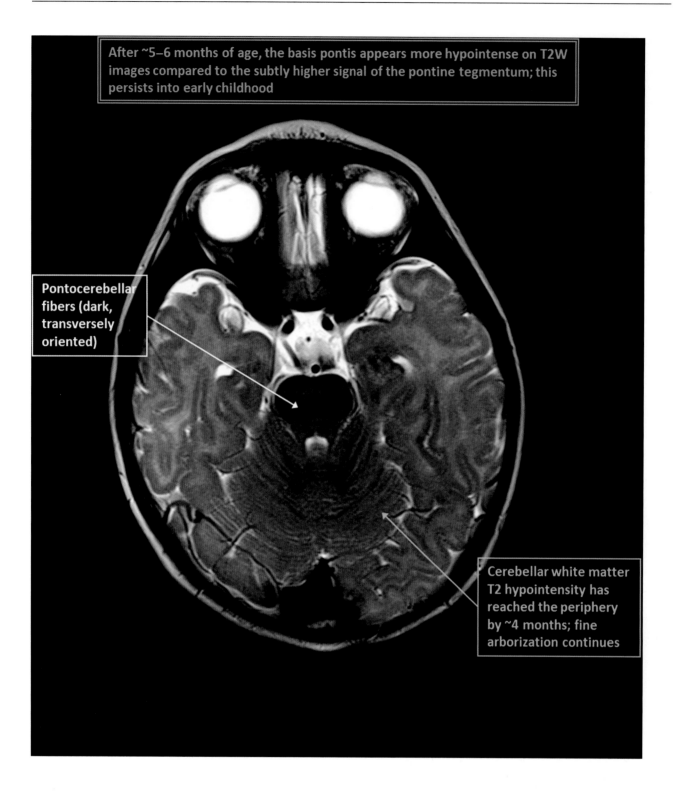

After ~5–6 months of age, the basis pontis appears more hypointense on T2W images compared to the subtly higher signal of the pontine tegmentum; this persists into early childhood

Pontocerebellar fibers (dark, transversely oriented)

Cerebellar white matter T2 hypointensity has reached the periphery by ~4 months; fine arborization continues

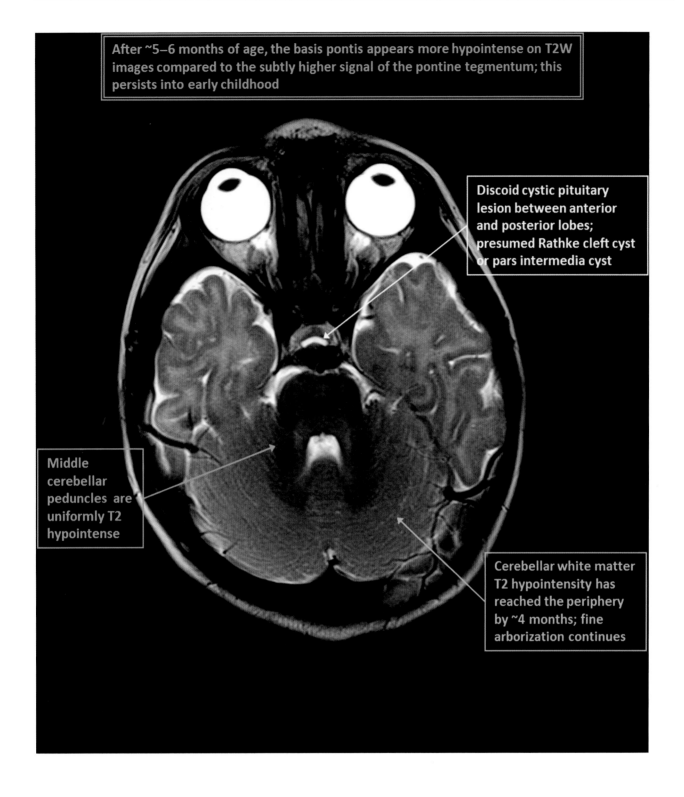

After ~5–6 months of age, the basis pontis appears more hypointense on T2W images compared to the subtly higher signal of the pontine tegmentum; this persists into early childhood

Discoid cystic pituitary lesion between anterior and posterior lobes; presumed Rathke cleft cyst or pars intermedia cyst

Middle cerebellar peduncles are uniformly T2 hypointense

Cerebellar white matter T2 hypointensity has reached the periphery by ~4 months; fine arborization continues

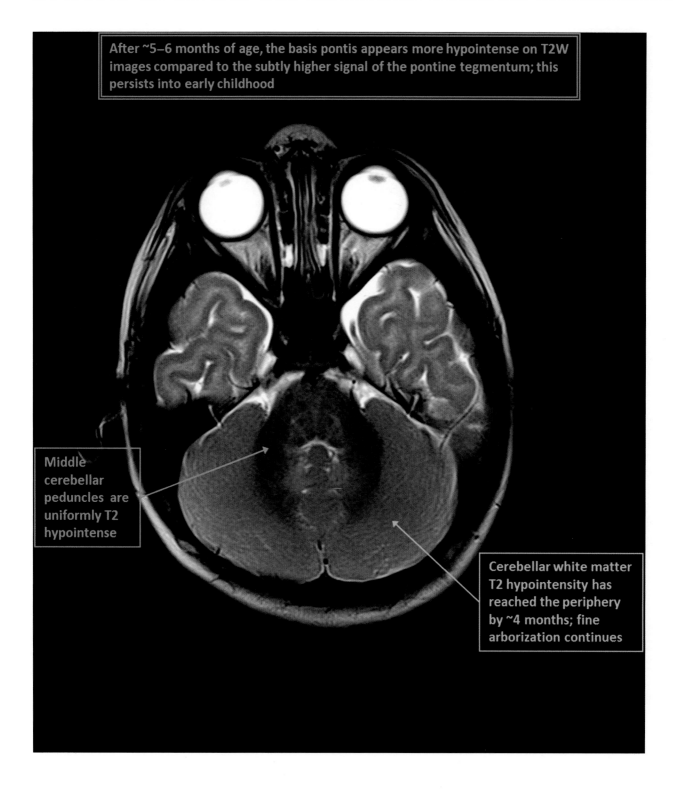

After ~5–6 months of age, the basis pontis appears more hypointense on T2W images compared to the subtly higher signal of the pontine tegmentum; this persists into early childhood

Middle cerebellar peduncles are uniformly T2 hypointense

Cerebellar white matter T2 hypointensity has reached the periphery by ~4 months; fine arborization continues

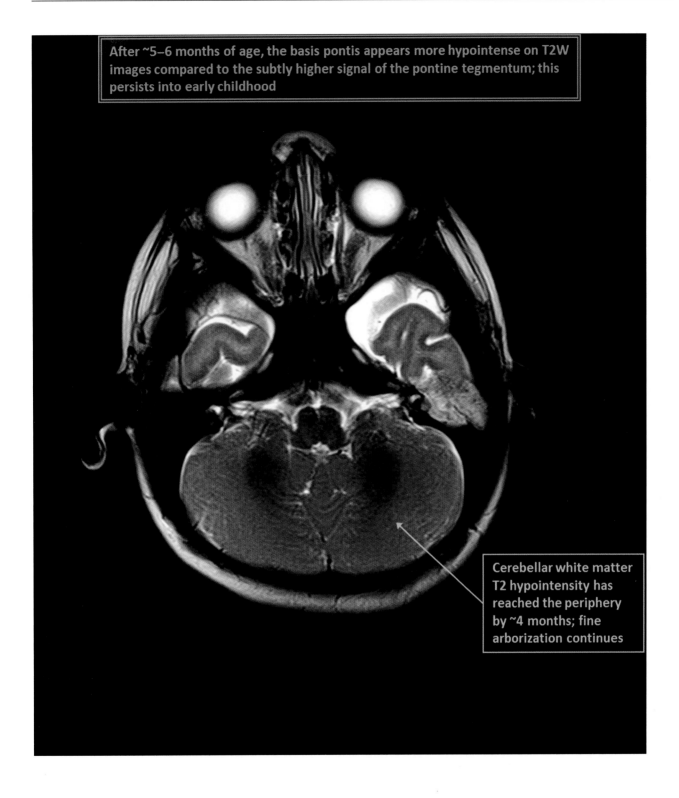

After ~5–6 months of age, the basis pontis appears more hypointense on T2W images compared to the subtly higher signal of the pontine tegmentum; this persists into early childhood

Cerebellar white matter T2 hypointensity has reached the periphery by ~4 months; fine arborization continues

6 Months, Diffusion Weighted Imaging (DWI) (b=1000 s/mm²)

Gray and white matter show increasing contrast on diffusion weighted images after ~5 months of age, with cerebral white matter eventually becoming hypointense to cortex and remaining so until late adulthood

Deep and periventricular WM, corpus callosum, and internal capsules are becoming increasingly hypointense. It remains difficult to distinguish subcortical WM from cortex at this age.

6 Months, Diffusion Weighted Imaging (DWI) (b=1000 s/mm²) Images 1-5

Gray and white matter show increasing contrast on diffusion weighted images after ~5 months of age, with cerebral white matter eventually becoming hypointense to cortex and remaining so until late adulthood

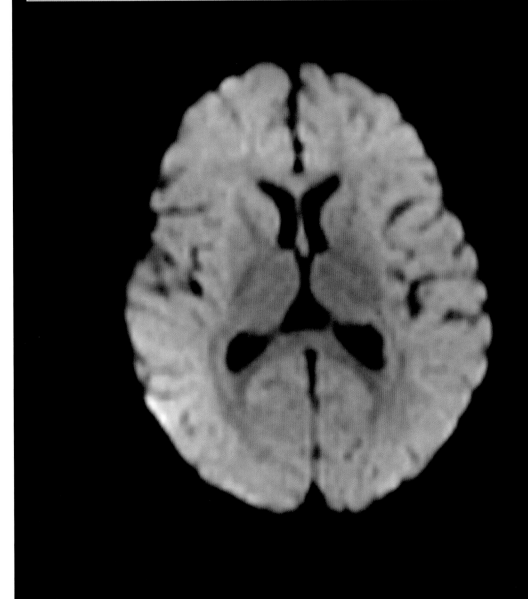

Deep and periventricular WM, corpus callosum, and internal capsules are becoming increasingly hypointense. It remains difficult to distinguish subcortical WM from cortex at this age.

Gray and white matter show increasing contrast on diffusion weighted images after ~5 months of age, with cerebral white matter eventually becoming hypointense to cortex and remaining so until late adulthood

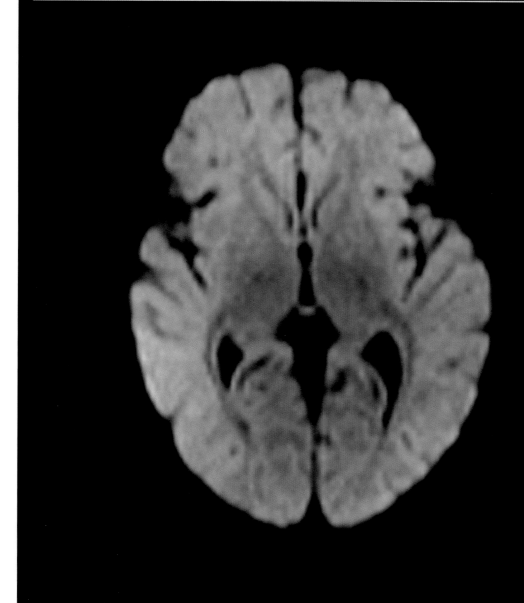

Deep and periventricular WM, corpus callosum, and internal capsules are becoming increasingly hypointense. It remains difficult to distinguish subcortical WM from cortex at this age.

For most of the first year of life, the cerebellum as a whole can have a noticeably more hypointense appearance on ADC than the cerebral hemispheres, while on DWI it is isointense to subtly hyperintense to the cerebrum

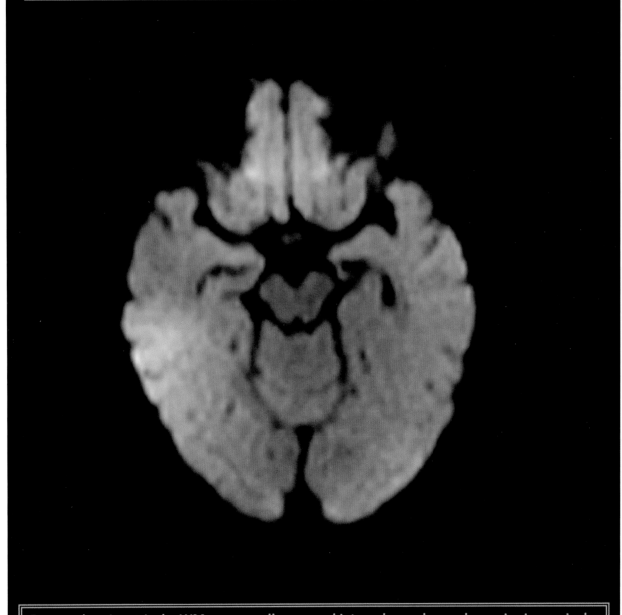

Deep and periventricular WM, corpus callosum, and internal capsules are becoming increasingly hypointense. It remains difficult to distinguish subcortical WM from cortex at this age.

For most of the first year of life, the cerebellum as a whole can have a noticeably more hypointense appearance on ADC than the cerebral hemispheres, while on DWI it is isointense to subtly hyperintense to the cerebrum

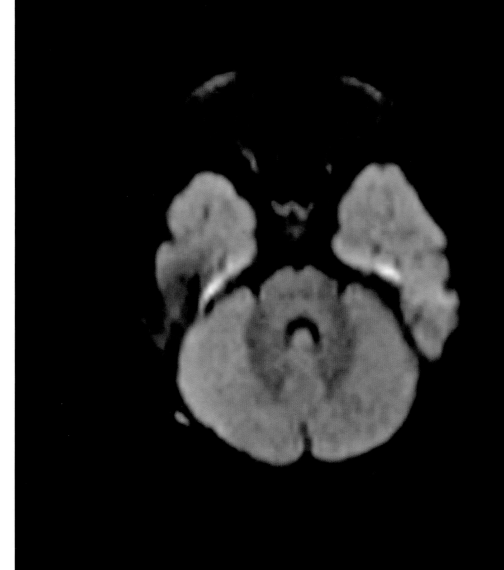

Deep and periventricular WM, corpus callosum, and internal capsules are becoming increasingly hypointense. It remains difficult to distinguish subcortical WM from cortex at this age.

6 Months, Apparent Diffusion Coefficient (ADC) Map

ADC values of WM continue to decrease, but at a slower rate after ~ age 5 months. Much of the cerebral gray and white matter will appear close to isointensity on ADC images by ~ age 1 year.

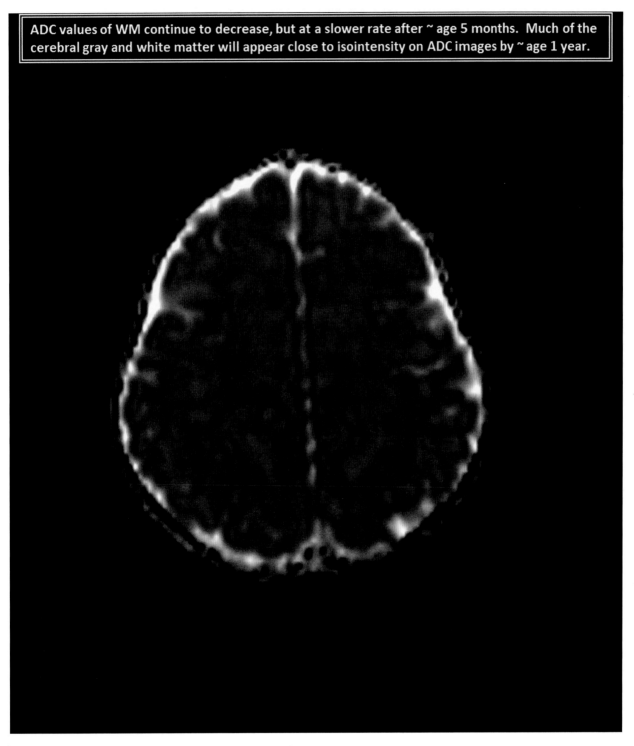

6 Months, Apparent Diffusion Coefficient (ADC) Map Images 1–5

ADC values of WM continue to decrease, but at a slower rate after ~ age 5 months. Much of the cerebral gray and white matter will appear close to isointensity on ADC images by ~ age 1 year.

ADC values of WM continue to decrease, but at a slower rate after ~ age 5 months. Much of the cerebral gray and white matter will appear close to isointensity on ADC images by ~ age 1 year.

For most of the first year of life, the cerebellum as a whole can have a noticeably more hypointense appearance on ADC than the cerebral hemispheres, while on DWI it is isointense to subtly hyperintense to the cerebrum

For most of the first year of life, the cerebellum as a whole can have a noticeably more hypointense appearance on ADC than the cerebral hemispheres, while on DWI it is isointense to subtly hyperintense to the cerebrum

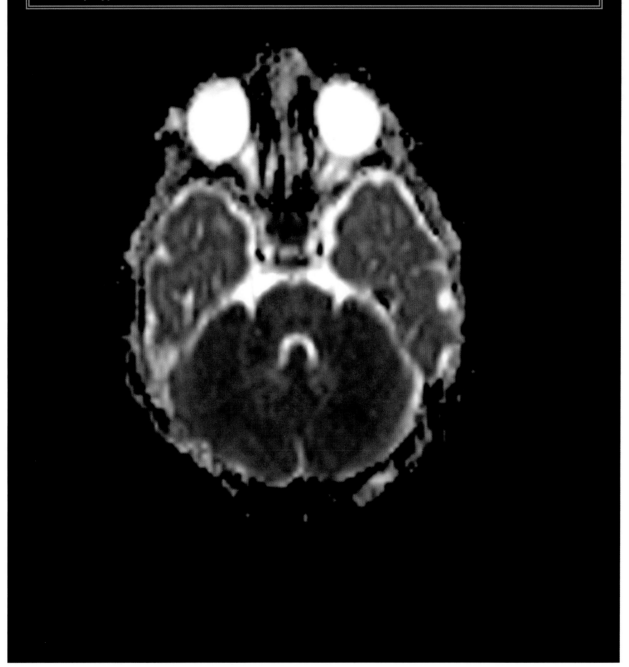

6 Months, Sagittal T1

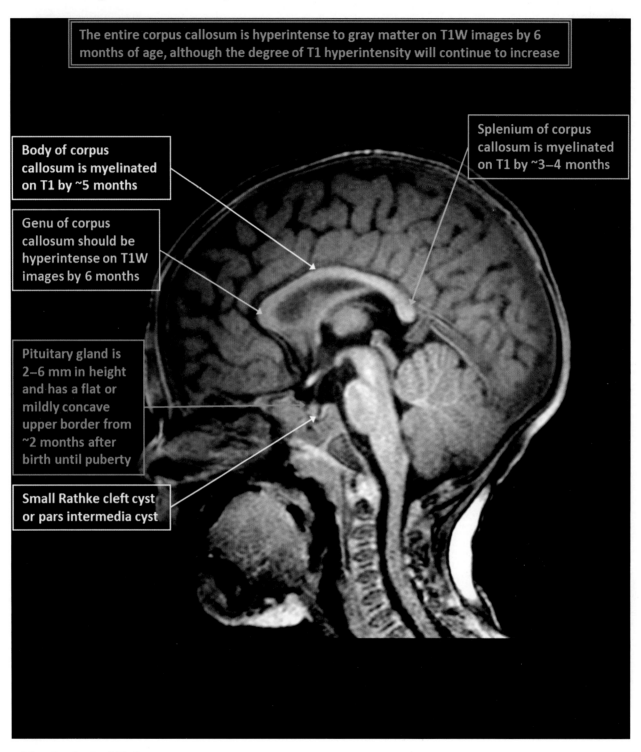

The entire corpus callosum is hyperintense to gray matter on T1W images by 6 months of age, although the degree of T1 hyperintensity will continue to increase

Splenium of corpus callosum is myelinated on T1 by ~3–4 months

Body of corpus callosum is myelinated on T1 by ~5 months

Genu of corpus callosum should be hyperintense on T1W images by 6 months

Pituitary gland is 2–6 mm in height and has a flat or mildly concave upper border from ~2 months after birth until puberty

Small Rathke cleft cyst or pars intermedia cyst

6 Months, Sagittal T1 Images 1–4

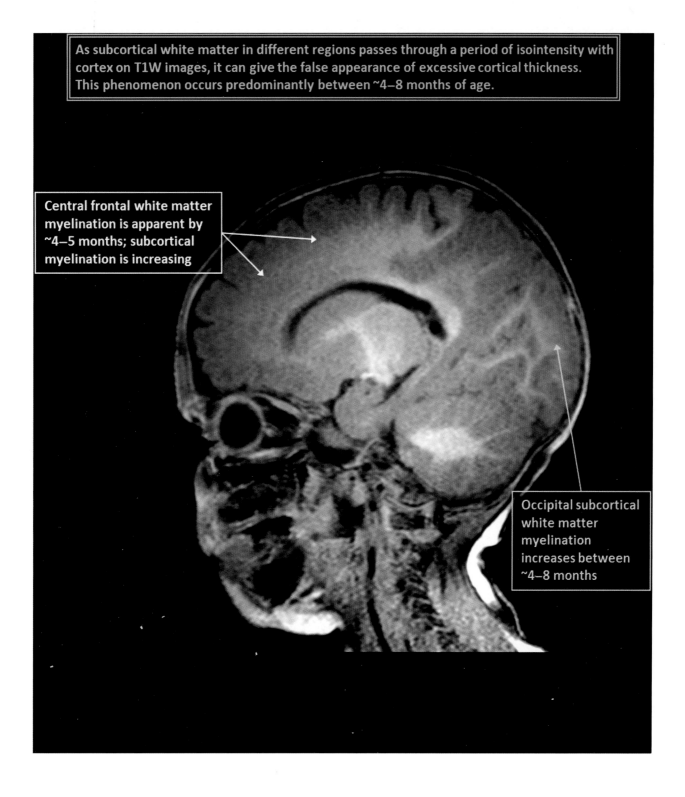

As subcortical white matter in different regions passes through a period of isointensity with cortex on T1W images, it can give the false appearance of excessive cortical thickness. This phenomenon occurs predominantly between ~4–8 months of age.

Central frontal white matter myelination is apparent by ~4–5 months; subcortical myelination is increasing

Occipital subcortical white matter myelination increases between ~4–8 months

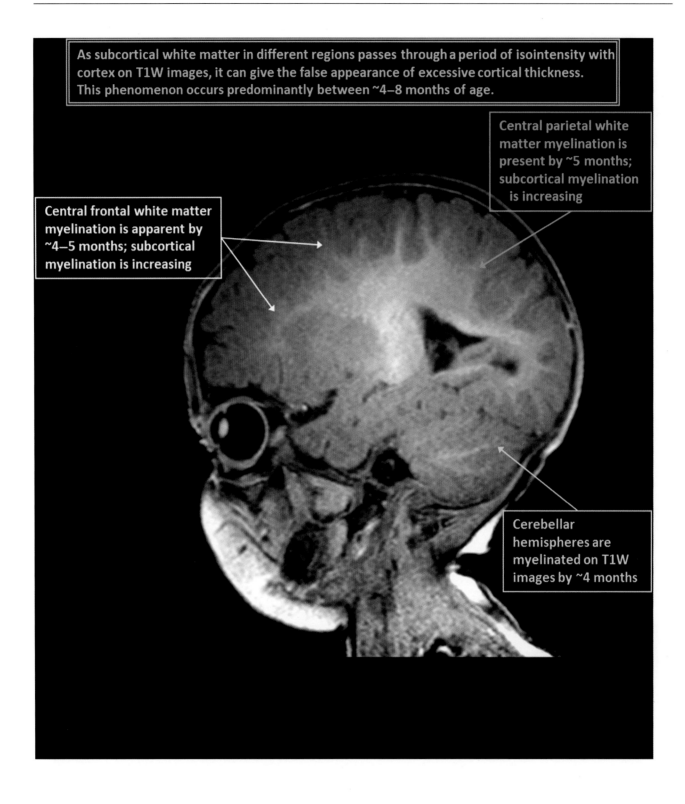

As subcortical white matter in different regions passes through a period of isointensity with cortex on T1W images, it can give the false appearance of excessive cortical thickness. This phenomenon occurs predominantly between ~4–8 months of age.

Central parietal white matter myelination is present by ~5 months; subcortical myelination is increasing

Central frontal white matter myelination is apparent by ~4–5 months; subcortical myelination is increasing

Cerebellar hemispheres are myelinated on T1W images by ~4 months

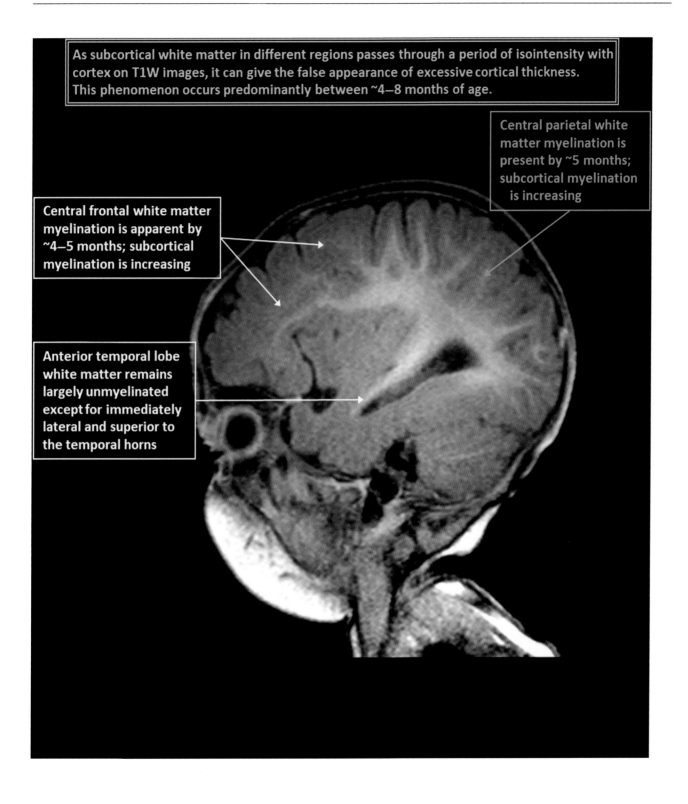

As subcortical white matter in different regions passes through a period of isointensity with cortex on T1W images, it can give the false appearance of excessive cortical thickness. This phenomenon occurs predominantly between ~4–8 months of age.

Central parietal white matter myelination is present by ~5 months; subcortical myelination is increasing

Central frontal white matter myelination is apparent by ~4–5 months; subcortical myelination is increasing

Anterior temporal lobe white matter remains largely unmyelinated except for immediately lateral and superior to the temporal horns

6 Months, Coronal TSE T2

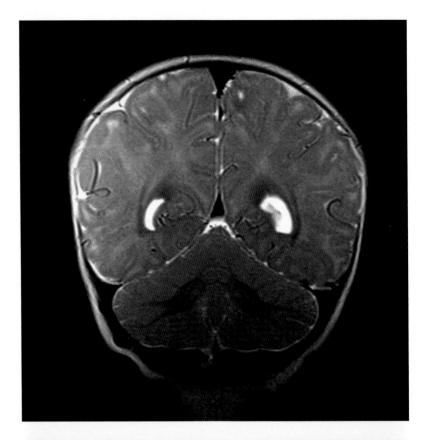

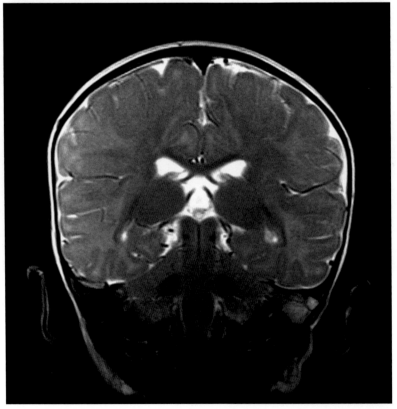

6 Months, Coronal TSE T2 Images 1–4

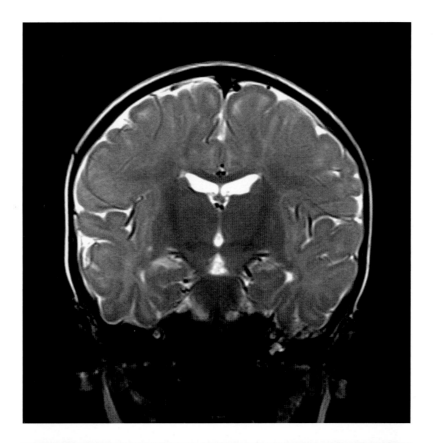

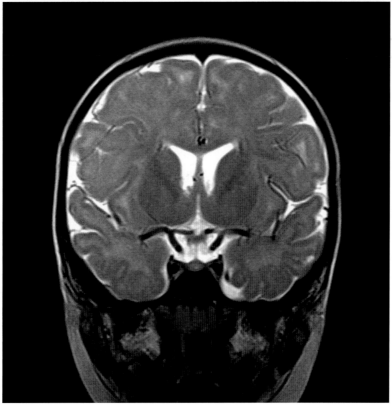

9 Months, Axial T1

At 9–10 months of age, myelination is approaching an adult pattern on T1W images except for some of the most peripheral subcortical white matter, mainly in the frontal and temporal lobes

Frontal subcortical white matter hyperintensity is present by ~8 months and will continue to subtly increase into the 2nd year

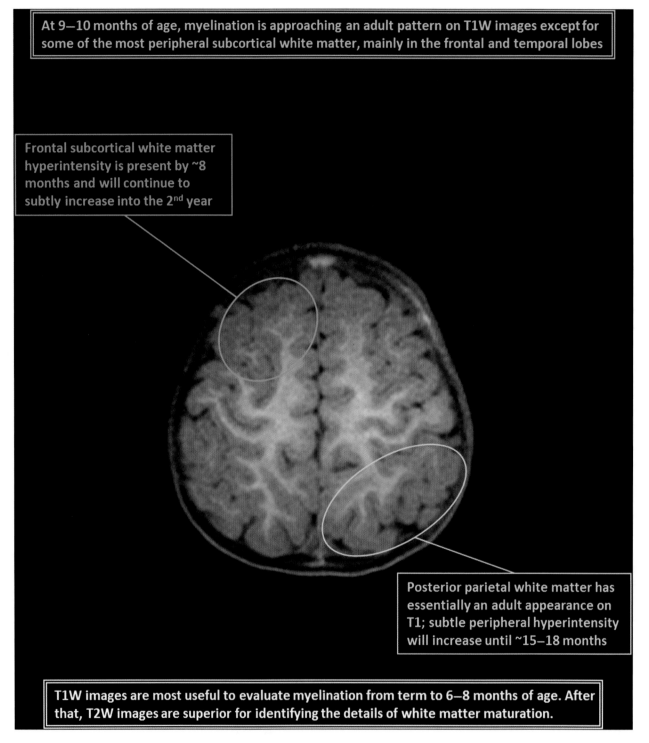

Posterior parietal white matter has essentially an adult appearance on T1; subtle peripheral hyperintensity will increase until ~15–18 months

T1W images are most useful to evaluate myelination from term to 6–8 months of age. After that, T2W images are superior for identifying the details of white matter maturation.

9 Months, Axial T1 Images 1–12

At 9–10 months of age, myelination is approaching an adult pattern on T1W images except for some of the most peripheral subcortical white matter, mainly in the frontal and temporal lobes

Frontal subcortical white matter hyperintensity is present by ~8 months and will continue to subtly increase into the 2nd year

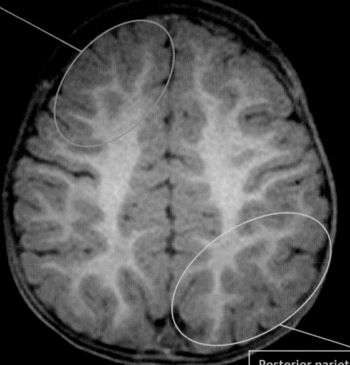

Posterior parietal white matter has essentially an adult appearance on T1; subtle peripheral hyperintensity will increase until ~15–18 months

T1W images are most useful to evaluate myelination from term to 6–8 months of age. After that, T2W images are superior for identifying the details of white matter maturation.

At 9–10 months of age, myelination is approaching an adult pattern on T1W images except for some of the most peripheral subcortical white matter, mainly in the frontal and temporal lobes

Frontal subcortical white matter hyperintensity is present by ~8 months and will continue to subtly increase into the 2nd year

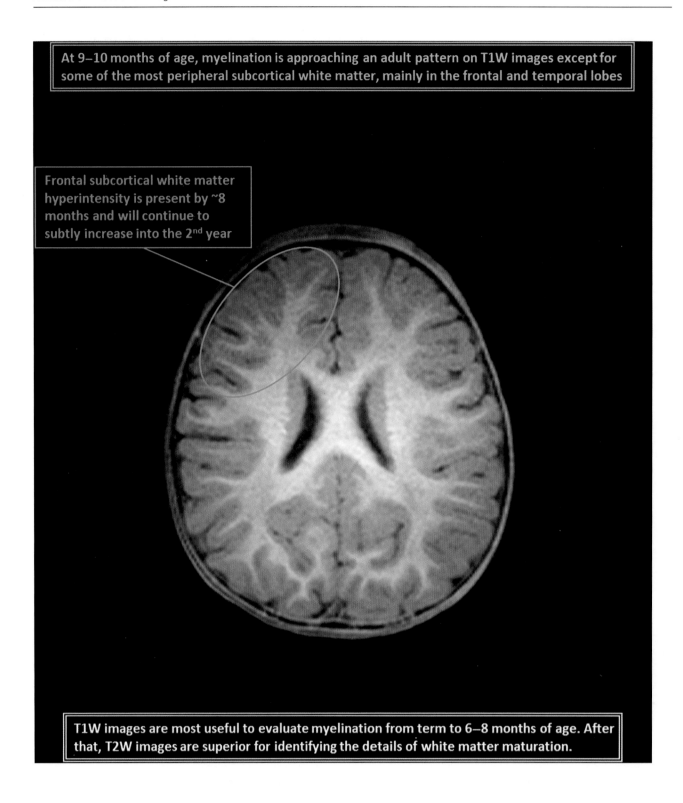

T1W images are most useful to evaluate myelination from term to 6–8 months of age. After that, T2W images are superior for identifying the details of white matter maturation.

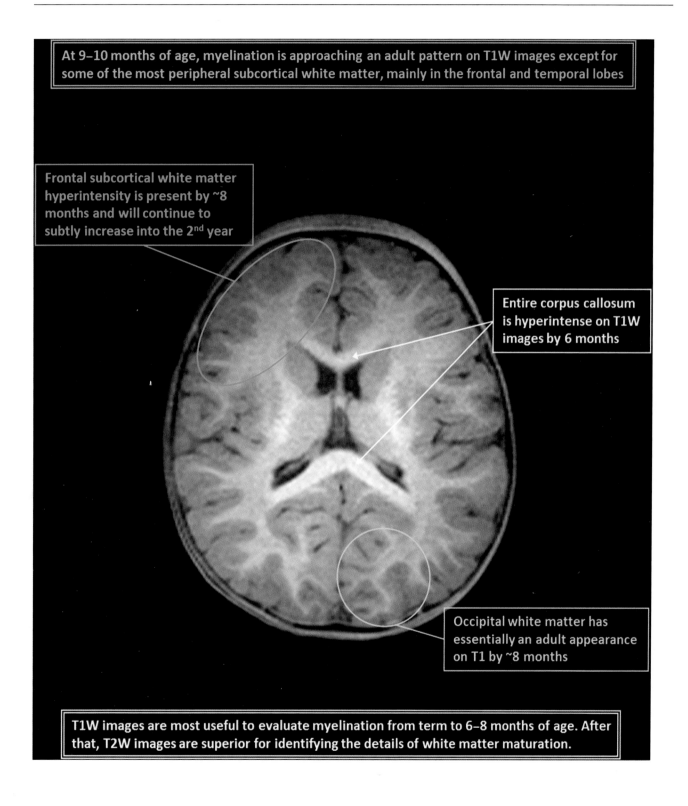

At 9–10 months of age, myelination is approaching an adult pattern on T1W images except for some of the most peripheral subcortical white matter, mainly in the frontal and temporal lobes

Frontal subcortical white matter hyperintensity is present by ~8 months and will continue to subtly increase into the 2nd year

Entire corpus callosum is hyperintense on T1W images by 6 months

Occipital white matter has essentially an adult appearance on T1 by ~8 months

T1W images are most useful to evaluate myelination from term to 6–8 months of age. After that, T2W images are superior for identifying the details of white matter maturation.

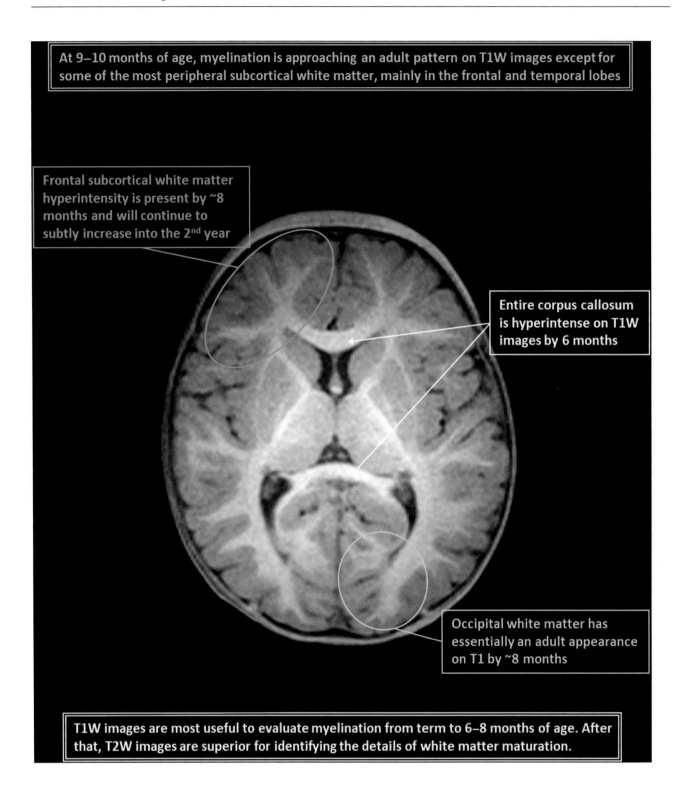

At 9–10 months of age, myelination is approaching an adult pattern on T1W images except for some of the most peripheral subcortical white matter, mainly in the frontal and temporal lobes

Frontal subcortical white matter hyperintensity is present by ~8 months and will continue to subtly increase into the 2nd year

Entire corpus callosum is hyperintense on T1W images by 6 months

Occipital white matter has essentially an adult appearance on T1 by ~8 months

T1W images are most useful to evaluate myelination from term to 6–8 months of age. After that, T2W images are superior for identifying the details of white matter maturation.

At 9-10 months of age, myelination is approaching an adult pattern on T1W images except for some of the most peripheral subcortical white matter, mainly in the frontal and temporal lobes

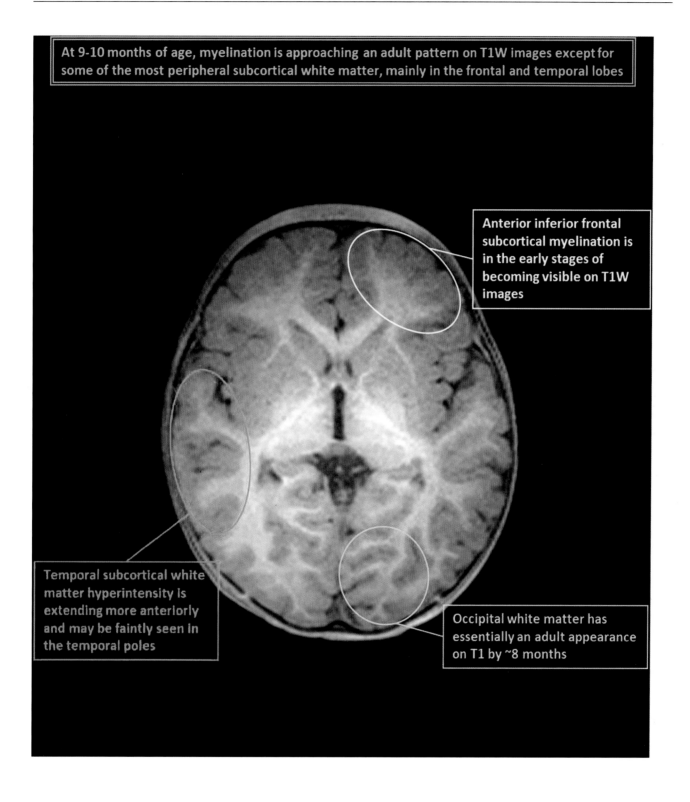

Anterior inferior frontal subcortical myelination is in the early stages of becoming visible on T1W images

Temporal subcortical white matter hyperintensity is extending more anteriorly and may be faintly seen in the temporal poles

Occipital white matter has essentially an adult appearance on T1 by ~8 months

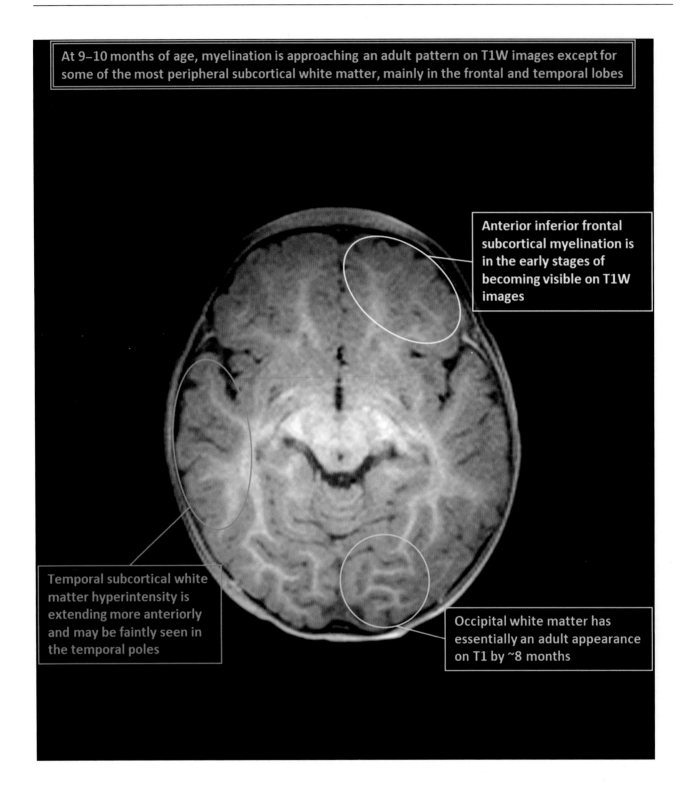

At 9–10 months of age, myelination is approaching an adult pattern on T1W images except for some of the most peripheral subcortical white matter, mainly in the frontal and temporal lobes

Anterior inferior frontal subcortical myelination is in the early stages of becoming visible on T1W images

Temporal subcortical white matter hyperintensity is extending more anteriorly and may be faintly seen in the temporal poles

Occipital white matter has essentially an adult appearance on T1 by ~8 months

At 9–10 months of age, myelination is approaching an adult pattern on T1W images except for some of the most peripheral subcortical white matter, mainly in the frontal and temporal lobes

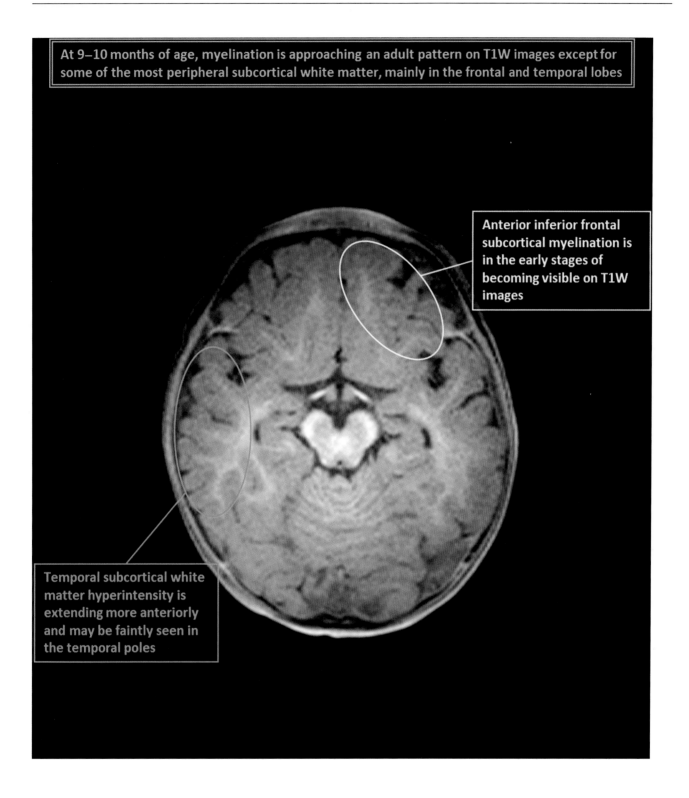

Anterior inferior frontal subcortical myelination is in the early stages of becoming visible on T1W images

Temporal subcortical white matter hyperintensity is extending more anteriorly and may be faintly seen in the temporal poles

At 9–10 months of age, myelination is approaching an adult pattern on T1W images except for some of the most peripheral subcortical white matter, mainly in the frontal and temporal lobes

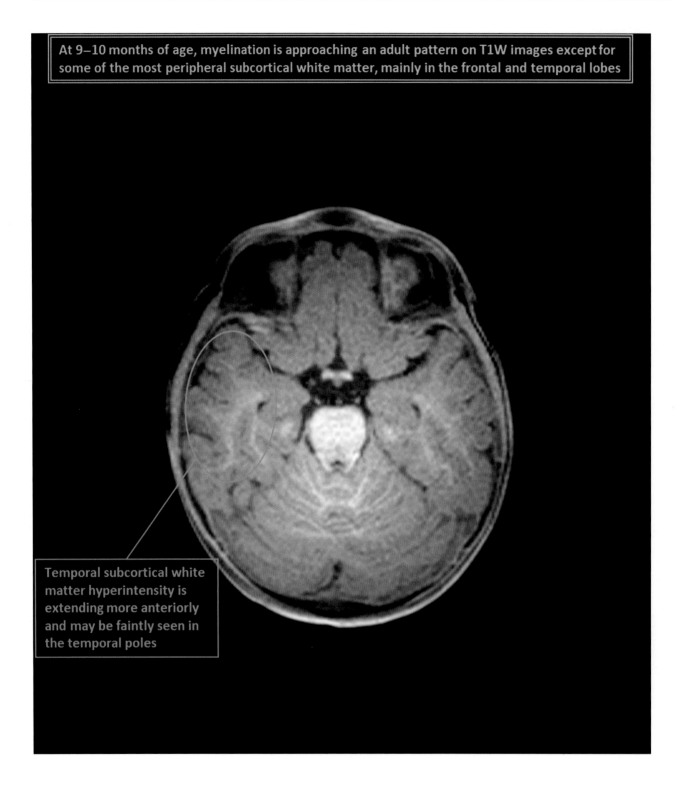

Temporal subcortical white matter hyperintensity is extending more anteriorly and may be faintly seen in the temporal poles

At 9–10 months of age, myelination is approaching an adult pattern on T1W images except for some of the most peripheral subcortical white matter, mainly in the frontal and temporal lobes

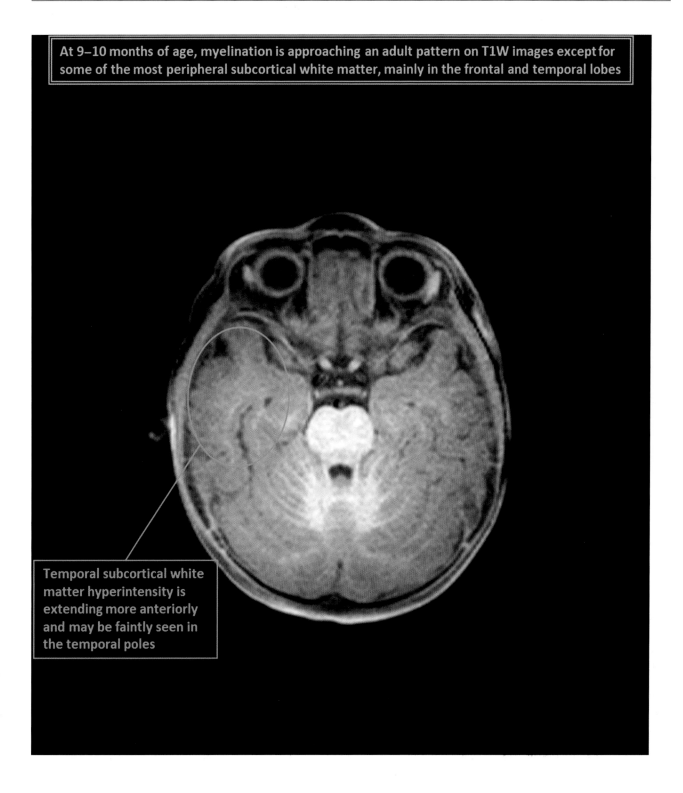

Temporal subcortical white matter hyperintensity is extending more anteriorly and may be faintly seen in the temporal poles

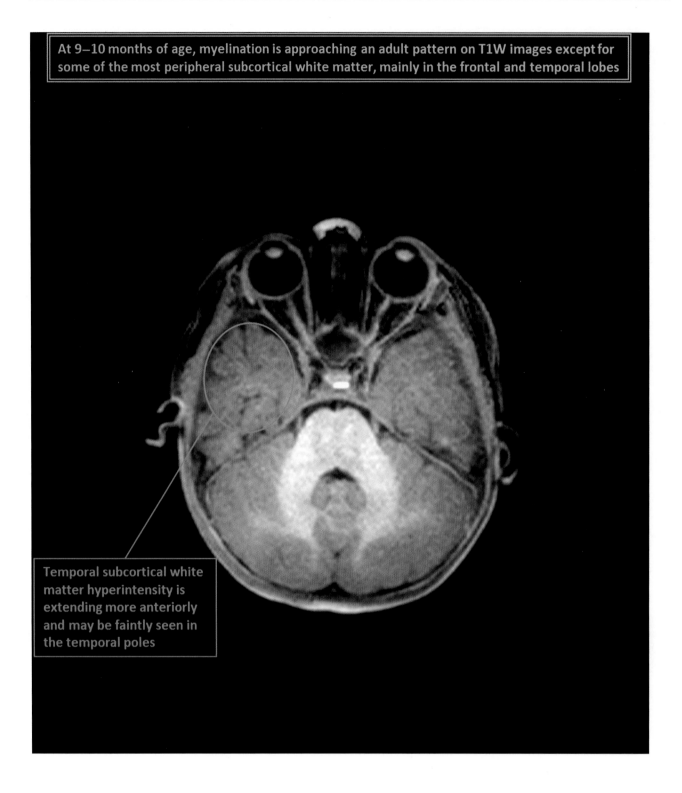

At 9–10 months of age, myelination is approaching an adult pattern on T1W images except for some of the most peripheral subcortical white matter, mainly in the frontal and temporal lobes

Temporal subcortical white matter hyperintensity is extending more anteriorly and may be faintly seen in the temporal poles

At 9–10 months of age, myelination is approaching an adult pattern on T1W images except for some of the most peripheral subcortical white matter, mainly in the frontal and temporal lobes

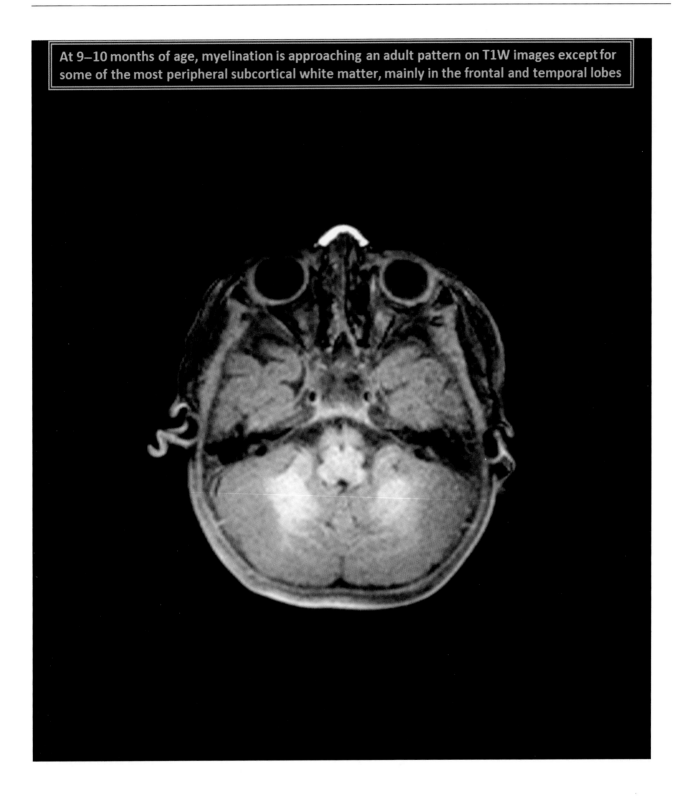

9 Months, Axial TSE T2

As cerebral hemispheric white matter is changing from hyperintensity to hypointensity on T2W images, gray-white matter differentiation can be poor in the 2nd half of the first year

Subcortical white matter in the perirolandic region is hypointense; fine arborization will continue into the second year

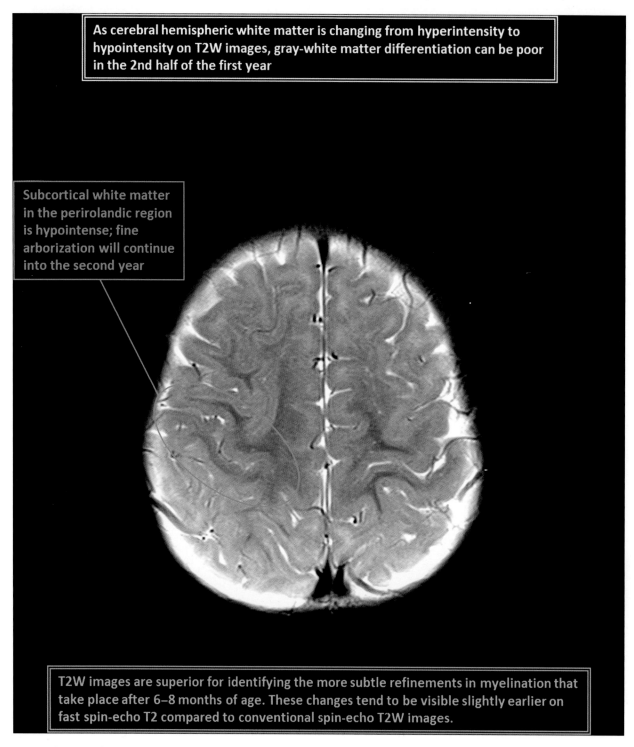

T2W images are superior for identifying the more subtle refinements in myelination that take place after 6–8 months of age. These changes tend to be visible slightly earlier on fast spin-echo T2 compared to conventional spin-echo T2W images.

9 Months, Axial TSE T2 Images 1–12

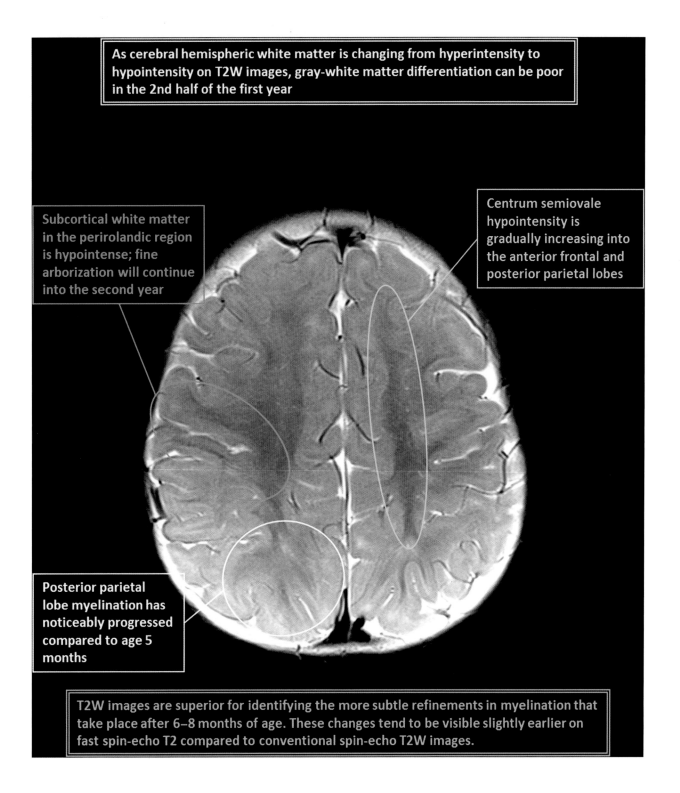

As cerebral hemispheric white matter is changing from hyperintensity to hypointensity on T2W images, gray-white matter differentiation can be poor in the 2nd half of the first year

Centrum semiovale hypointensity is gradually increasing into the anterior frontal and posterior parietal lobes

Subcortical white matter in the perirolandic region is hypointense; fine arborization will continue into the second year

Posterior parietal lobe myelination has noticeably progressed compared to age 5 months

T2W images are superior for identifying the more subtle refinements in myelination that take place after 6–8 months of age. These changes tend to be visible slightly earlier on fast spin-echo T2 compared to conventional spin-echo T2W images.

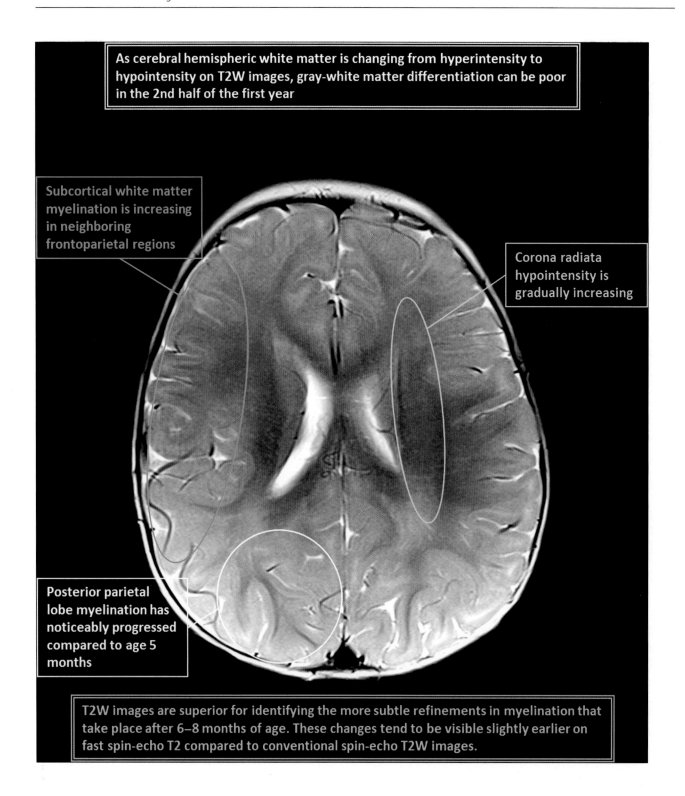

As cerebral hemispheric white matter is changing from hyperintensity to hypointensity on T2W images, gray-white matter differentiation can be poor in the 2nd half of the first year

Subcortical white matter myelination is increasing in neighboring frontoparietal regions

Corona radiata hypointensity is gradually increasing

Posterior parietal lobe myelination has noticeably progressed compared to age 5 months

T2W images are superior for identifying the more subtle refinements in myelination that take place after 6–8 months of age. These changes tend to be visible slightly earlier on fast spin-echo T2 compared to conventional spin-echo T2W images.

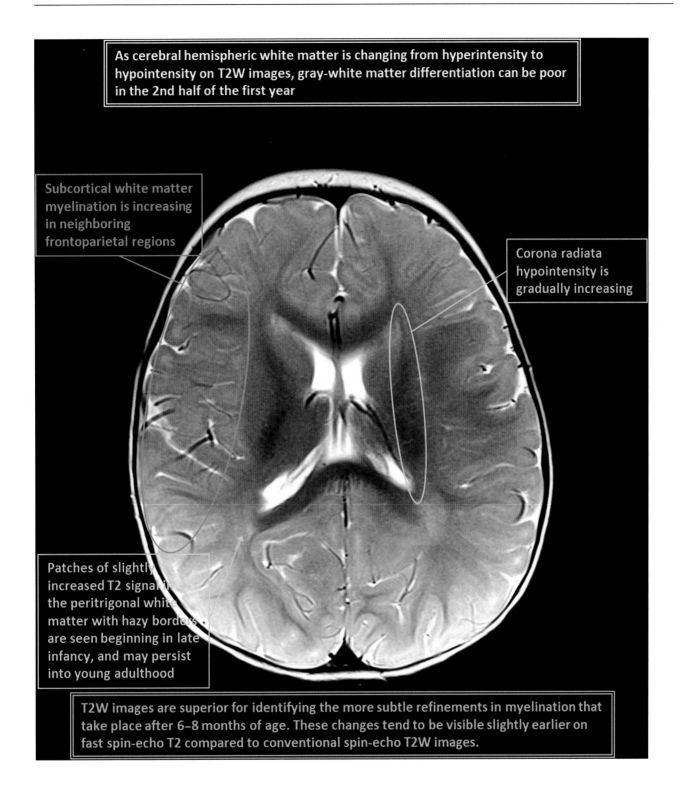

As cerebral hemispheric white matter is changing from hyperintensity to hypointensity on T2W images, gray-white matter differentiation can be poor in the 2nd half of the first year

Subcortical white matter myelination is increasing in neighboring frontoparietal regions

Corona radiata hypointensity is gradually increasing

Patches of slightly increased T2 signal in the peritrigonal white matter with hazy borders are seen beginning in late infancy, and may persist into young adulthood

T2W images are superior for identifying the more subtle refinements in myelination that take place after 6–8 months of age. These changes tend to be visible slightly earlier on fast spin-echo T2 compared to conventional spin-echo T2W images.

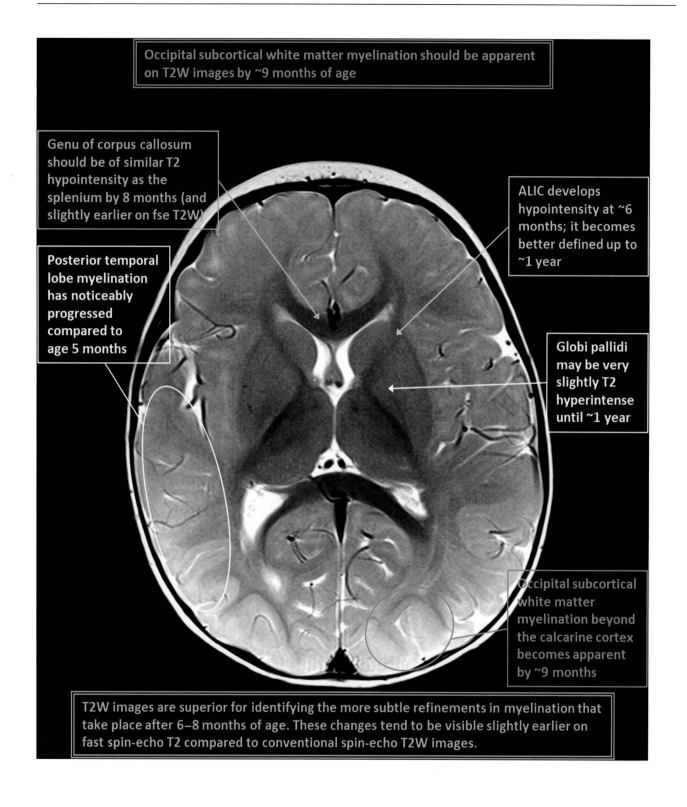

Occipital subcortical white matter myelination should be apparent on T2W images by ~9 months of age

Genu of corpus callosum should be of similar T2 hypointensity as the splenium by 8 months (and slightly earlier on fse T2W)

Posterior temporal lobe myelination has noticeably progressed compared to age 5 months

ALIC develops hypointensity at ~6 months; it becomes better defined up to ~1 year

Globi pallidi may be very slightly T2 hyperintense until ~1 year

Occipital subcortical white matter myelination beyond the calcarine cortex becomes apparent by ~9 months

T2W images are superior for identifying the more subtle refinements in myelination that take place after 6–8 months of age. These changes tend to be visible slightly earlier on fast spin-echo T2 compared to conventional spin-echo T2W images.

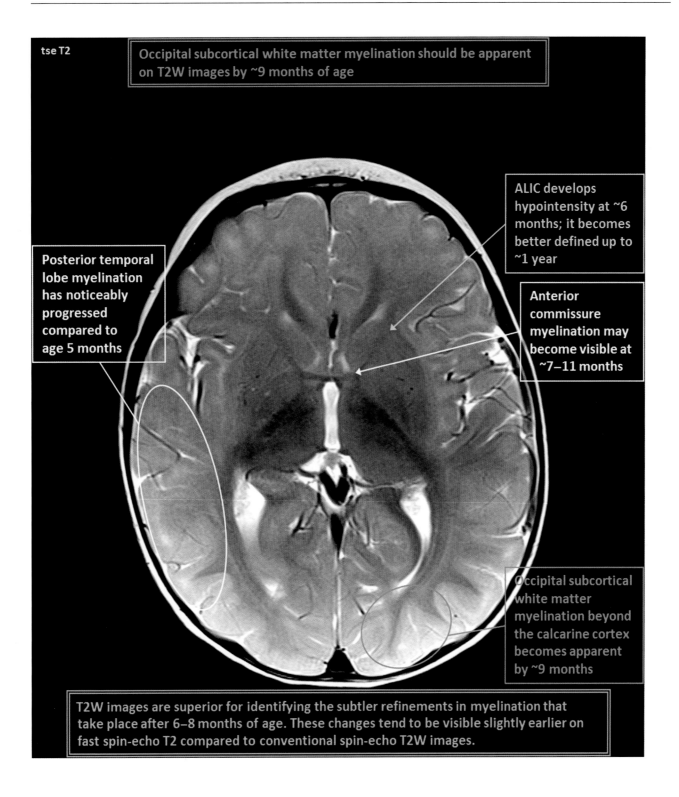

tse T2

Occipital subcortical white matter myelination should be apparent on T2W images by ~9 months of age

ALIC develops hypointensity at ~6 months; it becomes better defined up to ~1 year

Anterior commissure myelination may become visible at ~7–11 months

Posterior temporal lobe myelination has noticeably progressed compared to age 5 months

Occipital subcortical white matter myelination beyond the calcarine cortex becomes apparent by ~9 months

T2W images are superior for identifying the subtler refinements in myelination that take place after 6–8 months of age. These changes tend to be visible slightly earlier on fast spin-echo T2 compared to conventional spin-echo T2W images.

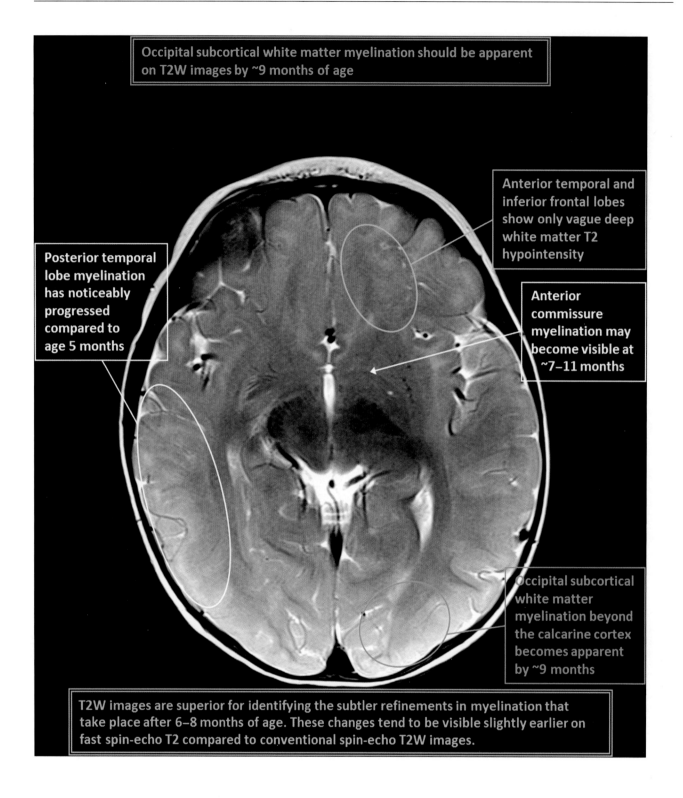

Occipital subcortical white matter myelination should be apparent on T2W images by ~9 months of age

Anterior temporal and inferior frontal lobes show only vague deep white matter T2 hypointensity

Anterior commissure myelination may become visible at ~7–11 months

Posterior temporal lobe myelination has noticeably progressed compared to age 5 months

Occipital subcortical white matter myelination beyond the calcarine cortex becomes apparent by ~9 months

T2W images are superior for identifying the subtler refinements in myelination that take place after 6–8 months of age. These changes tend to be visible slightly earlier on fast spin-echo T2 compared to conventional spin-echo T2W images.

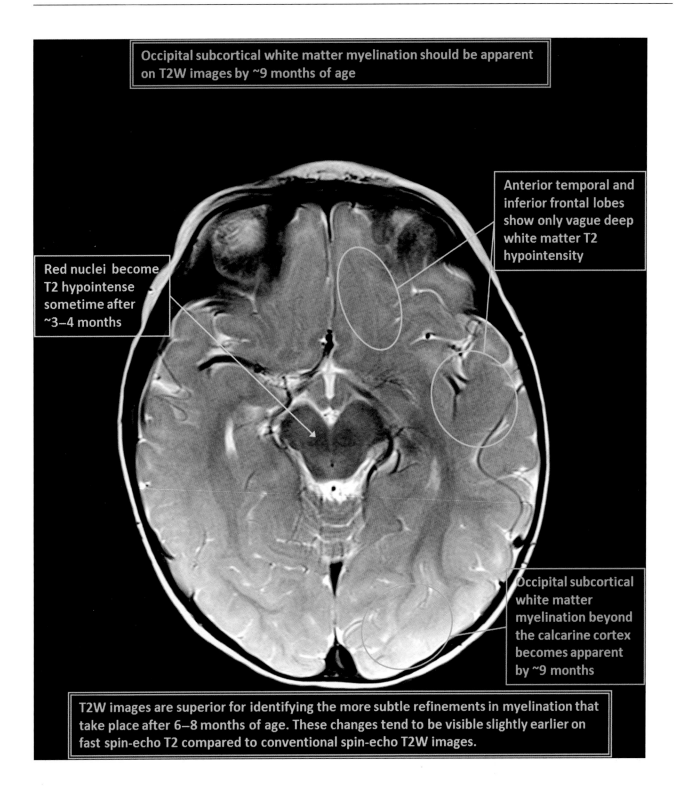

Occipital subcortical white matter myelination should be apparent on T2W images by ~9 months of age

Anterior temporal and inferior frontal lobes show only vague deep white matter T2 hypointensity

Red nuclei become T2 hypointense sometime after ~3–4 months

Occipital subcortical white matter myelination beyond the calcarine cortex becomes apparent by ~9 months

T2W images are superior for identifying the more subtle refinements in myelination that take place after 6–8 months of age. These changes tend to be visible slightly earlier on fast spin-echo T2 compared to conventional spin-echo T2W images.

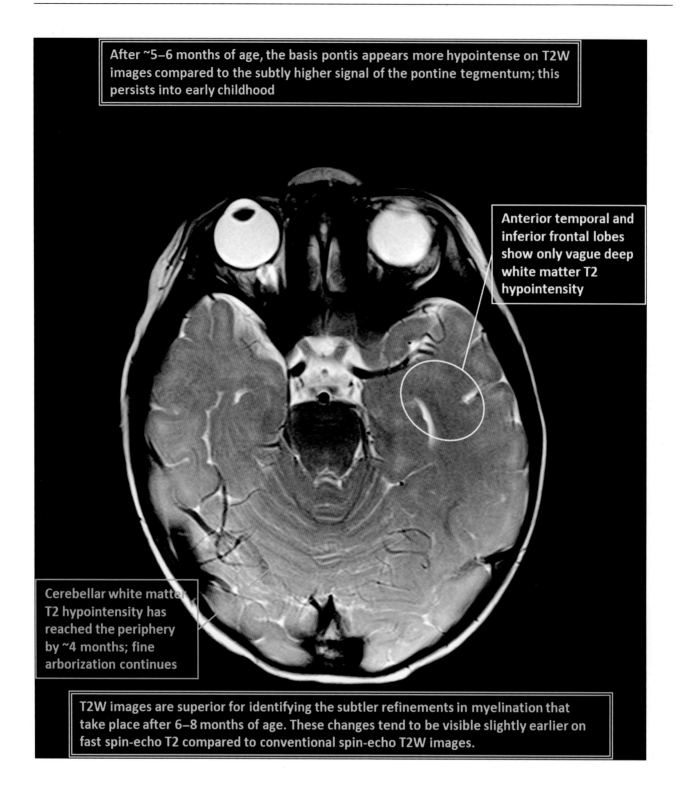

After ~5–6 months of age, the basis pontis appears more hypointense on T2W images compared to the subtly higher signal of the pontine tegmentum; this persists into early childhood

Anterior temporal and inferior frontal lobes show only vague deep white matter T2 hypointensity

Cerebellar white matter T2 hypointensity has reached the periphery by ~4 months; fine arborization continues

T2W images are superior for identifying the subtler refinements in myelination that take place after 6–8 months of age. These changes tend to be visible slightly earlier on fast spin-echo T2 compared to conventional spin-echo T2W images.

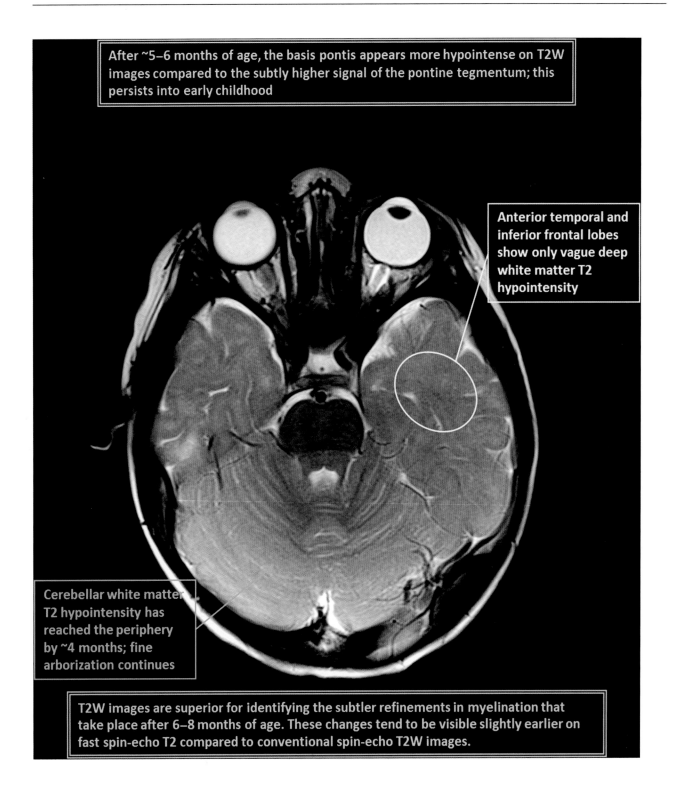

After ~5–6 months of age, the basis pontis appears more hypointense on T2W images compared to the subtly higher signal of the pontine tegmentum; this persists into early childhood

Anterior temporal and inferior frontal lobes show only vague deep white matter T2 hypointensity

Cerebellar white matter T2 hypointensity has reached the periphery by ~4 months; fine arborization continues

T2W images are superior for identifying the subtler refinements in myelination that take place after 6–8 months of age. These changes tend to be visible slightly earlier on fast spin-echo T2 compared to conventional spin-echo T2W images.

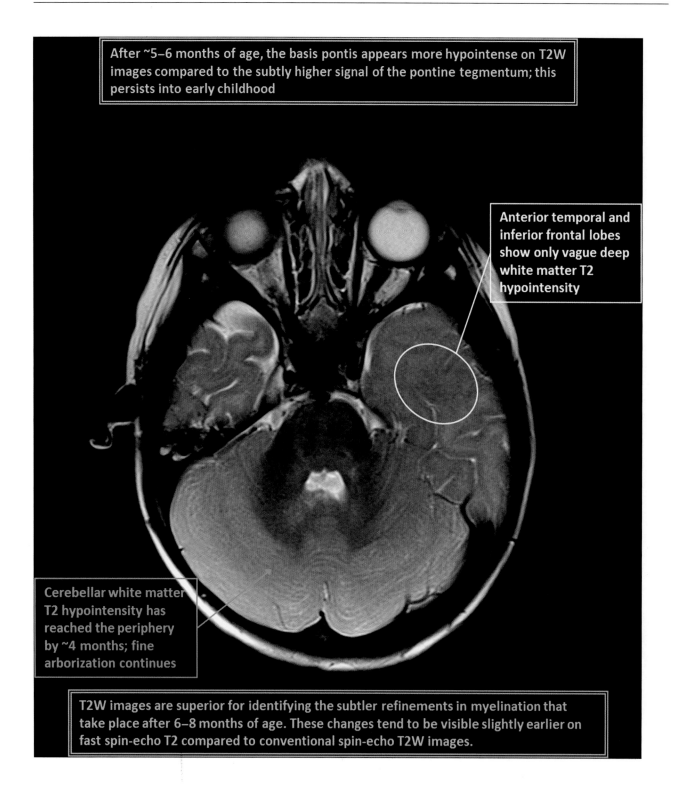

After ~5–6 months of age, the basis pontis appears more hypointense on T2W images compared to the subtly higher signal of the pontine tegmentum; this persists into early childhood

Anterior temporal and inferior frontal lobes show only vague deep white matter T2 hypointensity

Cerebellar white matter T2 hypointensity has reached the periphery by ~4 months; fine arborization continues

T2W images are superior for identifying the subtler refinements in myelination that take place after 6–8 months of age. These changes tend to be visible slightly earlier on fast spin-echo T2 compared to conventional spin-echo T2W images.

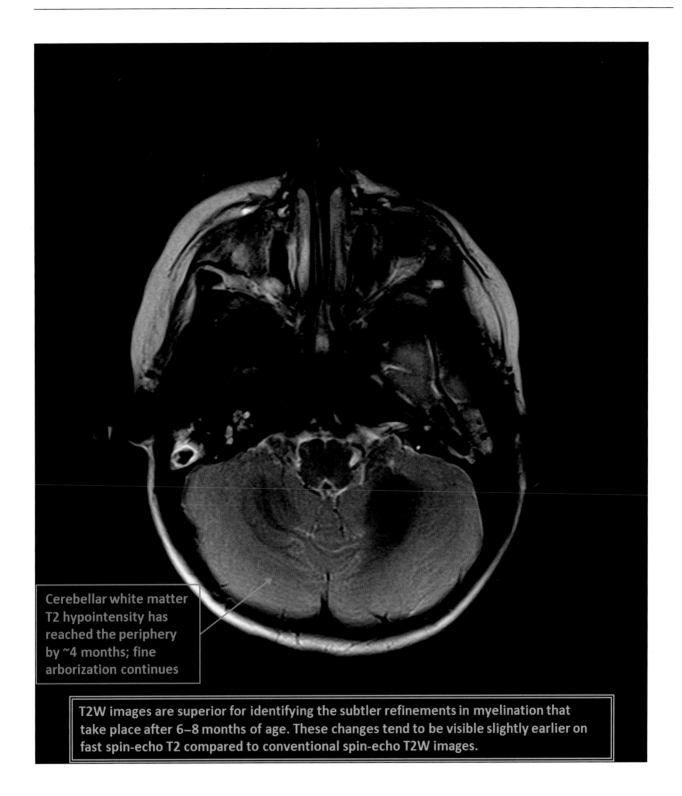

Cerebellar white matter T2 hypointensity has reached the periphery by ~4 months; fine arborization continues

T2W images are superior for identifying the subtler refinements in myelination that take place after 6–8 months of age. These changes tend to be visible slightly earlier on fast spin-echo T2 compared to conventional spin-echo T2W images.

9 Months, Diffusion Weighted Imaging (DWI) (b=1000 s/mm²)

> Cerebral white matter , including the subcortical regions, is hypointense to cortex on DWI after ~9 months of age and remains so into adulthood

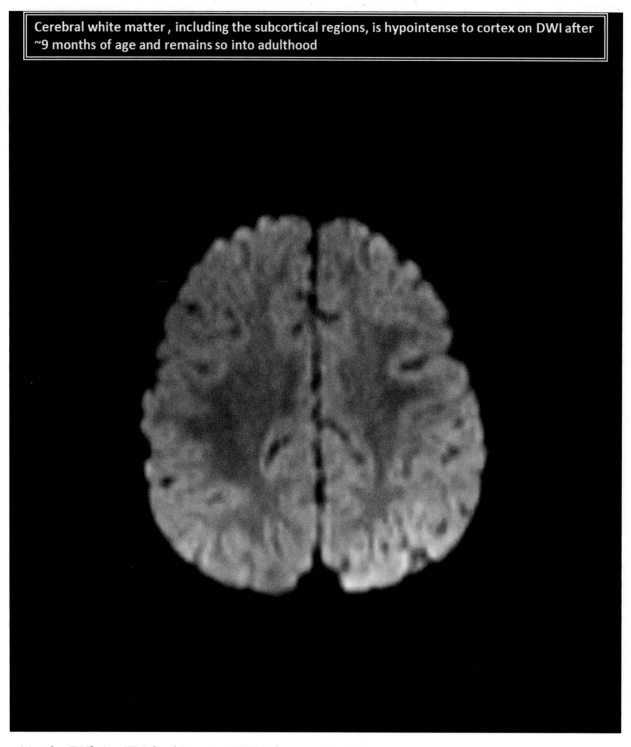

9 Months, Diffusion Weighted Imaging (DWI) (b=1000 s/mm²) Images 1–5

Cerebral white matter , including the subcortical regions, is hypointense to cortex on DWI after ~9 months of age and remains so into adulthood

Cerebral white matter , including the subcortical regions, is hypointense to cortex on DWI after ~9 months of age and remains so into adulthood

For most of the first year of life, the cerebellum as a whole can have a noticeably more hypointense appearance on ADC than the cerebral hemispheres, while on DWI it is isointense to subtly hyperintense to the cerebrum

For most of the first year of life, the cerebellum as a whole can have a noticeably more hypointense appearance on ADC than the cerebral hemispheres, while on DWI it is isointense to subtly hyperintense to the cerebrum

9 Months, Apparent Diffusion Coefficient (ADC) Map

> ADC values of WM continue to decrease, but at a slower rate after ~ age 5 months. Much of the cerebral gray and white matter will appear close to isointensity on ADC images by ~ age 1 year.

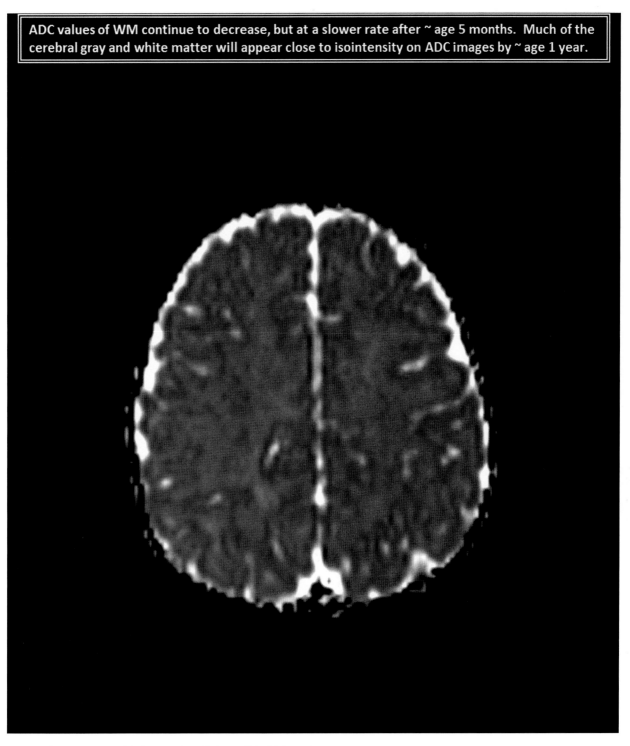

9 Months, Apparent Diffusion Coefficient (ADC) Map Images 1–5

ADC values of WM continue to decrease, but at a slower rate after ~ age 5 months. Much of the cerebral gray and white matter will appear close to isointensity on ADC images by ~ age 1 year.

ADC values of WM continue to decrease, but at a slower rate after ~ age 5 months. Much of the cerebral gray and white matter will appear close to isointensity on ADC images by ~ age 1 year.

For most of the first year of life, the cerebellum as a whole can have a noticeably more hypointense appearance on ADC than the cerebral hemispheres, while on DWI it is isointense to subtly hyperintense to the cerebrum

For most of the first year of life, the cerebellum as a whole can have a noticeably more hypointense appearance on ADC than the cerebral hemispheres, while on DWI it is isointense to subtly hyperintense to the cerebrum

9 Months, Sagittal T1

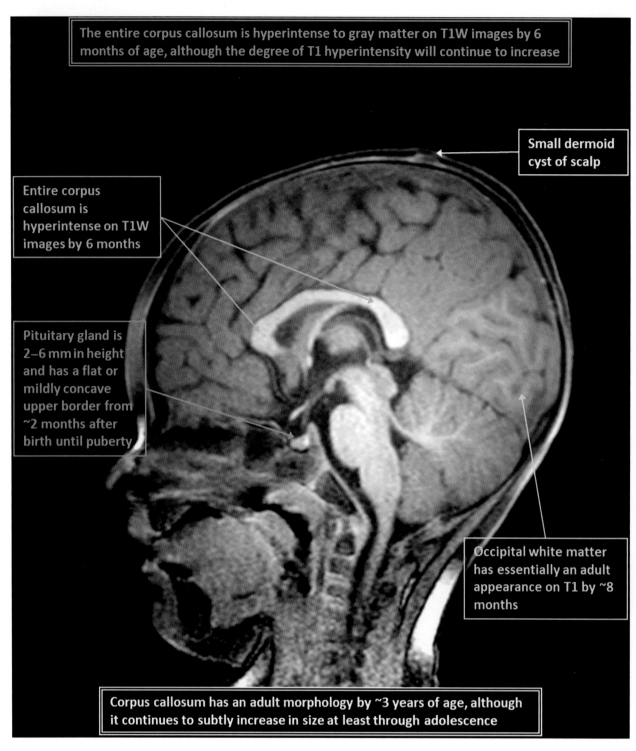

The entire corpus callosum is hyperintense to gray matter on T1W images by 6 months of age, although the degree of T1 hyperintensity will continue to increase

Small dermoid cyst of scalp

Entire corpus callosum is hyperintense on T1W images by 6 months

Pituitary gland is 2–6 mm in height and has a flat or mildly concave upper border from ~2 months after birth until puberty

Occipital white matter has essentially an adult appearance on T1 by ~8 months

Corpus callosum has an adult morphology by ~3 years of age, although it continues to subtly increase in size at least through adolescence

9 Months, Sagittal T1 Images 1–4

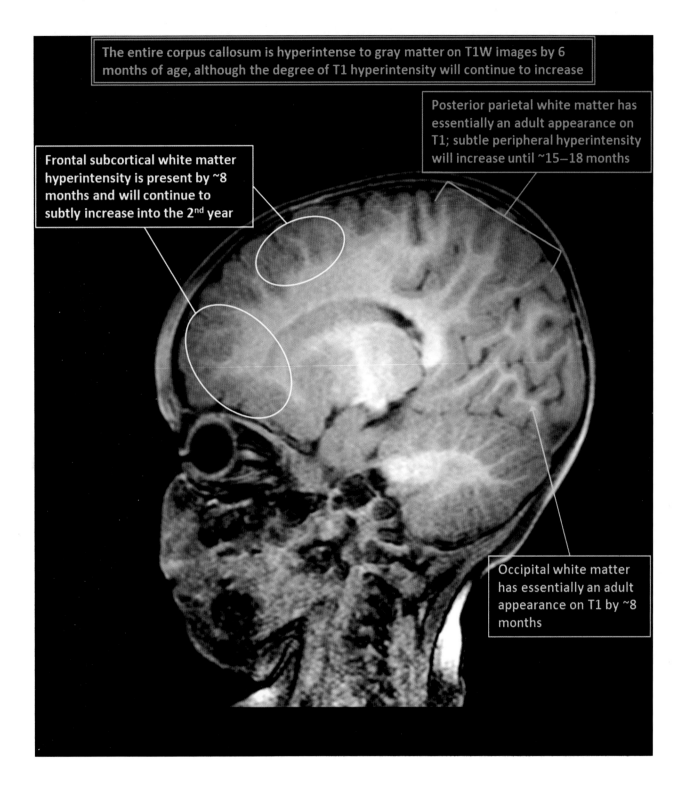

The entire corpus callosum is hyperintense to gray matter on T1W images by 6 months of age, although the degree of T1 hyperintensity will continue to increase

Posterior parietal white matter has essentially an adult appearance on T1; subtle peripheral hyperintensity will increase until ~15–18 months

Frontal subcortical white matter hyperintensity is present by ~8 months and will continue to subtly increase into the 2nd year

Occipital white matter has essentially an adult appearance on T1 by ~8 months

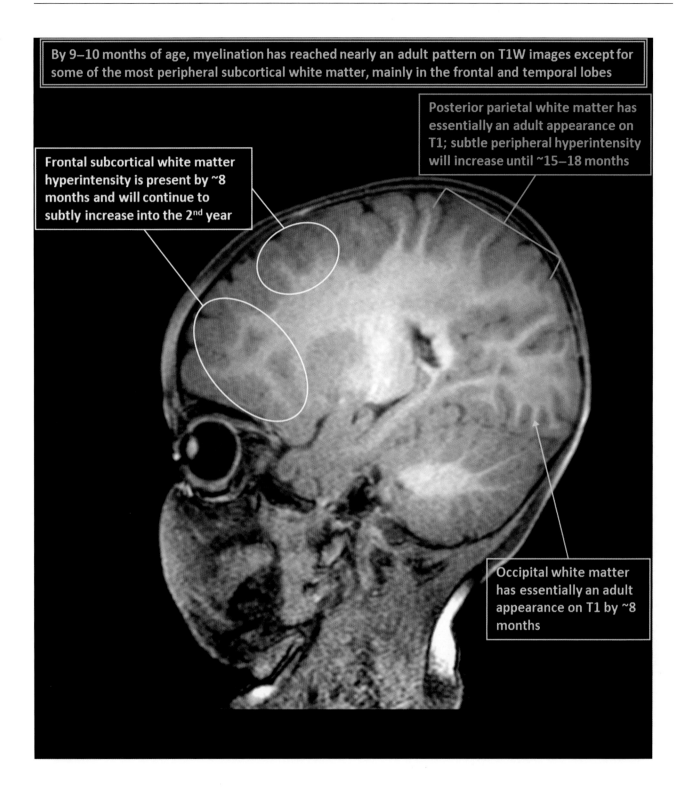

By 9–10 months of age, myelination has reached nearly an adult pattern on T1W images except for some of the most peripheral subcortical white matter, mainly in the frontal and temporal lobes

Posterior parietal white matter has essentially an adult appearance on T1; subtle peripheral hyperintensity will increase until ~15–18 months

Frontal subcortical white matter hyperintensity is present by ~8 months and will continue to subtly increase into the 2nd year

Occipital white matter has essentially an adult appearance on T1 by ~8 months

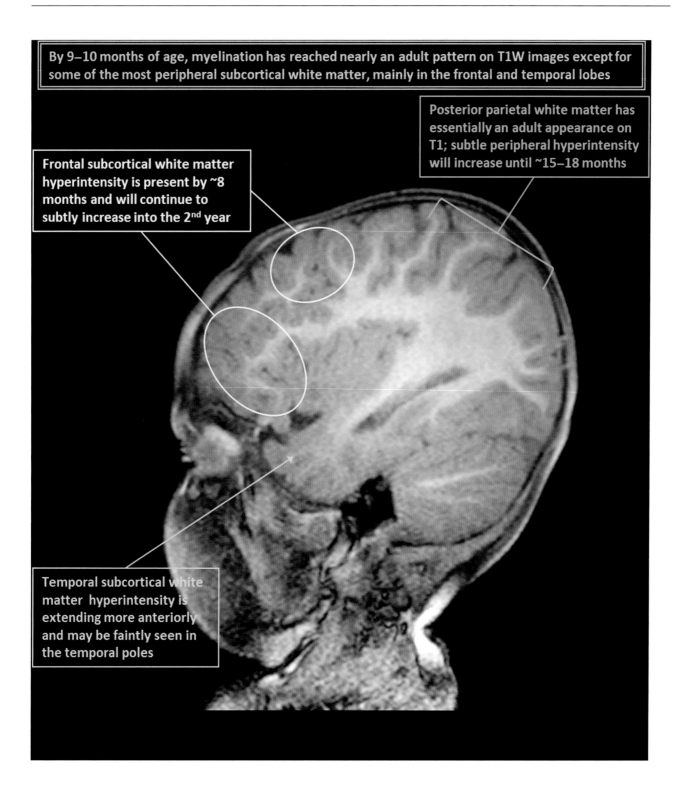

By 9–10 months of age, myelination has reached nearly an adult pattern on T1W images except for some of the most peripheral subcortical white matter, mainly in the frontal and temporal lobes

Posterior parietal white matter has essentially an adult appearance on T1; subtle peripheral hyperintensity will increase until ~15–18 months

Frontal subcortical white matter hyperintensity is present by ~8 months and will continue to subtly increase into the 2nd year

Temporal subcortical white matter hyperintensity is extending more anteriorly and may be faintly seen in the temporal poles

9 Months, Coronal TSE T2

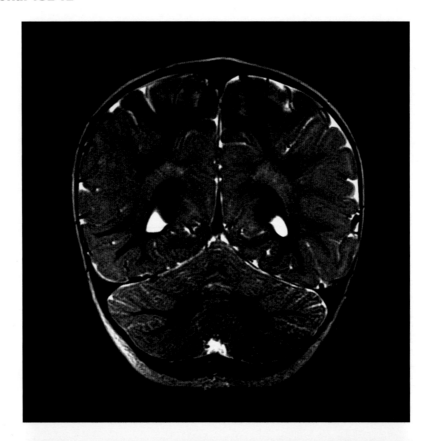

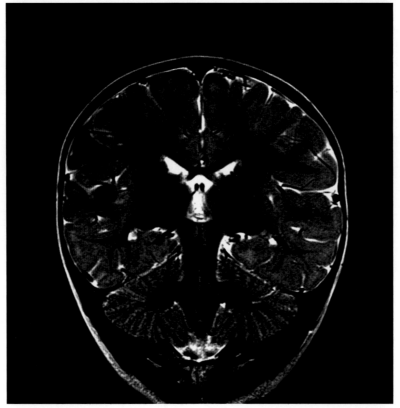

9 Months, Coronal TSE T2 Images 1–4

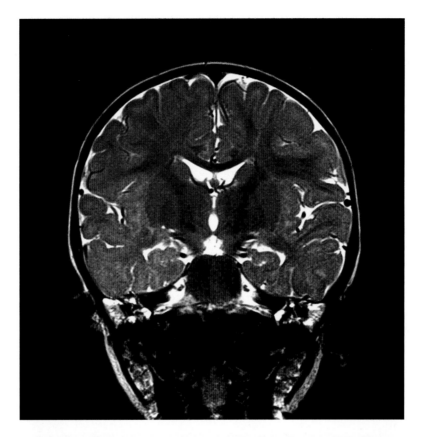

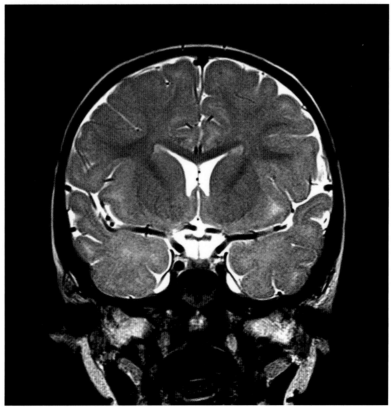

1 Year, Axial T1

Myelination essentially reaches an adult pattern on T1W images by 12–15 months, with minimal further T1 shortening occurring in subcortical U-fibers until approximately 18 months of age

Frontal subcortical white matter hyperintensity is present by ~8 months and will continue to subtly increase into the 2nd year

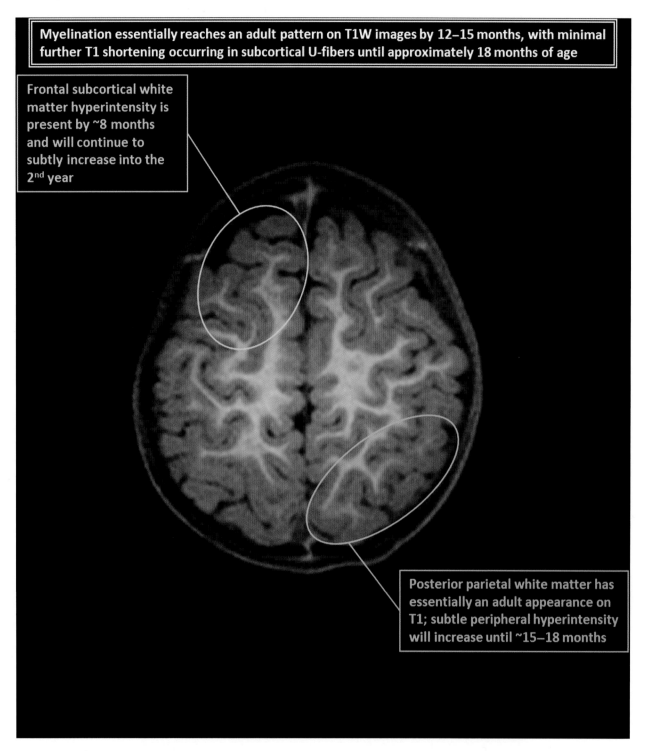

Posterior parietal white matter has essentially an adult appearance on T1; subtle peripheral hyperintensity will increase until ~15–18 months

1 Year, Axial T1 Images 1–12

Myelination essentially reaches an adult pattern on T1W images by 12–15 months, with minimal further T1 shortening occurring in subcortical U-fibers until approximately 18 months of age

Frontal subcortical white matter hyperintensity is present by ~8 months and will continue to subtly increase into the 2nd year

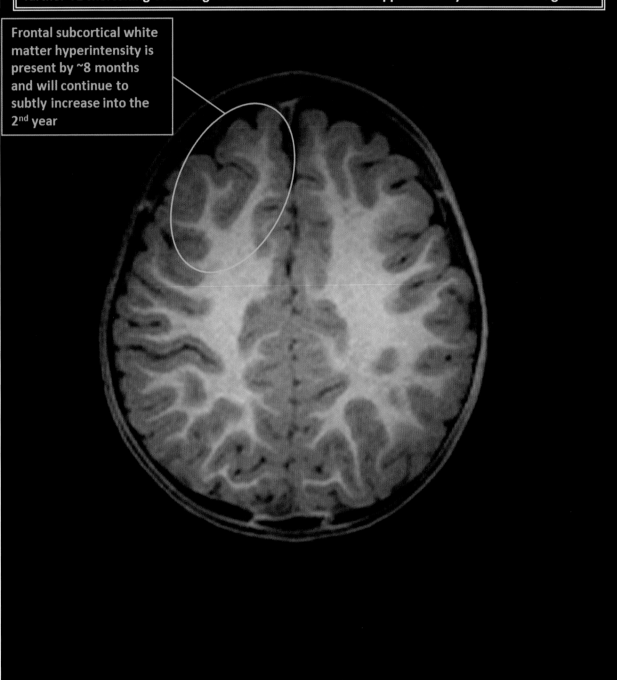

Myelination essentially reaches an adult pattern on T1W images by 12–15 months, with minimal further T1 shortening occurring in subcortical U-fibers until approximately 18 months of age

Frontal subcortical white matter hyperintensity is present by ~8 months and will continue to subtly increase into the 2nd year

Occipital white matter has essentially an adult appearance on T1 by ~8 months

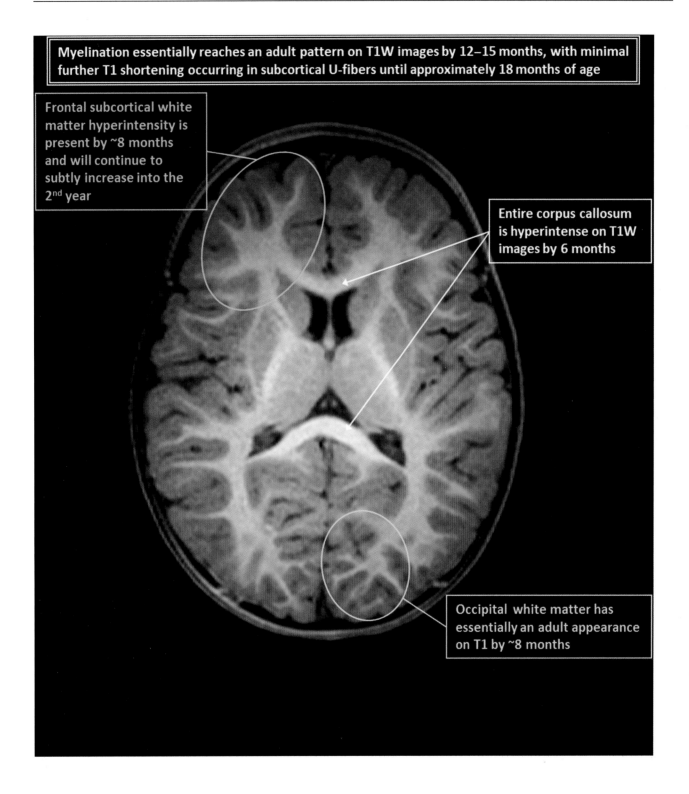

Myelination essentially reaches an adult pattern on T1W images by 12–15 months, with minimal further T1 shortening occurring in subcortical U-fibers until approximately 18 months of age

Frontal subcortical white matter hyperintensity is present by ~8 months and will continue to subtly increase into the 2nd year

Entire corpus callosum is hyperintense on T1W images by 6 months

Occipital white matter has essentially an adult appearance on T1 by ~8 months

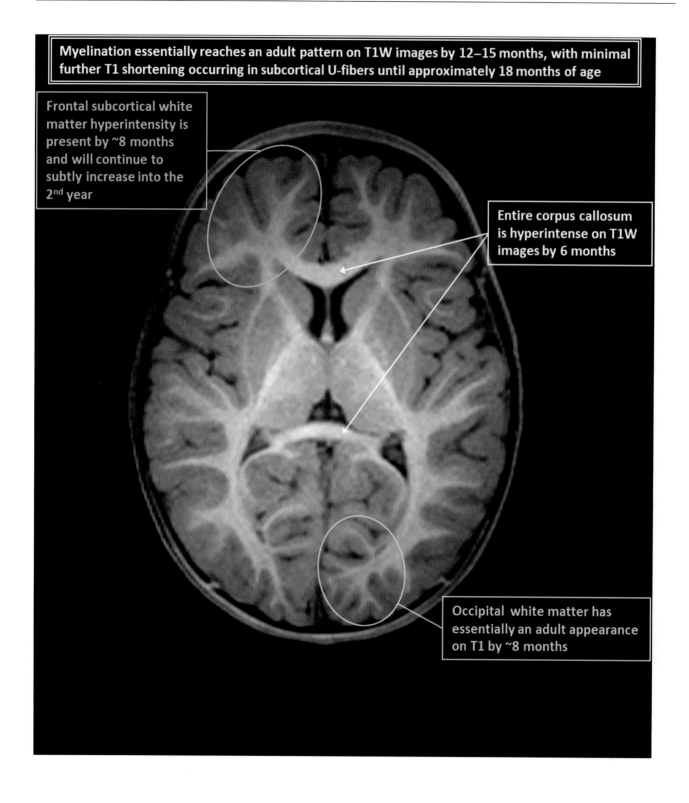

Myelination essentially reaches an adult pattern on T1W images by 12–15 months, with minimal further T1 shortening occurring in subcortical U-fibers until approximately 18 months of age

Frontal subcortical white matter hyperintensity is present by ~8 months and will continue to subtly increase into the 2nd year

Entire corpus callosum is hyperintense on T1W images by 6 months

Occipital white matter has essentially an adult appearance on T1 by ~8 months

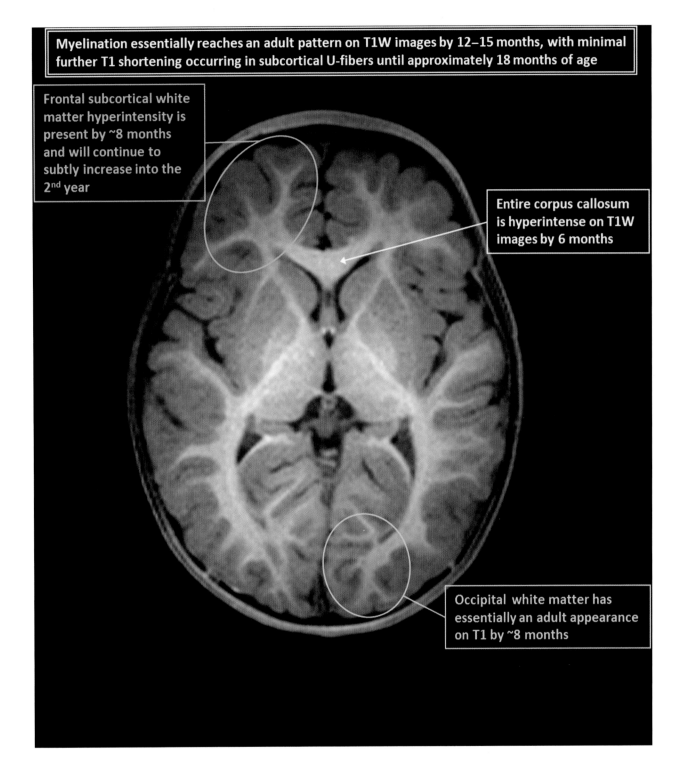

Myelination essentially reaches an adult pattern on T1W images by 12–15 months, with minimal further T1 shortening occurring in subcortical U-fibers until approximately 18 months of age

Frontal subcortical white matter hyperintensity is present by ~8 months and will continue to subtly increase into the 2nd year

Entire corpus callosum is hyperintense on T1W images by 6 months

Occipital white matter has essentially an adult appearance on T1 by ~8 months

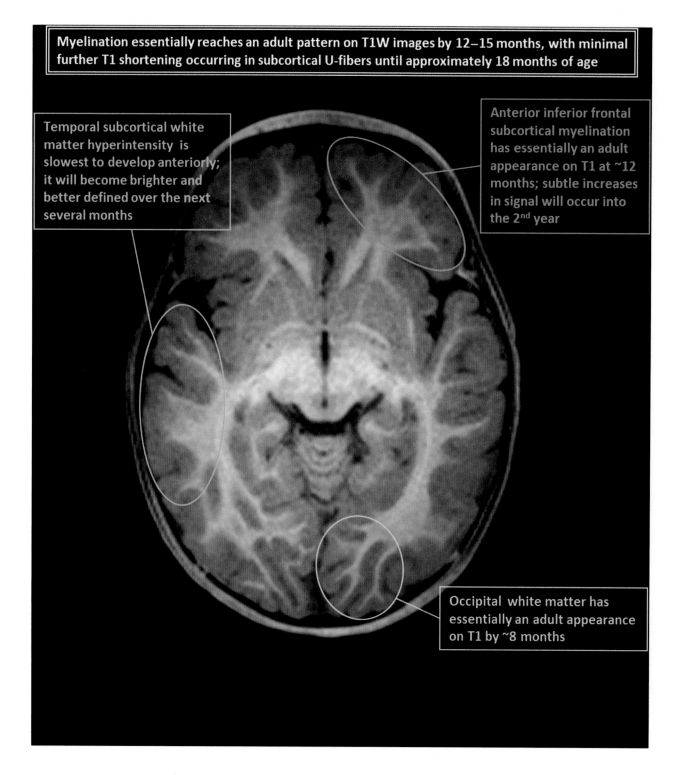

Myelination essentially reaches an adult pattern on T1W images by 12–15 months, with minimal further T1 shortening occurring in subcortical U-fibers until approximately 18 months of age

Temporal subcortical white matter hyperintensity is slowest to develop anteriorly; it will become brighter and better defined over the next several months

Anterior inferior frontal subcortical myelination has essentially an adult appearance on T1 at ~12 months; subtle increases in signal will occur into the 2nd year

Occipital white matter has essentially an adult appearance on T1 by ~8 months

Myelination essentially reaches an adult pattern on T1W images by 12–15 months, with minimal further T1 shortening occurring in subcortical U-fibers until approximately 18 months of age

Temporal subcortical white matter hyperintensity is slowest to develop anteriorly; it will become brighter and better defined over the next several months

Anterior inferior frontal subcortical myelination has essentially an adult appearance on T1 at ~12 months; subtle increases in signal will occur into the 2nd year

Occipital white matter has essentially an adult appearance on T1 by ~8 months

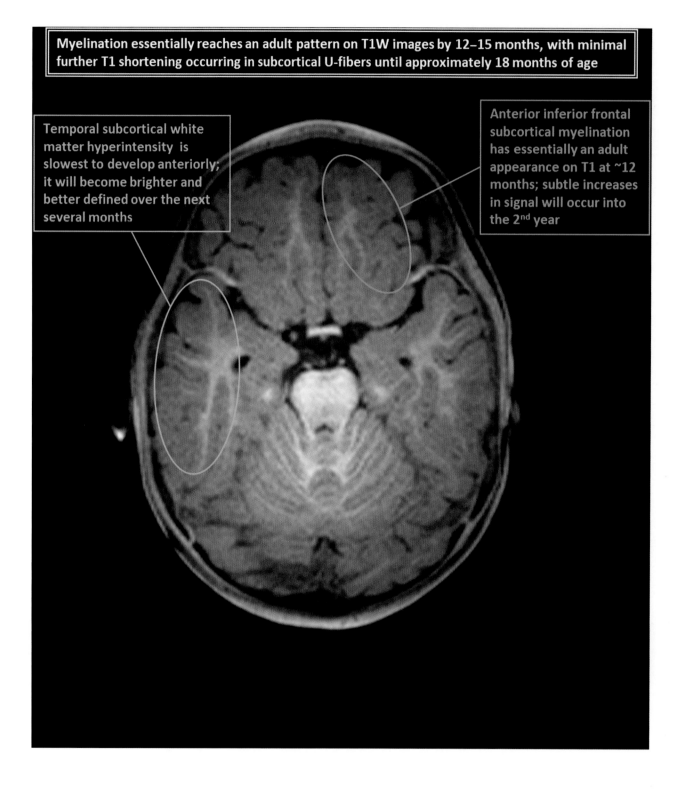

Myelination essentially reaches an adult pattern on T1W images by 12–15 months, with minimal further T1 shortening occurring in subcortical U-fibers until approximately 18 months of age

Temporal subcortical white matter hyperintensity is slowest to develop anteriorly; it will become brighter and better defined over the next several months

Anterior inferior frontal subcortical myelination has essentially an adult appearance on T1 at ~12 months; subtle increases in signal will occur into the 2nd year

Myelination essentially reaches an adult pattern on T1W images by 12–15 months, with minimal further T1 shortening occurring in subcortical U-fibers until approximately 18 months of age

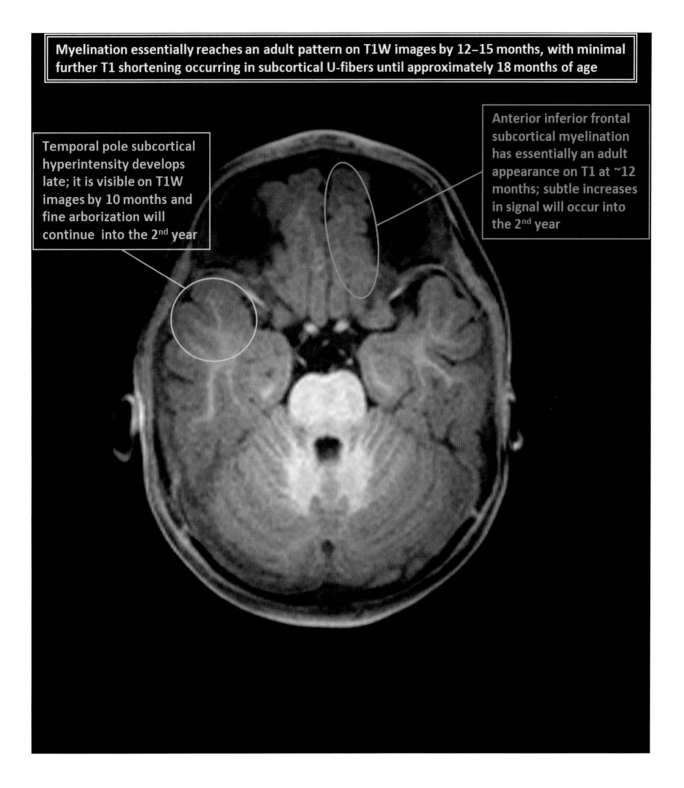

Temporal pole subcortical hyperintensity develops late; it is visible on T1W images by 10 months and fine arborization will continue into the 2nd year

Anterior inferior frontal subcortical myelination has essentially an adult appearance on T1 at ~12 months; subtle increases in signal will occur into the 2nd year

Myelination essentially reaches an adult pattern on T1W images by 12–15 months, with minimal further T1 shortening occurring in subcortical U-fibers until approximately 18 months of age

Temporal pole subcortical hyperintensity develops late; it is visible on T1W images by 10 months and fine arborization will continue into the 2nd year

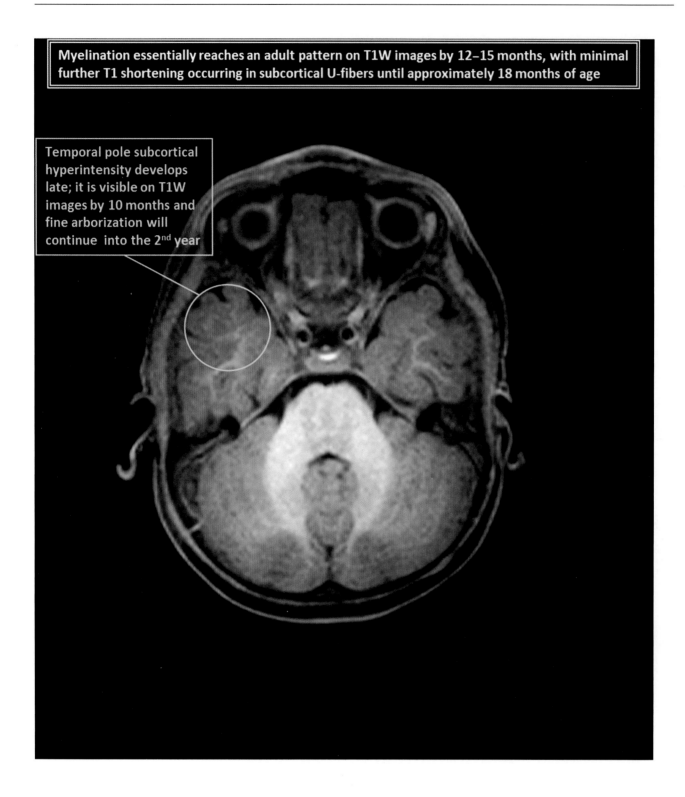

Myelination essentially reaches an adult pattern on T1W images by 12–15 months, with minimal further T1 shortening occurring in subcortical U-fibers until approximately 18 months of age

Temporal pole subcortical hyperintensity develops late; it is visible on T1W images by 10 months and fine arborization will continue into the 2nd year

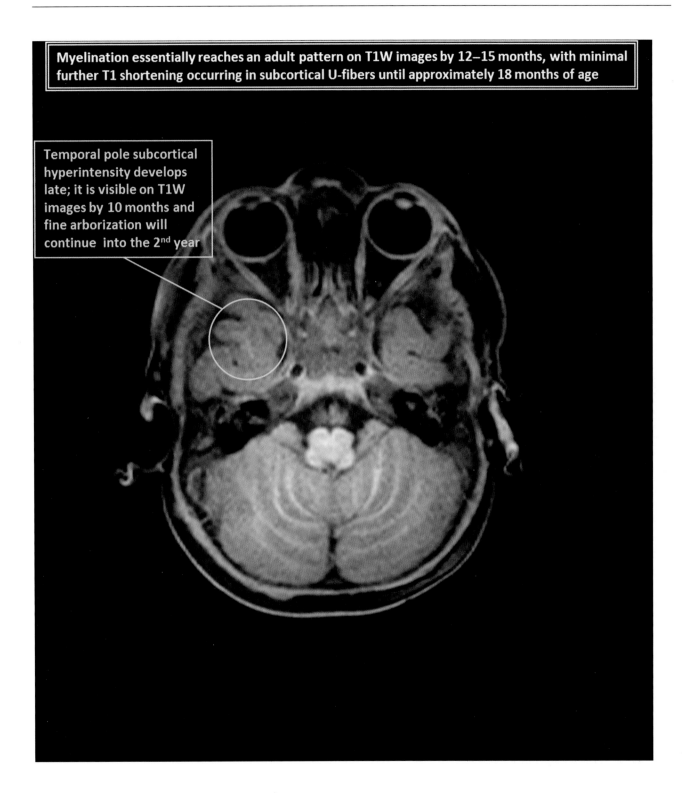

1 Year, Axial TSE T2

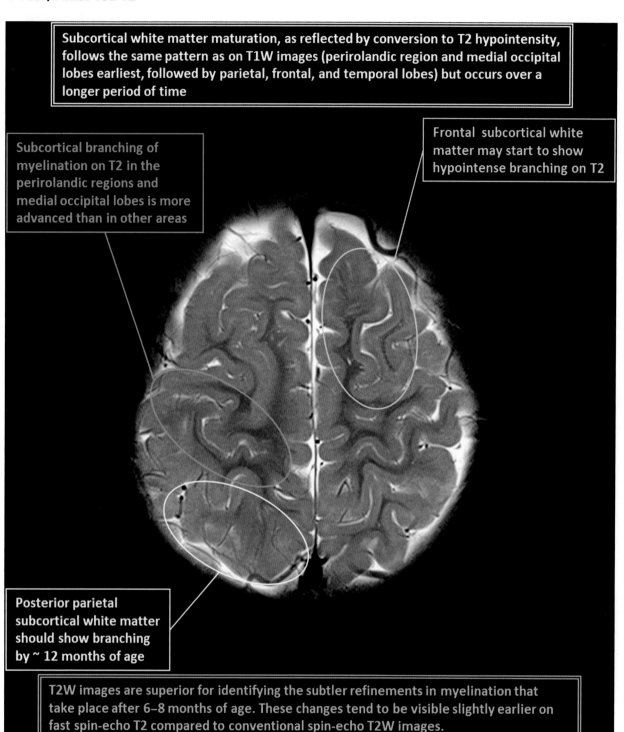

Subcortical white matter maturation, as reflected by conversion to T2 hypointensity, follows the same pattern as on T1W images (perirolandic region and medial occipital lobes earliest, followed by parietal, frontal, and temporal lobes) but occurs over a longer period of time

Frontal subcortical white matter may start to show hypointense branching on T2

Subcortical branching of myelination on T2 in the perirolandic regions and medial occipital lobes is more advanced than in other areas

Posterior parietal subcortical white matter should show branching by ~ 12 months of age

T2W images are superior for identifying the subtler refinements in myelination that take place after 6–8 months of age. These changes tend to be visible slightly earlier on fast spin-echo T2 compared to conventional spin-echo T2W images.

1 Year, Axial TSE T2 Images 1–12

Subcortical white matter maturation, as reflected by conversion to T2 hypointensity, follows the same pattern as on T1W images (perirolandic region and medial occipital lobes earliest, followed by parietal, frontal, and temporal lobes) but occurs over a longer period of time

Frontal subcortical white matter may start to show hypointense branching on T2

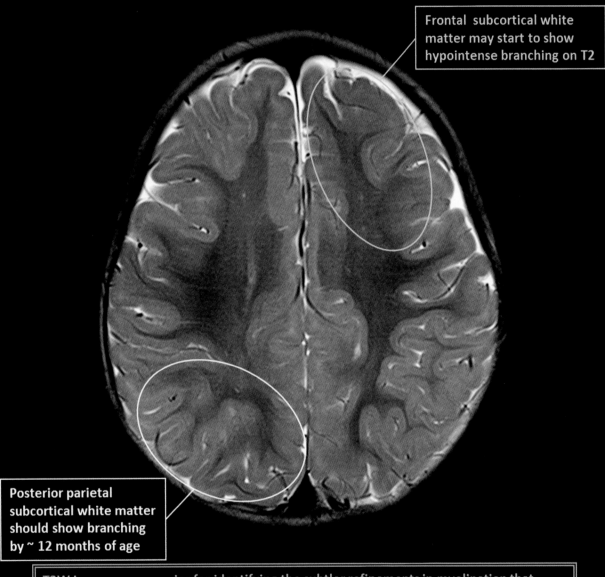

Posterior parietal subcortical white matter should show branching by ~ 12 months of age

T2W images are superior for identifying the subtler refinements in myelination that take place after 6–8 months of age. These changes tend to be visible slightly earlier on fast spin-echo T2 compared to conventional spin-echo T2W images.

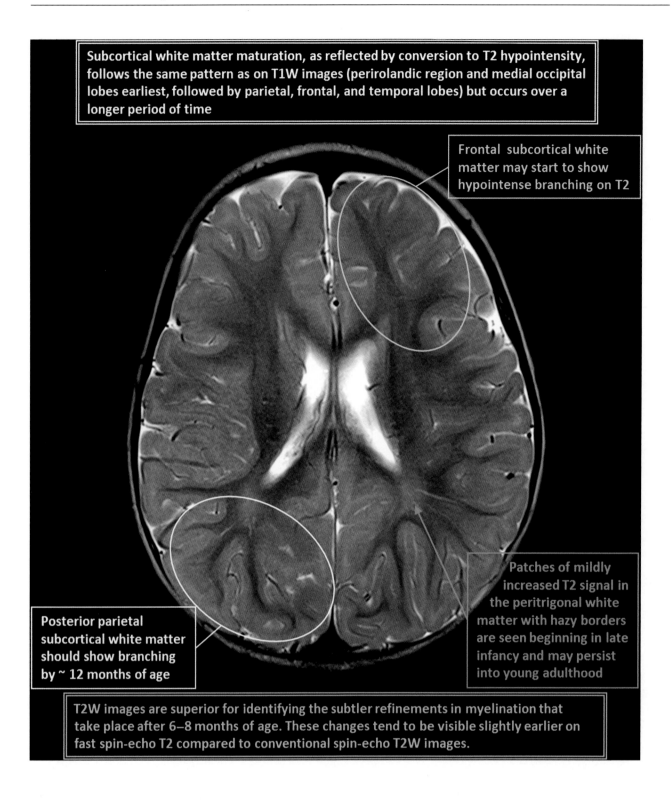

Subcortical white matter maturation, as reflected by conversion to T2 hypointensity, follows the same pattern as on T1W images (perirolandic region and medial occipital lobes earliest, followed by parietal, frontal, and temporal lobes) but occurs over a longer period of time

Frontal subcortical white matter may start to show hypointense branching on T2

Patches of mildly increased T2 signal in the peritrigonal white matter with hazy borders are seen beginning in late infancy and may persist into young adulthood

Posterior parietal subcortical white matter should show branching by ~ 12 months of age

T2W images are superior for identifying the subtler refinements in myelination that take place after 6–8 months of age. These changes tend to be visible slightly earlier on fast spin-echo T2 compared to conventional spin-echo T2W images.

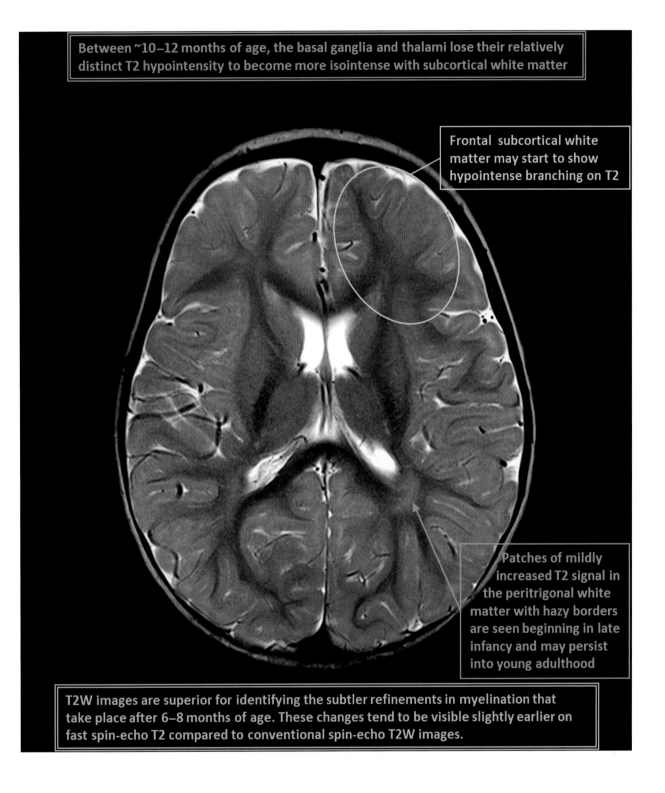

Between ~10–12 months of age, the basal ganglia and thalami lose their relatively distinct T2 hypointensity to become more isointense with subcortical white matter

Frontal subcortical white matter may start to show hypointense branching on T2

Patches of mildly increased T2 signal in the peritrigonal white matter with hazy borders are seen beginning in late infancy and may persist into young adulthood

T2W images are superior for identifying the subtler refinements in myelination that take place after 6–8 months of age. These changes tend to be visible slightly earlier on fast spin-echo T2 compared to conventional spin-echo T2W images.

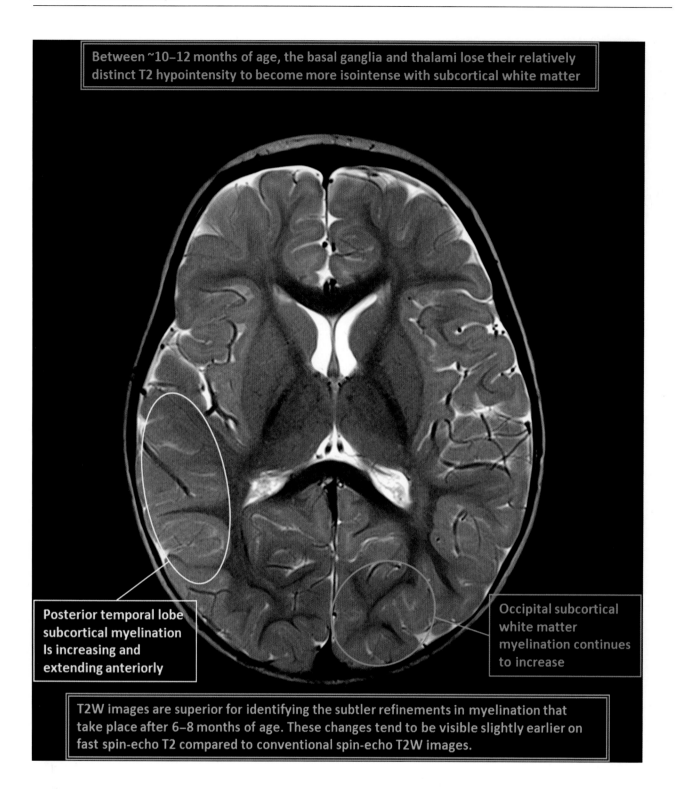

Between ~10–12 months of age, the basal ganglia and thalami lose their relatively distinct T2 hypointensity to become more isointense with subcortical white matter

Posterior temporal lobe subcortical myelination Is increasing and extending anteriorly

Occipital subcortical white matter myelination continues to increase

T2W images are superior for identifying the subtler refinements in myelination that take place after 6–8 months of age. These changes tend to be visible slightly earlier on fast spin-echo T2 compared to conventional spin-echo T2W images.

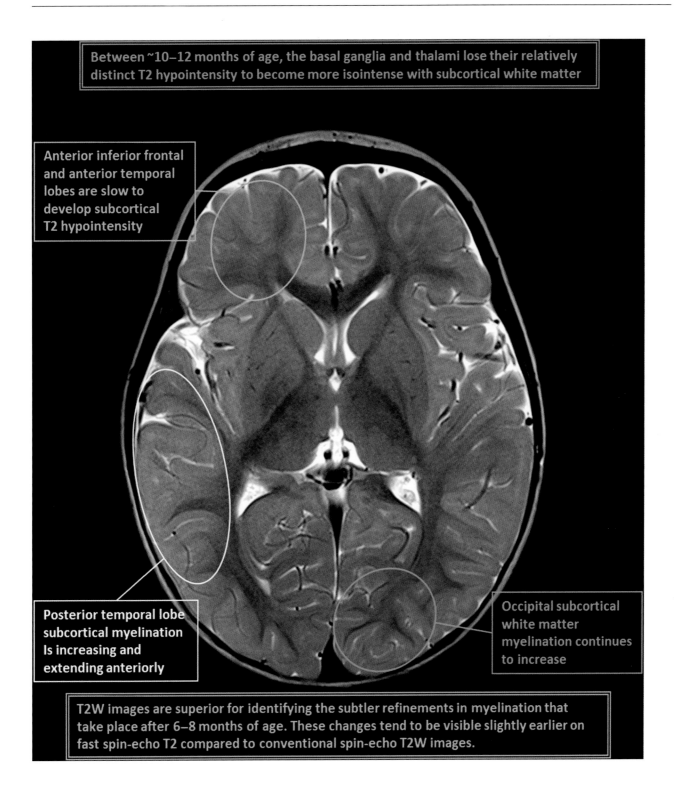

Between ~10–12 months of age, the basal ganglia and thalami lose their relatively distinct T2 hypointensity to become more isointense with subcortical white matter

Anterior inferior frontal and anterior temporal lobes are slow to develop subcortical T2 hypointensity

Posterior temporal lobe subcortical myelination is increasing and extending anteriorly

Occipital subcortical white matter myelination continues to increase

T2W images are superior for identifying the subtler refinements in myelination that take place after 6–8 months of age. These changes tend to be visible slightly earlier on fast spin-echo T2 compared to conventional spin-echo T2W images.

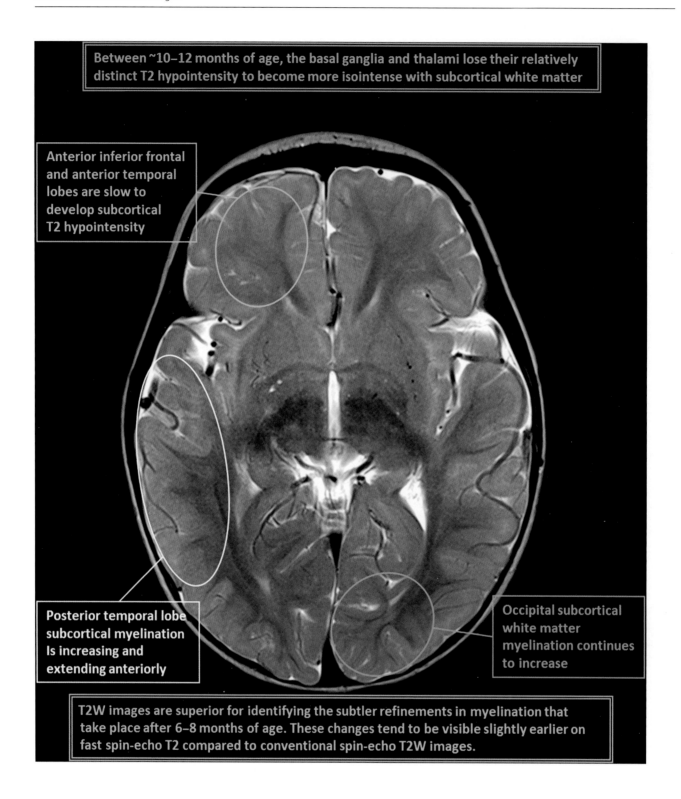

Between ~10–12 months of age, the basal ganglia and thalami lose their relatively distinct T2 hypointensity to become more isointense with subcortical white matter

Anterior inferior frontal and anterior temporal lobes are slow to develop subcortical T2 hypointensity

Posterior temporal lobe subcortical myelination Is increasing and extending anteriorly

Occipital subcortical white matter myelination continues to increase

T2W images are superior for identifying the subtler refinements in myelination that take place after 6–8 months of age. These changes tend to be visible slightly earlier on fast spin-echo T2 compared to conventional spin-echo T2W images.

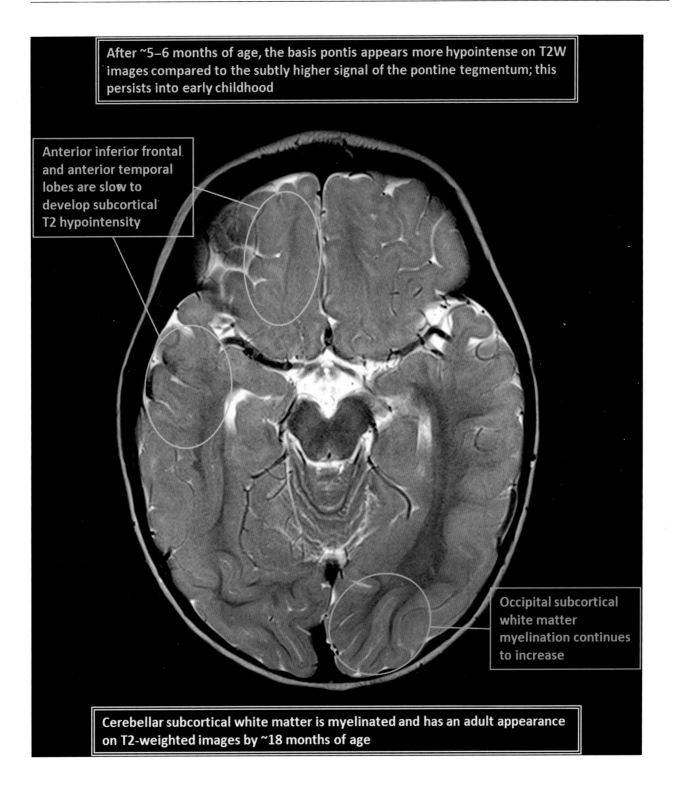

After ~5–6 months of age, the basis pontis appears more hypointense on T2W images compared to the subtly higher signal of the pontine tegmentum; this persists into early childhood

Anterior inferior frontal and anterior temporal lobes are slow to develop subcortical T2 hypointensity

Occipital subcortical white matter myelination continues to increase

Cerebellar subcortical white matter is myelinated and has an adult appearance on T2-weighted images by ~18 months of age

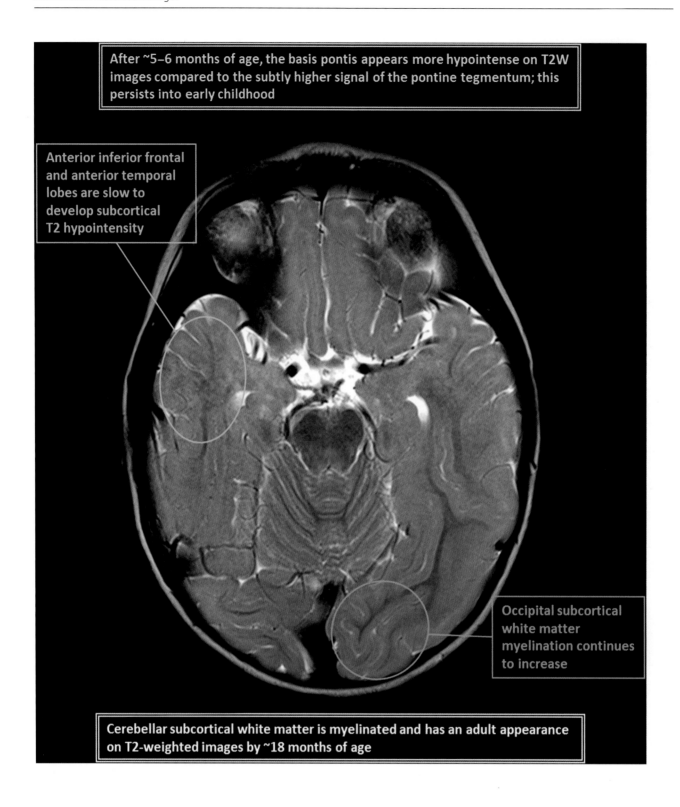

After ~5–6 months of age, the basis pontis appears more hypointense on T2W images compared to the subtly higher signal of the pontine tegmentum; this persists into early childhood

Anterior inferior frontal and anterior temporal lobes are slow to develop subcortical T2 hypointensity

Occipital subcortical white matter myelination continues to increase

Cerebellar subcortical white matter is myelinated and has an adult appearance on T2-weighted images by ~18 months of age

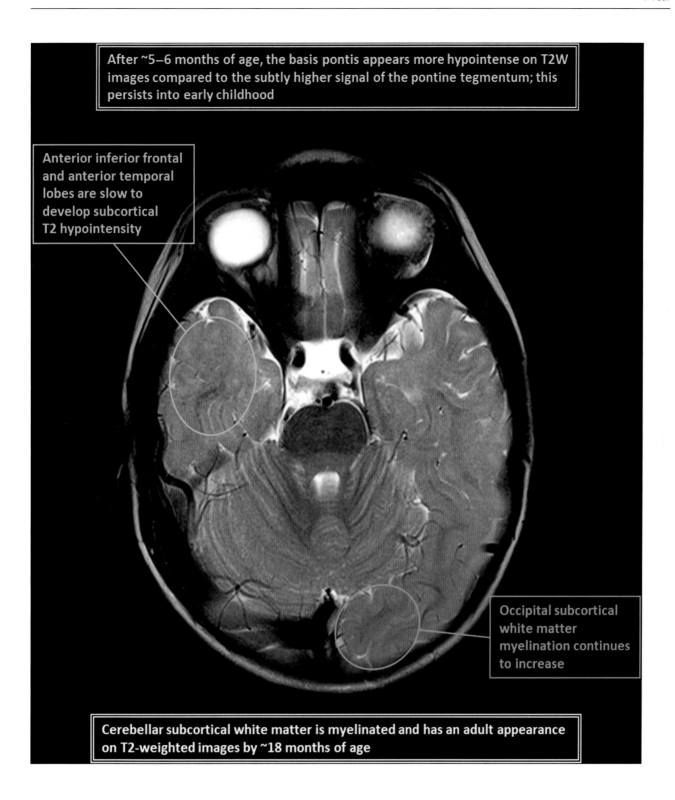

After ~5–6 months of age, the basis pontis appears more hypointense on T2W images compared to the subtly higher signal of the pontine tegmentum; this persists into early childhood

Anterior inferior frontal and anterior temporal lobes are slow to develop subcortical T2 hypointensity

Occipital subcortical white matter myelination continues to increase

Cerebellar subcortical white matter is myelinated and has an adult appearance on T2-weighted images by ~18 months of age

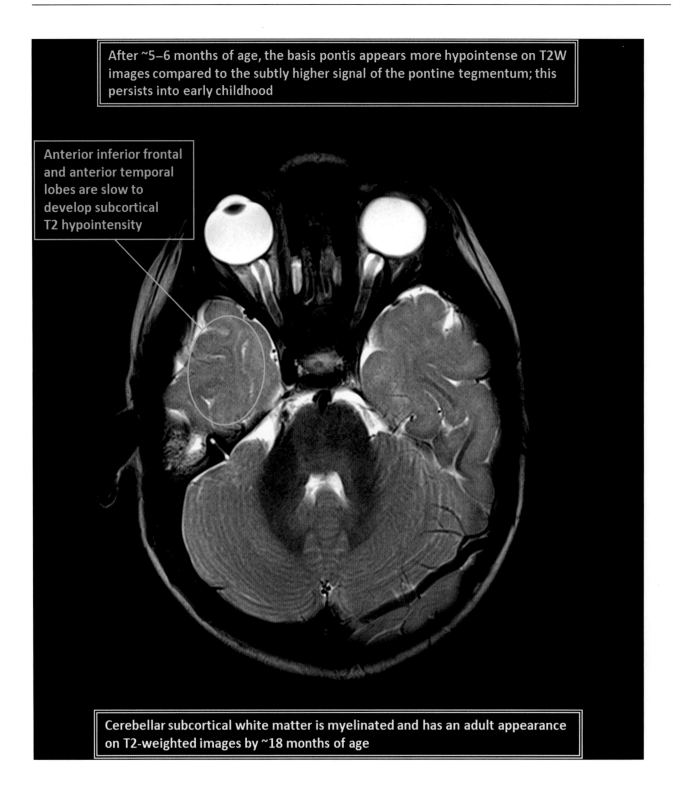

After ~5–6 months of age, the basis pontis appears more hypointense on T2W images compared to the subtly higher signal of the pontine tegmentum; this persists into early childhood

Anterior inferior frontal and anterior temporal lobes are slow to develop subcortical T2 hypointensity

Cerebellar subcortical white matter is myelinated and has an adult appearance on T2-weighted images by ~18 months of age

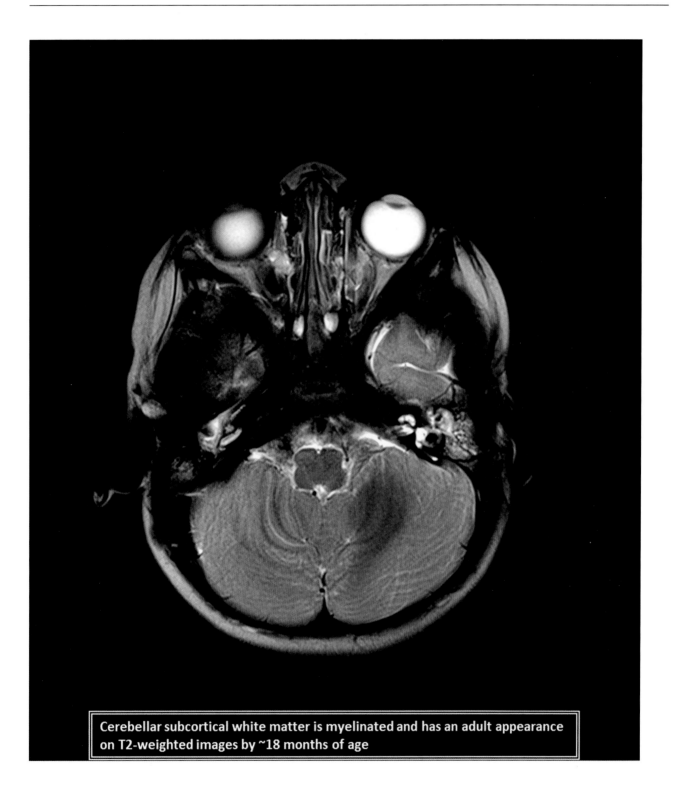

Cerebellar subcortical white matter is myelinated and has an adult appearance on T2-weighted images by ~18 months of age

1 Year, Axial FLAIR

On FLAIR images beyond the neonatal period, the conversion of deep and subcortical white matter from hyperintensity to hypointensity relative to cortex generally follows the same pattern as on spin-echo T2W images, but occurs more slowly. The mild delay is probably due to the T1 weighting inherent in the FLAIR technique.

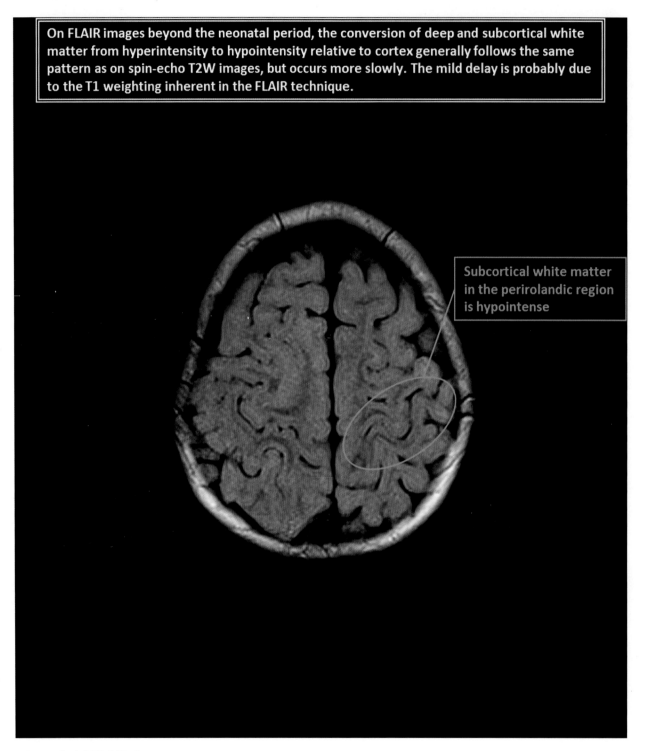

Subcortical white matter in the perirolandic region is hypointense

1 Year, Axial FLAIR Images 1–12

On FLAIR images beyond the neonatal period, the conversion of deep and subcortical white matter from hyperintensity to hypointensity relative to cortex generally follows the same pattern as on spin-echo T2W images, but occurs more slowly. The mild delay is probably due to the T1 weighting inherent in the FLAIR technique.

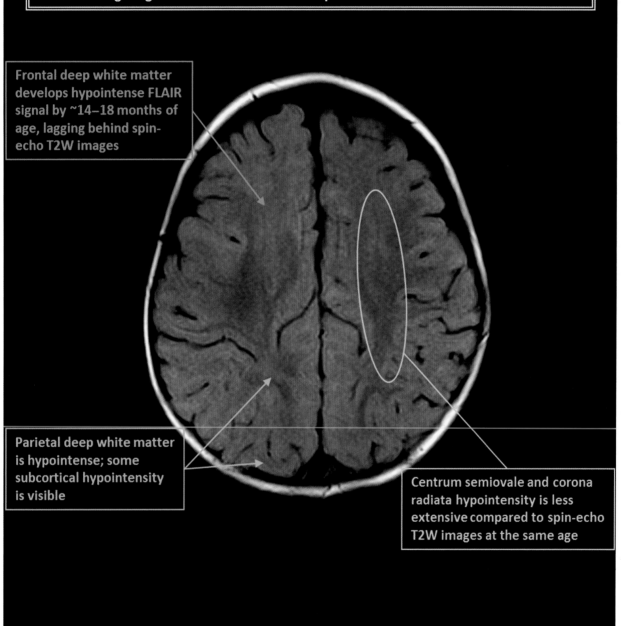

Frontal deep white matter develops hypointense FLAIR signal by ~14–18 months of age, lagging behind spin-echo T2W images

Parietal deep white matter is hypointense; some subcortical hypointensity is visible

Centrum semiovale and corona radiata hypointensity is less extensive compared to spin-echo T2W images at the same age

On FLAIR images beyond the neonatal period, the conversion of deep and subcortical white matter from hyperintensity to hypointensity relative to cortex generally follows the same pattern as on spin-echo T2W images, but occurs more slowly. The mild delay is probably due to the T1 weighting inherent in the FLAIR technique.

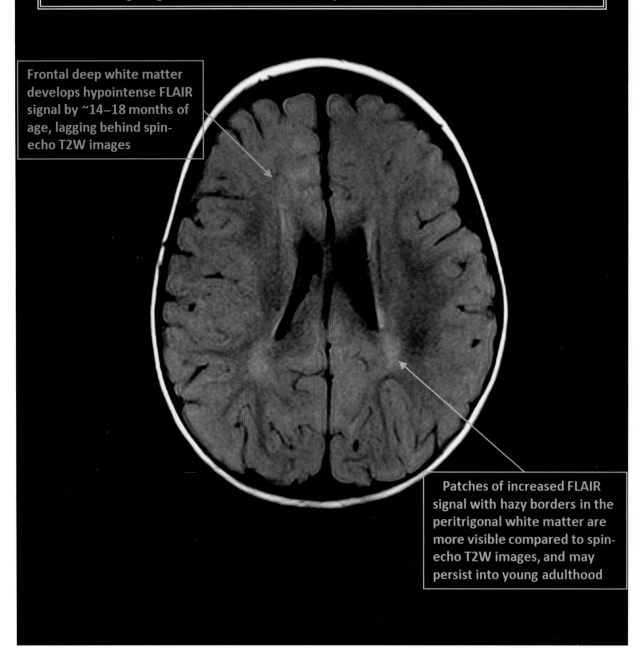

Frontal deep white matter develops hypointense FLAIR signal by ~14–18 months of age, lagging behind spin-echo T2W images

Patches of increased FLAIR signal with hazy borders in the peritrigonal white matter are more visible compared to spin-echo T2W images, and may persist into young adulthood

On FLAIR images beyond the neonatal period, the conversion of deep and subcortical white matter from hyperintensity to hypointensity relative to cortex generally follows the same pattern as on spin-echo T2W images, but occurs more slowly. The mild delay is probably due to the T1 weighting inherent in the FLAIR technique.

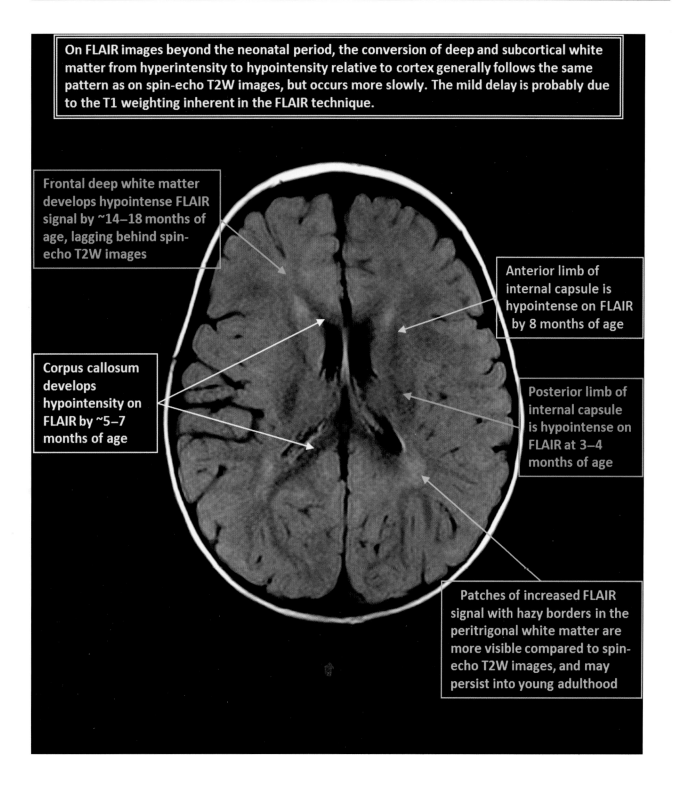

Frontal deep white matter develops hypointense FLAIR signal by ~14–18 months of age, lagging behind spin-echo T2W images

Corpus callosum develops hypointensity on FLAIR by ~5–7 months of age

Anterior limb of internal capsule is hypointense on FLAIR by 8 months of age

Posterior limb of internal capsule is hypointense on FLAIR at 3–4 months of age

Patches of increased FLAIR signal with hazy borders in the peritrigonal white matter are more visible compared to spin-echo T2W images, and may persist into young adulthood

On FLAIR images beyond the neonatal period, the conversion of deep and subcortical white matter from hyperintensity to hypointensity relative to cortex generally follows the same pattern as on spin-echo T2W images, but occurs more slowly. The mild delay is probably due to the T1 weighting inherent in the FLAIR technique.

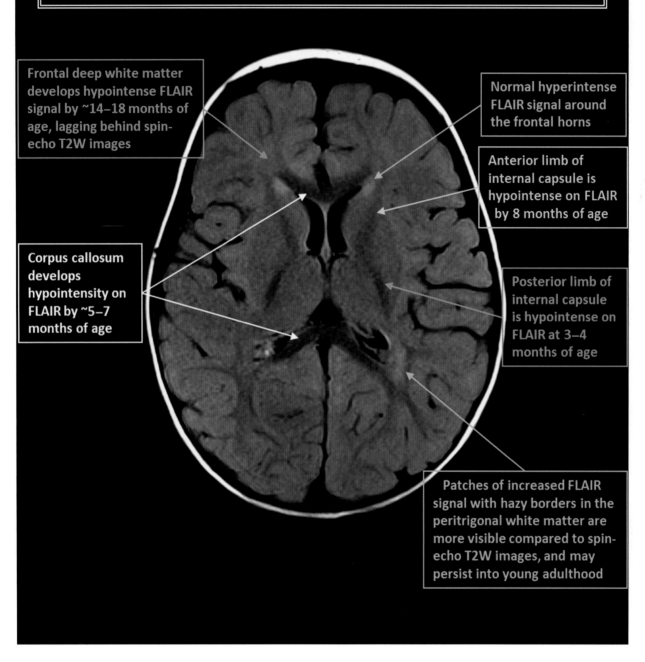

Frontal deep white matter develops hypointense FLAIR signal by ~14–18 months of age, lagging behind spin-echo T2W images

Corpus callosum develops hypointensity on FLAIR by ~5–7 months of age

Normal hyperintense FLAIR signal around the frontal horns

Anterior limb of internal capsule is hypointense on FLAIR by 8 months of age

Posterior limb of internal capsule is hypointense on FLAIR at 3–4 months of age

Patches of increased FLAIR signal with hazy borders in the peritrigonal white matter are more visible compared to spin-echo T2W images, and may persist into young adulthood

On FLAIR images beyond the neonatal period, the conversion of deep and subcortical white matter from hyperintensity to hypointensity relative to cortex generally follows the same pattern as on spin-echo T2W images, but occurs more slowly. The mild delay is probably due to the T1 weighting inherent in the FLAIR technique.

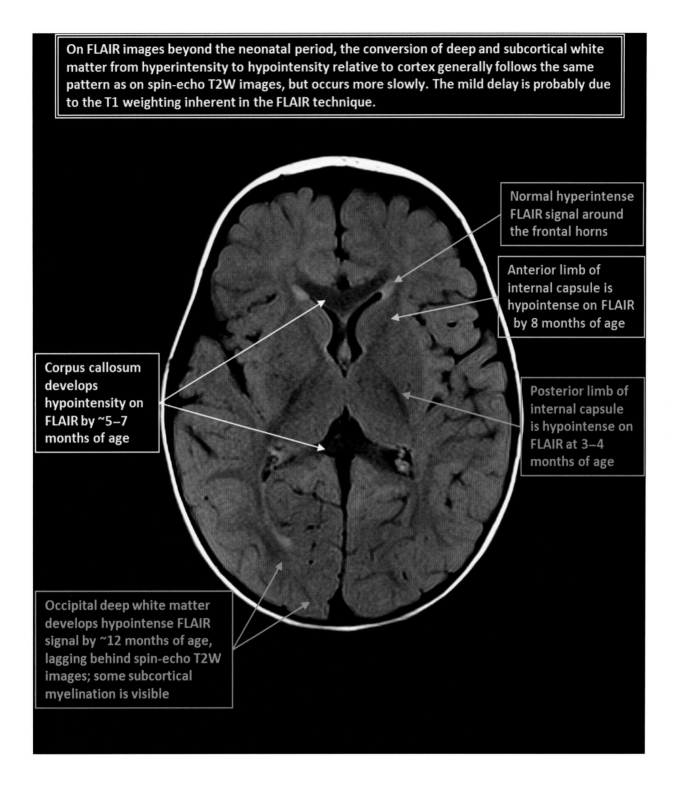

Normal hyperintense FLAIR signal around the frontal horns

Anterior limb of internal capsule is hypointense on FLAIR by 8 months of age

Corpus callosum develops hypointensity on FLAIR by ~5–7 months of age

Posterior limb of internal capsule is hypointense on FLAIR at 3–4 months of age

Occipital deep white matter develops hypointense FLAIR signal by ~12 months of age, lagging behind spin-echo T2W images; some subcortical myelination is visible

On FLAIR images beyond the neonatal period, the conversion of deep and subcortical white matter from hyperintensity to hypointensity relative to cortex generally follows the same pattern as on spin-echo T2W images, but occurs more slowly. The mild delay is probably due to the T1 weighting inherent in the FLAIR technique.

Normal hyperintense FLAIR signal around the frontal horns

Anterior limb of internal capsule is hypointense on FLAIR by 8 months of age

Posterior limb of internal capsule is hypointense on FLAIR at 3–4 months of age

Occipital deep white matter develops hypointense FLAIR signal by ~12 months of age, lagging behind spin-echo T2W images; some subcortical myelination is visible

Normal hyperintense FLAIR signal around the occipital horns is more visible than on spin-echo T2W images

On FLAIR images beyond the neonatal period, the conversion of deep and subcortical white matter from hyperintensity to hypointensity relative to cortex generally follows the same pattern as on spin-echo T2W images, but occurs more slowly. The mild delay is probably due to the T1 weighting inherent in the FLAIR technique.

Anterior temporal white matter is not yet hypointense on FLAIR

Occipital deep white matter develops hypointense FLAIR signal by ~12 months of age, lagging behind spin-echo T2W images; some subcortical myelination is visible

Normal hyperintense FLAIR signal around the occipital horns is more visible than on spin-echo T2W images

On FLAIR images beyond the neonatal period, the conversion of deep and subcortical white matter from hyperintensity to hypointensity relative to cortex generally follows the same pattern as on spin-echo T2W images, but occurs more slowly. The mild delay is probably due to the T1 weighting inherent in the FLAIR technique.

Anterior temporal white matter is not yet hypointense on FLAIR

On FLAIR images beyond the neonatal period, the conversion of deep and subcortical white matter from hyperintensity to hypointensity relative to cortex generally follows the same pattern as on spin-echo T2W images, but occurs more slowly. The mild delay is probably due to the T1 weighting inherent in the FLAIR technique.

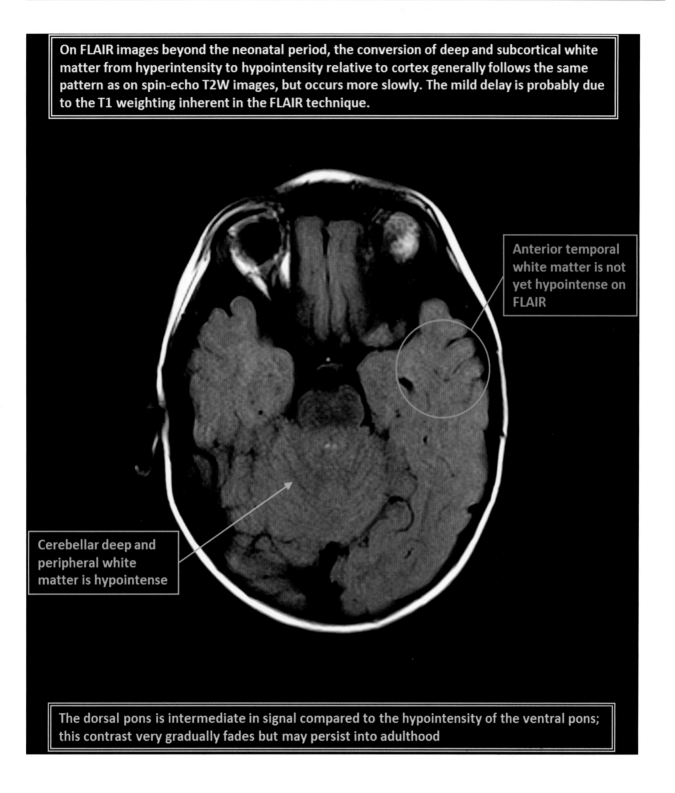

Anterior temporal white matter is not yet hypointense on FLAIR

Cerebellar deep and peripheral white matter is hypointense

The dorsal pons is intermediate in signal compared to the hypointensity of the ventral pons; this contrast very gradually fades but may persist into adulthood

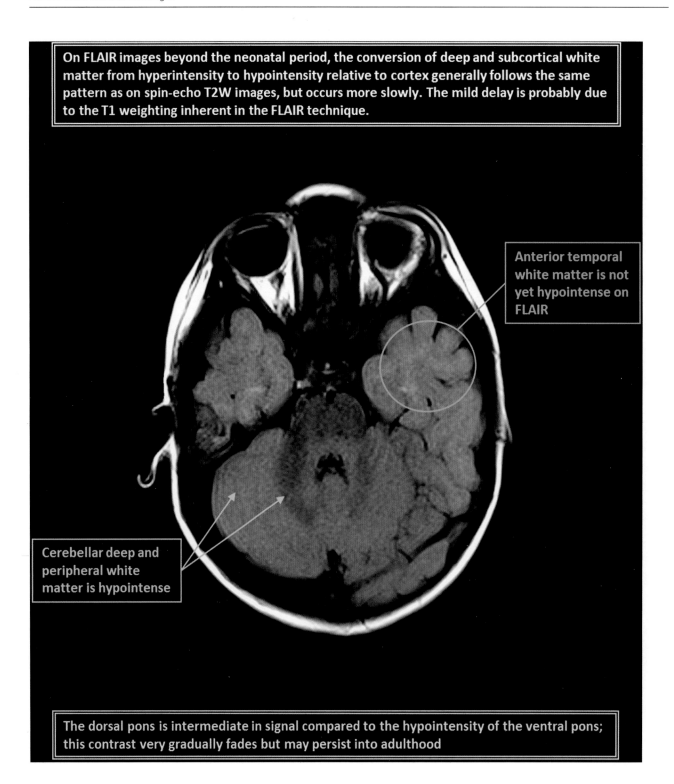

On FLAIR images beyond the neonatal period, the conversion of deep and subcortical white matter from hyperintensity to hypointensity relative to cortex generally follows the same pattern as on spin-echo T2W images, but occurs more slowly. The mild delay is probably due to the T1 weighting inherent in the FLAIR technique.

Anterior temporal white matter is not yet hypointense on FLAIR

Cerebellar deep and peripheral white matter is hypointense

The dorsal pons is intermediate in signal compared to the hypointensity of the ventral pons; this contrast very gradually fades but may persist into adulthood

On FLAIR images beyond the neonatal period, the conversion of deep and subcortical white matter from hyperintensity to hypointensity relative to cortex generally follows the same pattern as on spin-echo T2W images, but occurs more slowly. The mild delay is probably due to the T1 weighting inherent in the FLAIR technique.

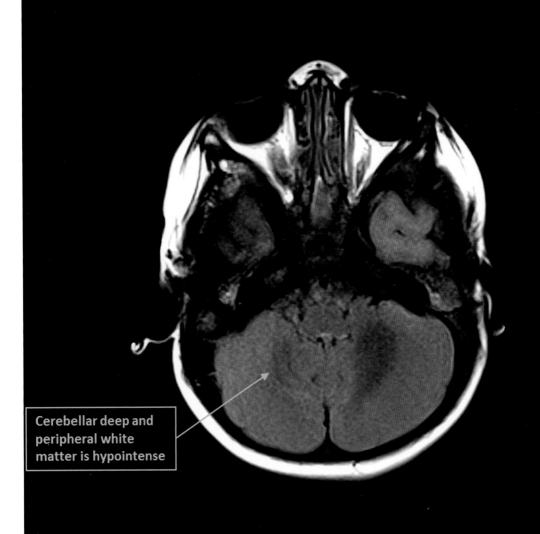

Cerebellar deep and peripheral white matter is hypointense

The dorsal pons is intermediate in signal compared to the hypointensity of the ventral pons; this contrast very gradually fades but may persist into adulthood

1 Year, Diffusion Weighted Imaging (DWI) (b=1000 s/mm²)

> **Cerebral white matter , including the subcortical regions, is hypointense to cortex on DWI after ~9 months of age and remains so into adulthood**

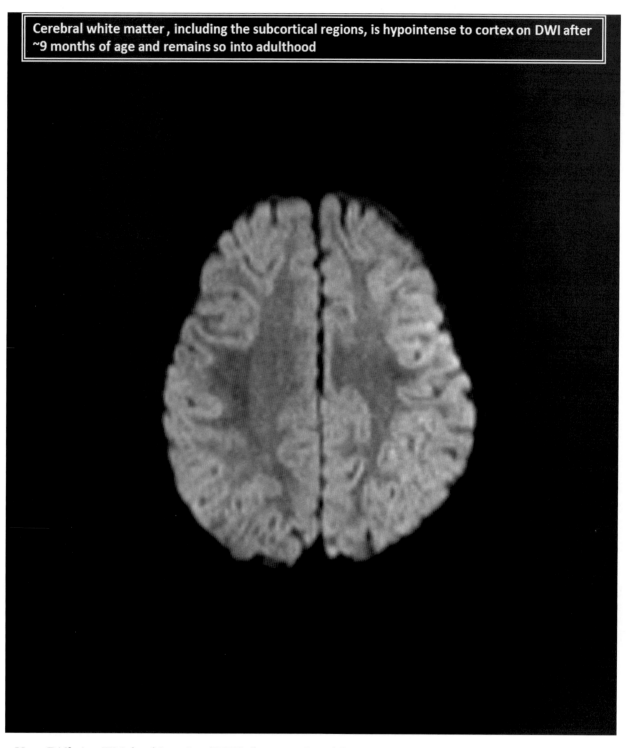

1 Year, Diffusion Weighted Imaging (DWI) (b=1000 s/mm²) Images 1–5

Cerebral white matter , including the subcortical regions, is hypointense to cortex on DWI after ~9 months of age and remains so into adulthood

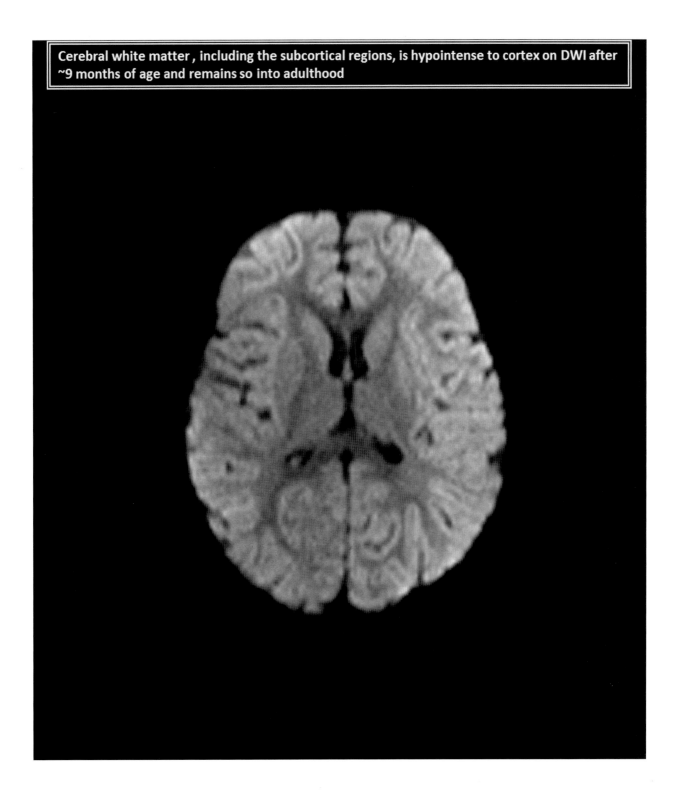

Cerebral white matter , including the subcortical regions, is hypointense to cortex on DWI after ~9 months of age and remains so into adulthood

For most of the first year of life, the cerebellum as a whole can have a noticeably more hypointense appearance on ADC than the cerebral hemispheres, while on DWI it is isointense to subtly hyperintense to the cerebrum

For most of the first year of life, the cerebellum as a whole can have a noticeably more hypointense appearance on ADC than the cerebral hemispheres, while on DWI it is isointense to subtly hyperintense to the cerebrum

1 Year, Apparent Diffusion Coefficient (ADC) Map

Cerebral gray matter and white matter are close to isointensity on ADC images by ~1 year of age, except for mild residual hyperintensity in the peritrigonal regions and some subcortical white matter

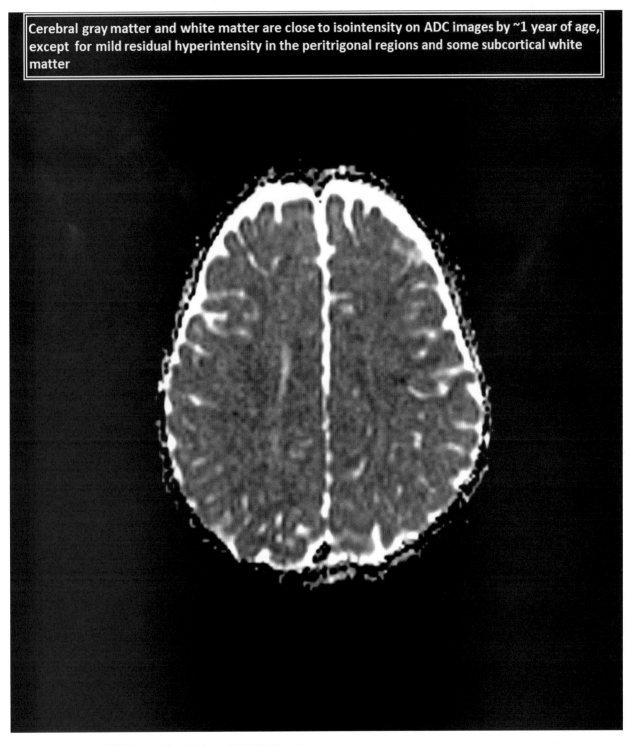

1 Year, Apparent Diffusion Coefficient (ADC) Map Images 1–5

Cerebral gray matter and white matter are close to isointensity on ADC images by ~1 year of age, except for mild residual hyperintensity in the peritrigonal regions and some subcortical white matter

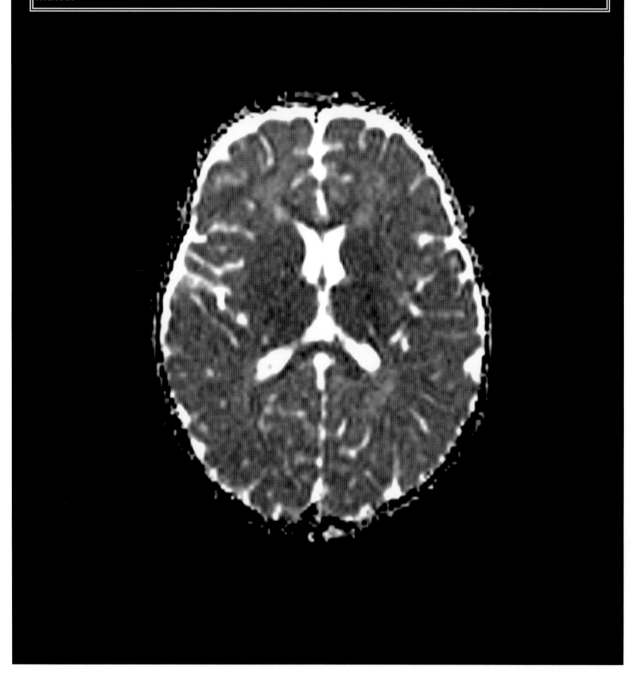

Cerebral gray matter and white matter are close to isointensity on ADC images by ~1 year of age, except for mild residual hyperintensity in the peritrigonal regions and some subcortical white matter

For most of the first year of life, the cerebellum as a whole can have a noticeably more hypointense appearance on ADC than the cerebral hemispheres, while on DWI it is isointense to subtly hyperintense to the cerebrum

For most of the first year of life, the cerebellum as a whole can have a noticeably more hypointense appearance on ADC than the cerebral hemispheres, while on DWI it is isointense to subtly hyperintense to the cerebrum

1 Year, Sagittal T1

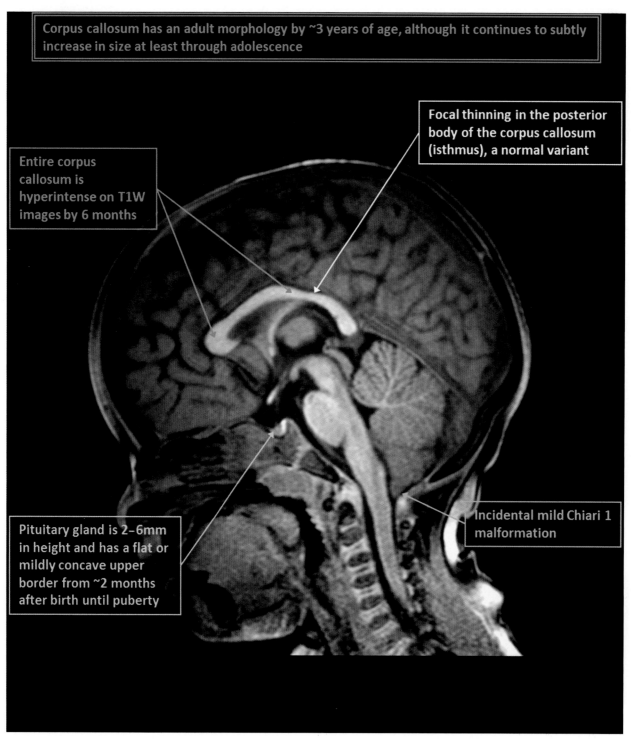

Corpus callosum has an adult morphology by ~3 years of age, although it continues to subtly increase in size at least through adolescence

Focal thinning in the posterior body of the corpus callosum (isthmus), a normal variant

Entire corpus callosum is hyperintense on T1W images by 6 months

Pituitary gland is 2–6mm in height and has a flat or mildly concave upper border from ~2 months after birth until puberty

Incidental mild Chiari 1 malformation

1 Year, Sagittal T1 Images 1–4

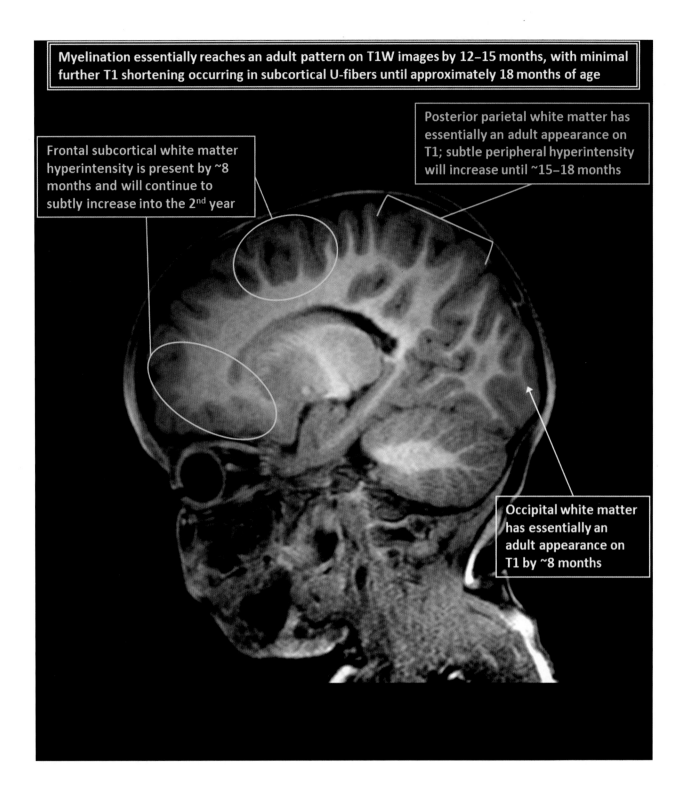

Myelination essentially reaches an adult pattern on T1W images by 12–15 months, with minimal further T1 shortening occurring in subcortical U-fibers until approximately 18 months of age

Frontal subcortical white matter hyperintensity is present by ~8 months and will continue to subtly increase into the 2nd year

Posterior parietal white matter has essentially an adult appearance on T1; subtle peripheral hyperintensity will increase until ~15–18 months

Occipital white matter has essentially an adult appearance on T1 by ~8 months

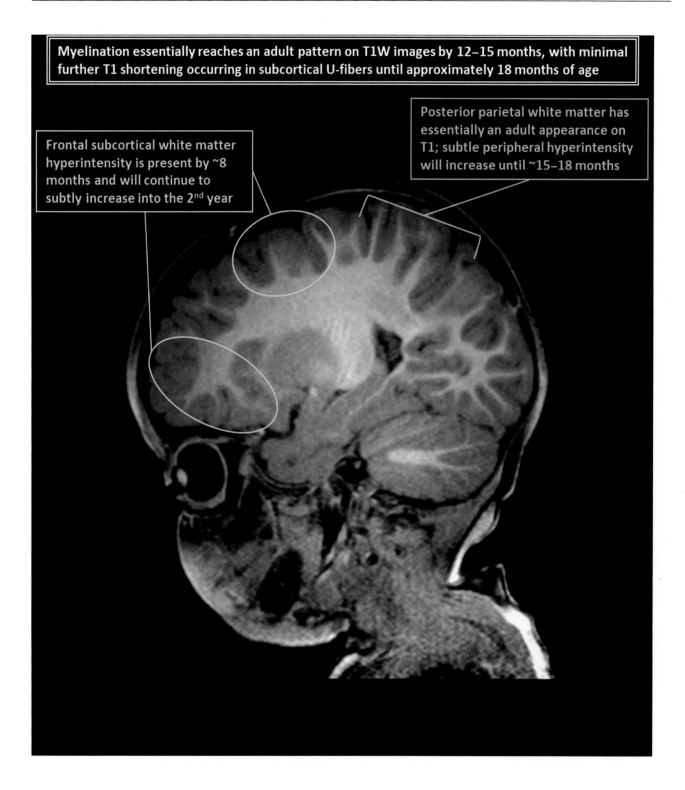

Myelination essentially reaches an adult pattern on T1W images by 12–15 months, with minimal further T1 shortening occurring in subcortical U-fibers until approximately 18 months of age

Posterior parietal white matter has essentially an adult appearance on T1; subtle peripheral hyperintensity will increase until ~15–18 months

Frontal subcortical white matter hyperintensity is present by ~8 months and will continue to subtly increase into the 2nd year

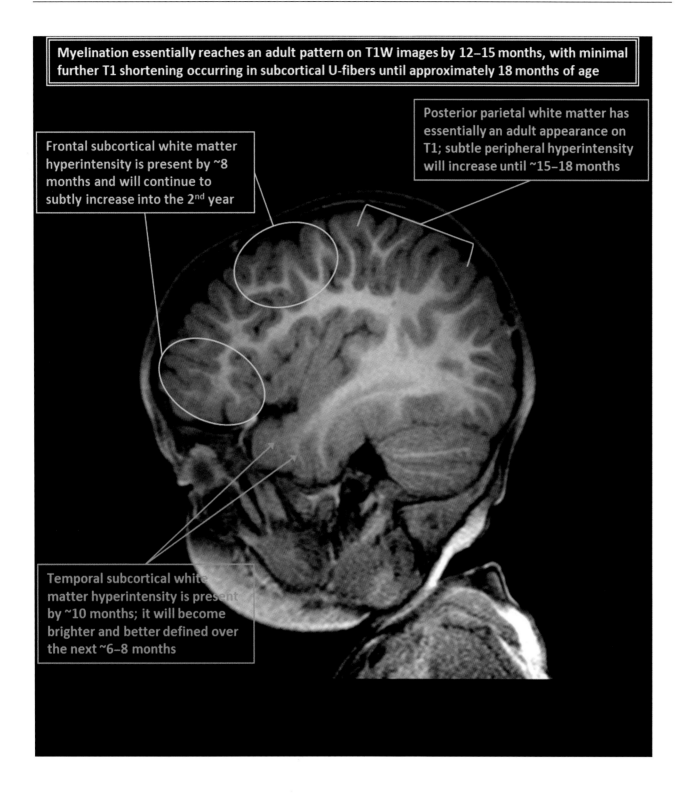

Myelination essentially reaches an adult pattern on T1W images by 12–15 months, with minimal further T1 shortening occurring in subcortical U-fibers until approximately 18 months of age

Frontal subcortical white matter hyperintensity is present by ~8 months and will continue to subtly increase into the 2nd year

Posterior parietal white matter has essentially an adult appearance on T1; subtle peripheral hyperintensity will increase until ~15–18 months

Temporal subcortical white matter hyperintensity is present by ~10 months; it will become brighter and better defined over the next ~6–8 months

1 Year, Coronal TSE T2

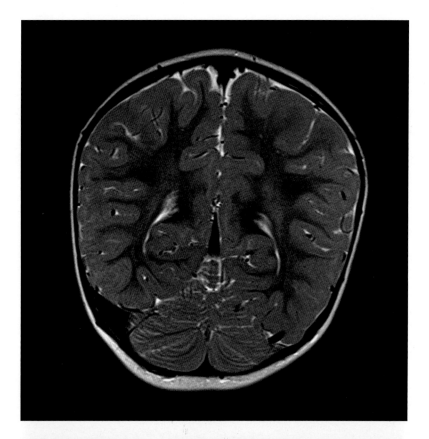

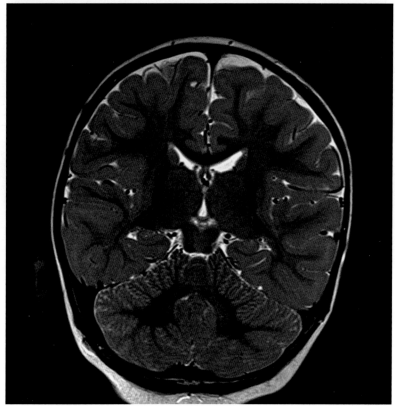

1 Year, Coronal TSE T2 Images 1–4

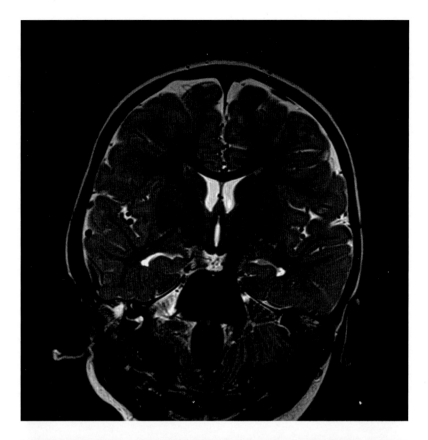

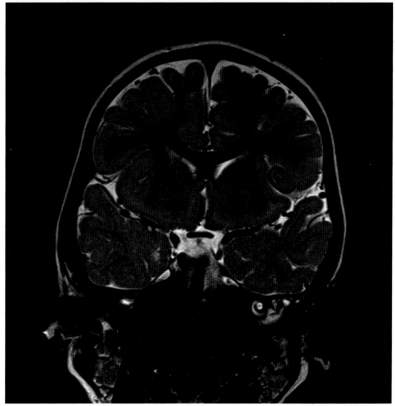

1 Year 6 Months, Axial TSE T2

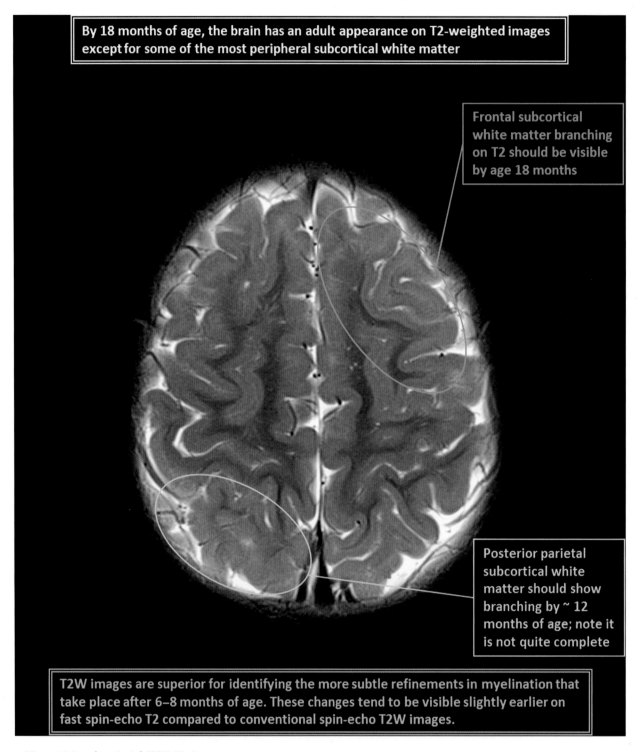

By 18 months of age, the brain has an adult appearance on T2-weighted images except for some of the most peripheral subcortical white matter

Frontal subcortical white matter branching on T2 should be visible by age 18 months

Posterior parietal subcortical white matter should show branching by ~ 12 months of age; note it is not quite complete

T2W images are superior for identifying the more subtle refinements in myelination that take place after 6–8 months of age. These changes tend to be visible slightly earlier on fast spin-echo T2 compared to conventional spin-echo T2W images.

1 Year 6 Months, Axial TSE T2 Images 1–10

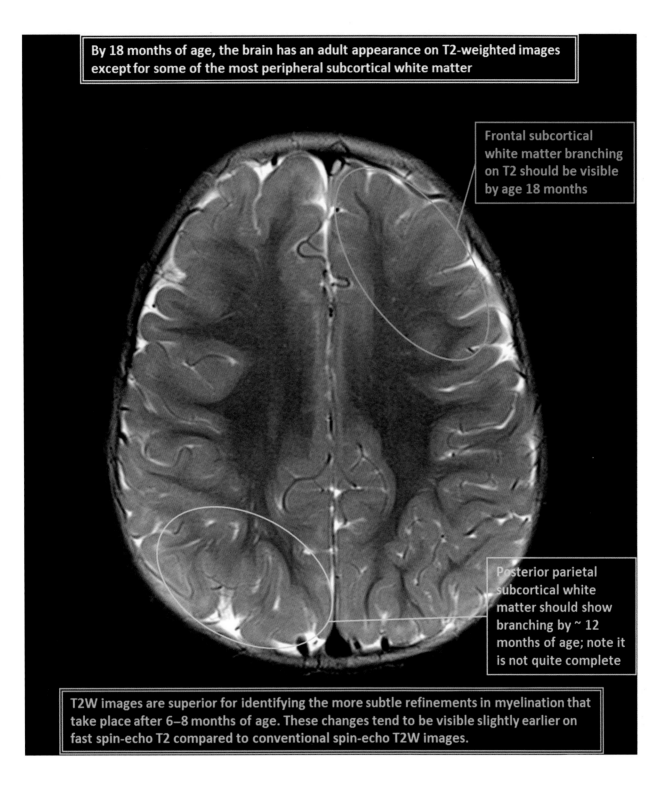

By 18 months of age, the brain has an adult appearance on T2-weighted images except for some of the most peripheral subcortical white matter

Frontal subcortical white matter branching on T2 should be visible by age 18 months

Posterior parietal subcortical white matter should show branching by ~ 12 months of age; note it is not quite complete

T2W images are superior for identifying the more subtle refinements in myelination that take place after 6–8 months of age. These changes tend to be visible slightly earlier on fast spin-echo T2 compared to conventional spin-echo T2W images.

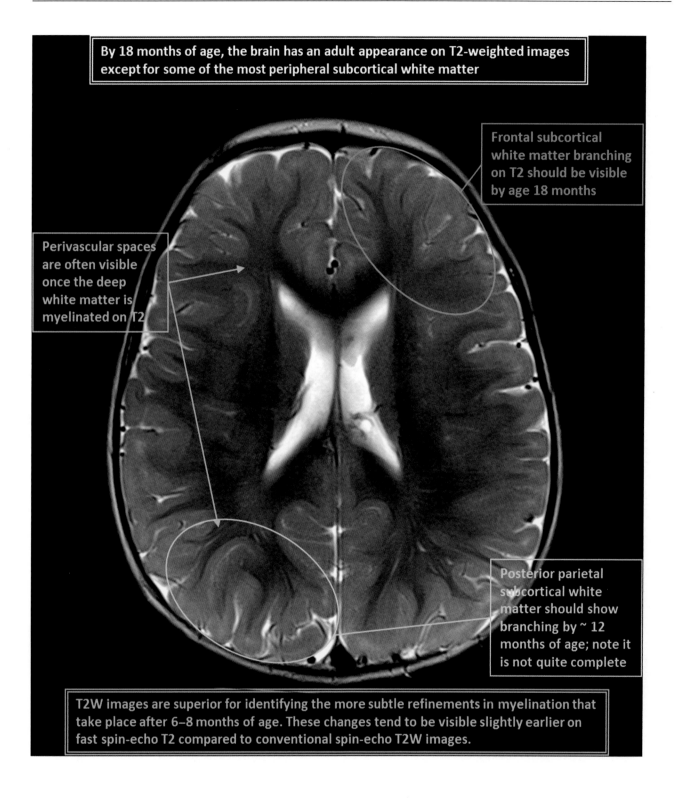

By 18 months of age, the brain has an adult appearance on T2-weighted images except for some of the most peripheral subcortical white matter

Frontal subcortical white matter branching on T2 should be visible by age 18 months

Perivascular spaces are often visible once the deep white matter is myelinated on T2

Posterior parietal subcortical white matter should show branching by ~ 12 months of age; note it is not quite complete

T2W images are superior for identifying the more subtle refinements in myelination that take place after 6–8 months of age. These changes tend to be visible slightly earlier on fast spin-echo T2 compared to conventional spin-echo T2W images.

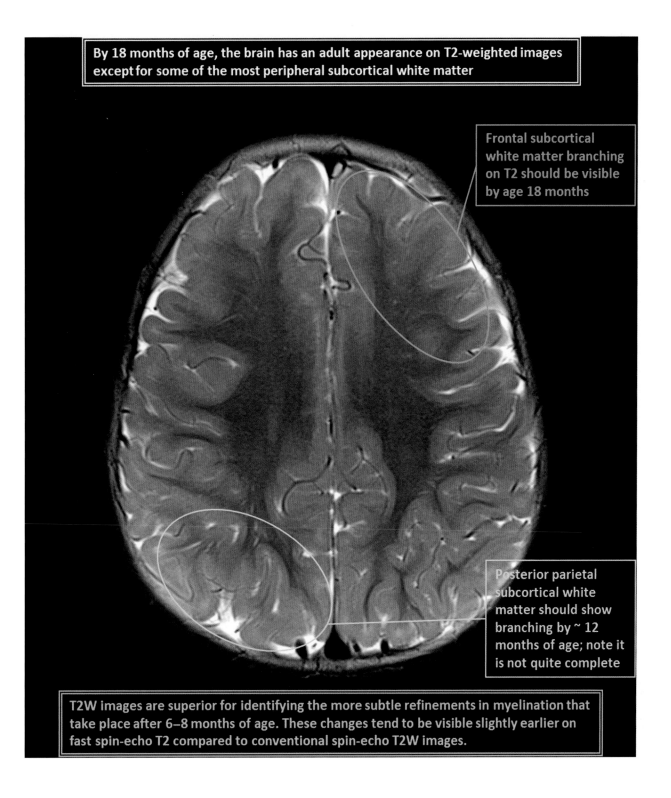

By 18 months of age, the brain has an adult appearance on T2-weighted images except for some of the most peripheral subcortical white matter

Frontal subcortical white matter branching on T2 should be visible by age 18 months

Posterior parietal subcortical white matter should show branching by ~ 12 months of age; note it is not quite complete

T2W images are superior for identifying the more subtle refinements in myelination that take place after 6–8 months of age. These changes tend to be visible slightly earlier on fast spin-echo T2 compared to conventional spin-echo T2W images.

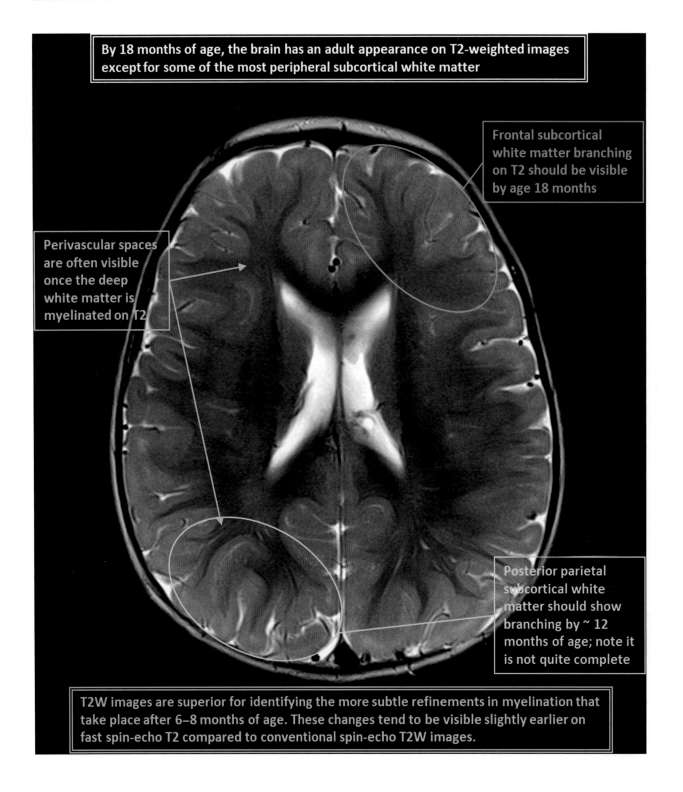

By 18 months of age, the brain has an adult appearance on T2-weighted images except for some of the most peripheral subcortical white matter

Frontal subcortical white matter branching on T2 should be visible by age 18 months

Perivascular spaces are often visible once the deep white matter is myelinated on T2

Posterior parietal subcortical white matter should show branching by ~ 12 months of age; note it is not quite complete

T2W images are superior for identifying the more subtle refinements in myelination that take place after 6–8 months of age. These changes tend to be visible slightly earlier on fast spin-echo T2 compared to conventional spin-echo T2W images.

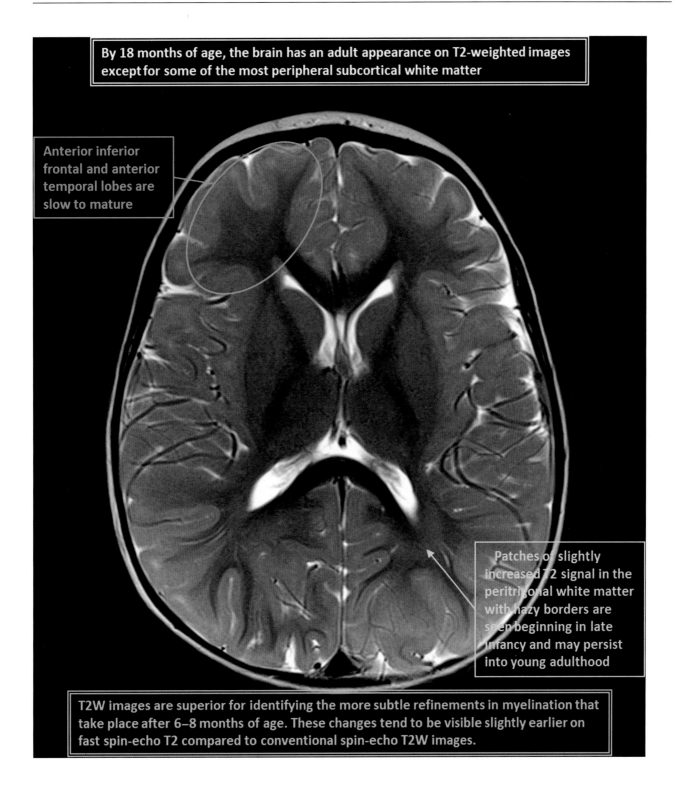

By 18 months of age, the brain has an adult appearance on T2-weighted images except for some of the most peripheral subcortical white matter

Anterior inferior frontal and anterior temporal lobes are slow to mature

Patches of slightly increased T2 signal in the peritrigonal white matter with hazy borders are seen beginning in late infancy and may persist into young adulthood

T2W images are superior for identifying the more subtle refinements in myelination that take place after 6–8 months of age. These changes tend to be visible slightly earlier on fast spin-echo T2 compared to conventional spin-echo T2W images.

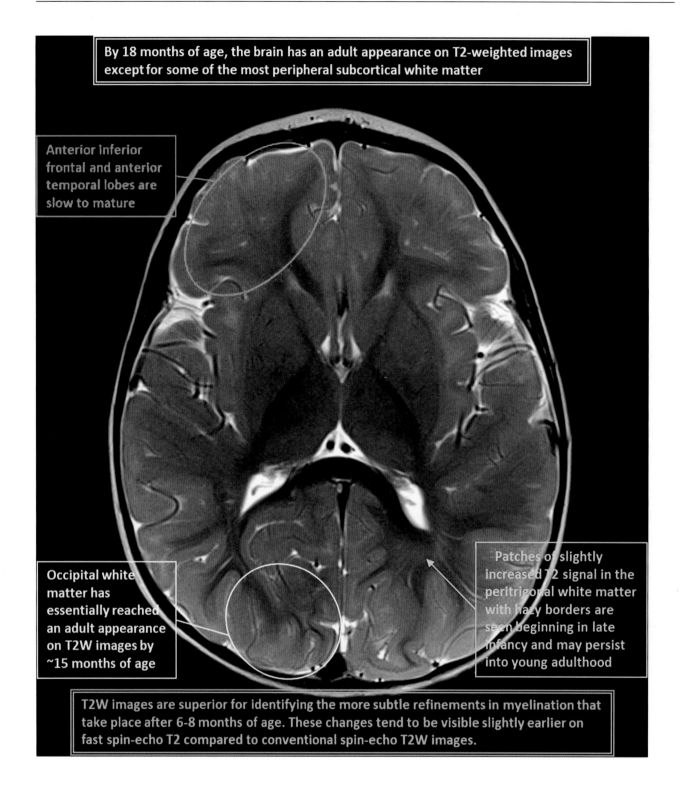

By 18 months of age, the brain has an adult appearance on T2-weighted images except for some of the most peripheral subcortical white matter

Anterior Inferior frontal and anterior temporal lobes are slow to mature

Occipital white matter has essentially reached an adult appearance on T2W images by ~15 months of age

Patches of slightly increased T2 signal in the peritrigonal white matter with hazy borders are seen beginning in late infancy and may persist into young adulthood

T2W images are superior for identifying the more subtle refinements in myelination that take place after 6-8 months of age. These changes tend to be visible slightly earlier on fast spin-echo T2 compared to conventional spin-echo T2W images.

By 18 months of age, the brain has an adult appearance on T2-weighted images except for some of the most peripheral subcortical white matter

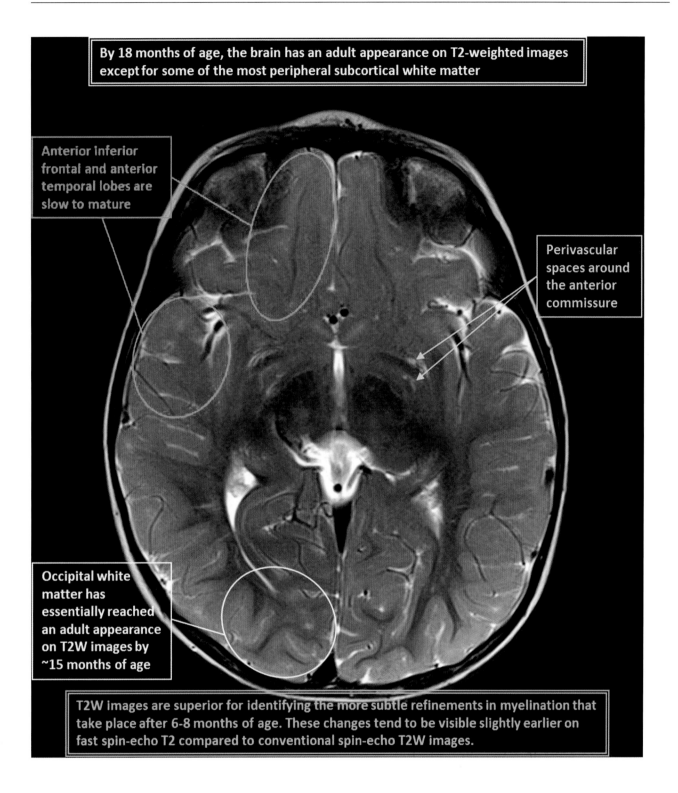

Anterior Inferior frontal and anterior temporal lobes are slow to mature

Perivascular spaces around the anterior commissure

Occipital white matter has essentially reached an adult appearance on T2W images by ~15 months of age

T2W images are superior for identifying the more subtle refinements in myelination that take place after 6-8 months of age. These changes tend to be visible slightly earlier on fast spin-echo T2 compared to conventional spin-echo T2W images.

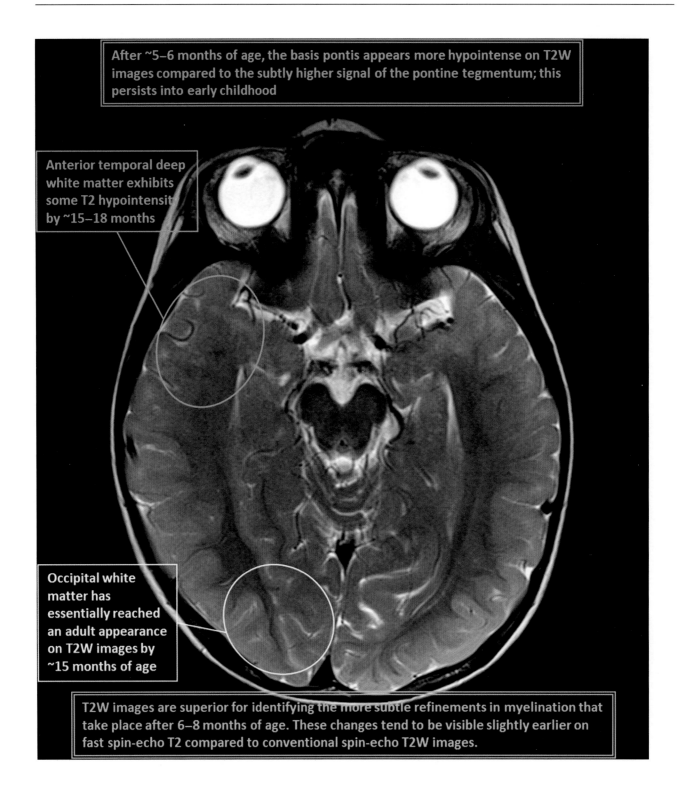

After ~5–6 months of age, the basis pontis appears more hypointense on T2W images compared to the subtly higher signal of the pontine tegmentum; this persists into early childhood

Anterior temporal deep white matter exhibits some T2 hypointensity by ~15–18 months

Occipital white matter has essentially reached an adult appearance on T2W images by ~15 months of age

T2W images are superior for identifying the more subtle refinements in myelination that take place after 6–8 months of age. These changes tend to be visible slightly earlier on fast spin-echo T2 compared to conventional spin-echo T2W images.

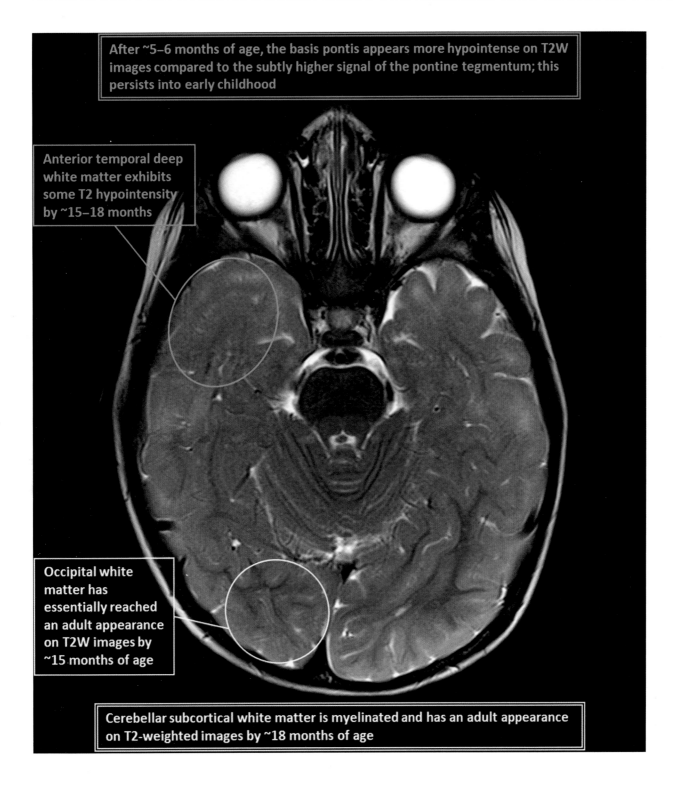

After ~5–6 months of age, the basis pontis appears more hypointense on T2W images compared to the subtly higher signal of the pontine tegmentum; this persists into early childhood

Anterior temporal deep white matter exhibits some T2 hypointensity by ~15–18 months

Occipital white matter has essentially reached an adult appearance on T2W images by ~15 months of age

Cerebellar subcortical white matter is myelinated and has an adult appearance on T2-weighted images by ~18 months of age

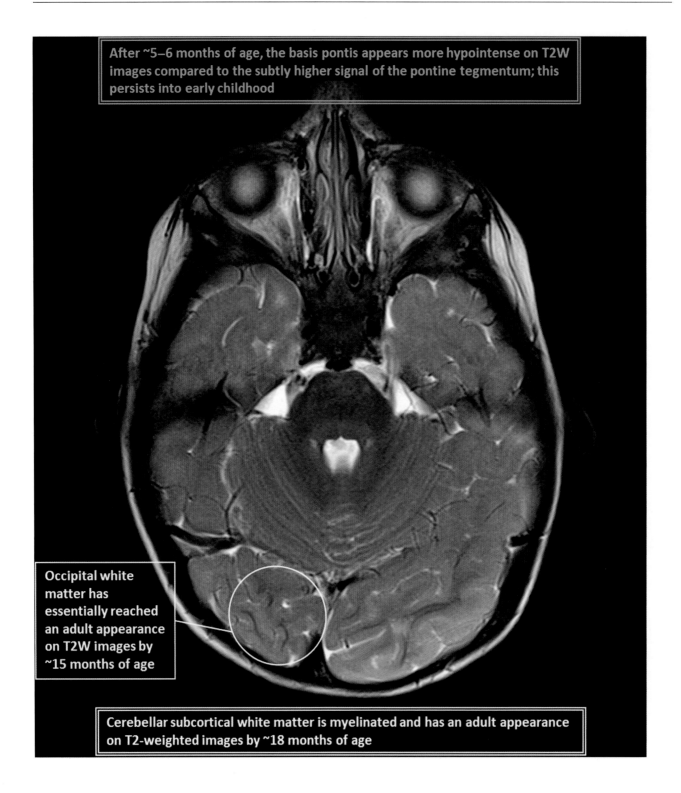

After ~5–6 months of age, the basis pontis appears more hypointense on T2W images compared to the subtly higher signal of the pontine tegmentum; this persists into early childhood

Occipital white matter has essentially reached an adult appearance on T2W images by ~15 months of age

Cerebellar subcortical white matter is myelinated and has an adult appearance on T2-weighted images by ~18 months of age

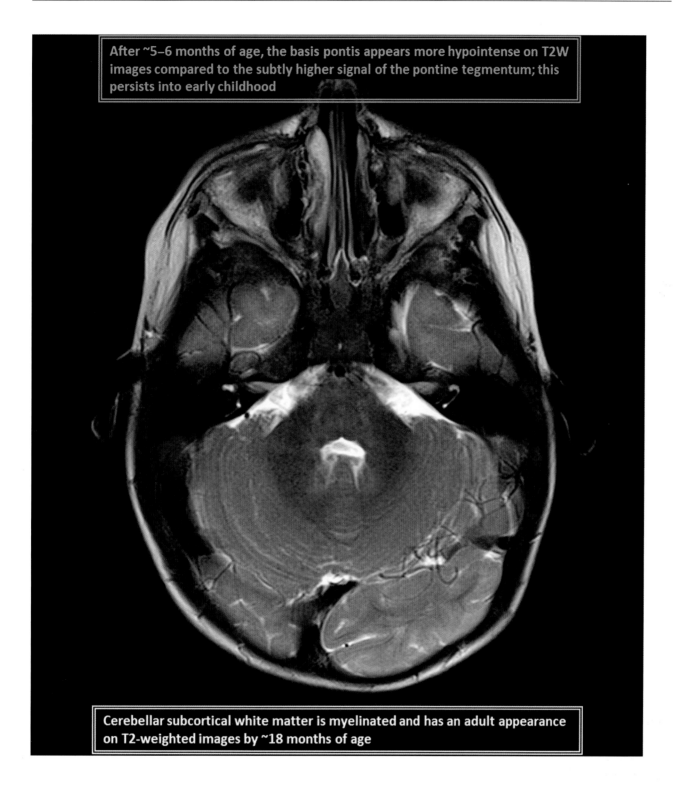

After ~5–6 months of age, the basis pontis appears more hypointense on T2W images compared to the subtly higher signal of the pontine tegmentum; this persists into early childhood

Cerebellar subcortical white matter is myelinated and has an adult appearance on T2-weighted images by ~18 months of age

1 Year 6 Months, Axial FLAIR

On FLAIR images beyond the neonatal period, the conversion of deep and subcortical white matter from hyperintensity to hypointensity relative to cortex generally follows the same pattern as on spin-echo T2W images, but occurs more slowly. The mild delay is probably due to the T1 weighting inherent in the FLAIR technique.

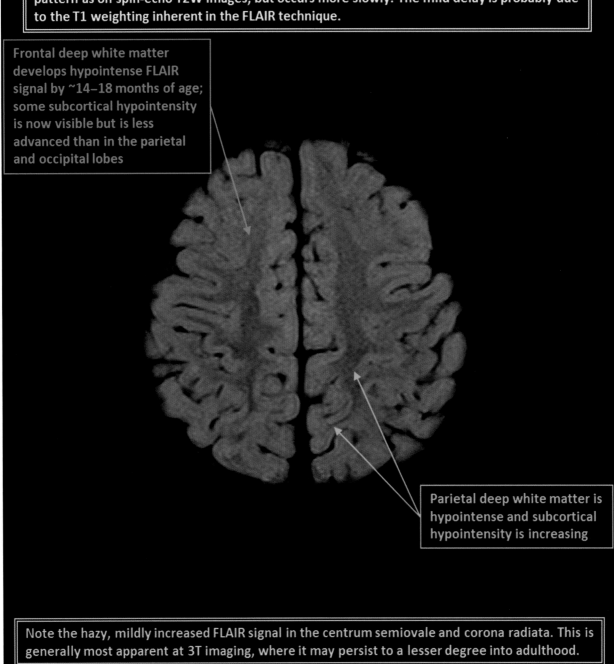

Frontal deep white matter develops hypointense FLAIR signal by ~14–18 months of age; some subcortical hypointensity is now visible but is less advanced than in the parietal and occipital lobes

Parietal deep white matter is hypointense and subcortical hypointensity is increasing

Note the hazy, mildly increased FLAIR signal in the centrum semiovale and corona radiata. This is generally most apparent at 3T imaging, where it may persist to a lesser degree into adulthood.

1 Year 6 Months, Axial FLAIR Images 1–10

On FLAIR images beyond the neonatal period, the conversion of deep and subcortical white matter from hyperintensity to hypointensity relative to cortex generally follows the same pattern as on spin-echo T2W images, but occurs more slowly. The mild delay is probably due to the T1 weighting inherent in the FLAIR technique.

Frontal deep white matter develops hypointense FLAIR signal by ~14–18 months of age; some subcortical hypointensity is now visible but is less advanced than in the parietal and occipital lobes

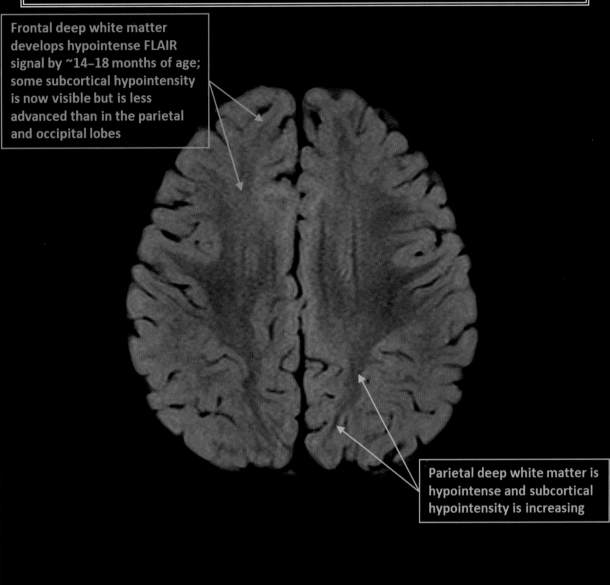

Parietal deep white matter is hypointense and subcortical hypointensity is increasing

Note the hazy, mildly increased FLAIR signal in the centrum semiovale and corona radiata. This is generally most apparent at 3T imaging, where it may persist to a lesser degree into adulthood.

On FLAIR images beyond the neonatal period, the conversion of deep and subcortical white matter from hyperintensity to hypointensity relative to cortex generally follows the same pattern as on spin-echo T2W images, but occurs more slowly. The mild delay is probably due to the T1 weighting inherent in the FLAIR technique.

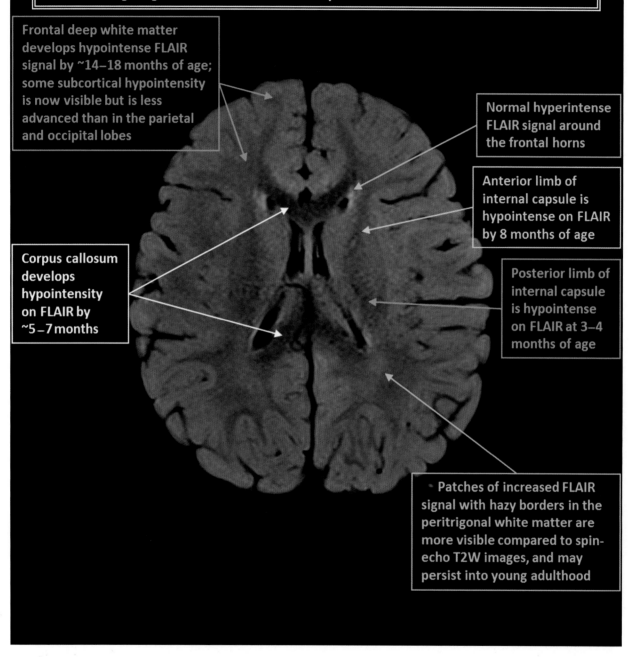

Frontal deep white matter develops hypointense FLAIR signal by ~14–18 months of age; some subcortical hypointensity is now visible but is less advanced than in the parietal and occipital lobes

Normal hyperintense FLAIR signal around the frontal horns

Anterior limb of internal capsule is hypointense on FLAIR by 8 months of age

Corpus callosum develops hypointensity on FLAIR by ~5–7 months

Posterior limb of internal capsule is hypointense on FLAIR at 3–4 months of age

Patches of increased FLAIR signal with hazy borders in the peritrigonal white matter are more visible compared to spin-echo T2W images, and may persist into young adulthood

On FLAIR images beyond the neonatal period, the conversion of deep and subcortical white matter from hyperintensity to hypointensity relative to cortex generally follows the same pattern as on spin-echo T2W images, but occurs more slowly. The mild delay is probably due to the T1 weighting inherent in the FLAIR technique.

Frontal deep white matter develops hypointense FLAIR signal by ~14–18 months of age; some subcortical hypointensity is now visible but is less advanced than in the parietal and occipital lobes

Normal hyperintense FLAIR signal around the frontal horns

Anterior limb of internal capsule is hypointense on FLAIR by 8 months of age

Corpus callosum develops hypointensity on FLAIR by ~5–7 months

Posterior limb of internal capsule is hypointense on FLAIR at 3–4 months of age

Patches of increased FLAIR signal with hazy borders in the peritrigonal white matter are more visible compared to spin-echo T2W images, and may persist into young adulthood

On FLAIR images beyond the neonatal period, the conversion of deep and subcortical white matter from hyperintensity to hypointensity relative to cortex generally follows the same pattern as on spin-echo T2W images, but occurs more slowly. The mild delay is probably due to the T1 weighting inherent in the FLAIR technique.

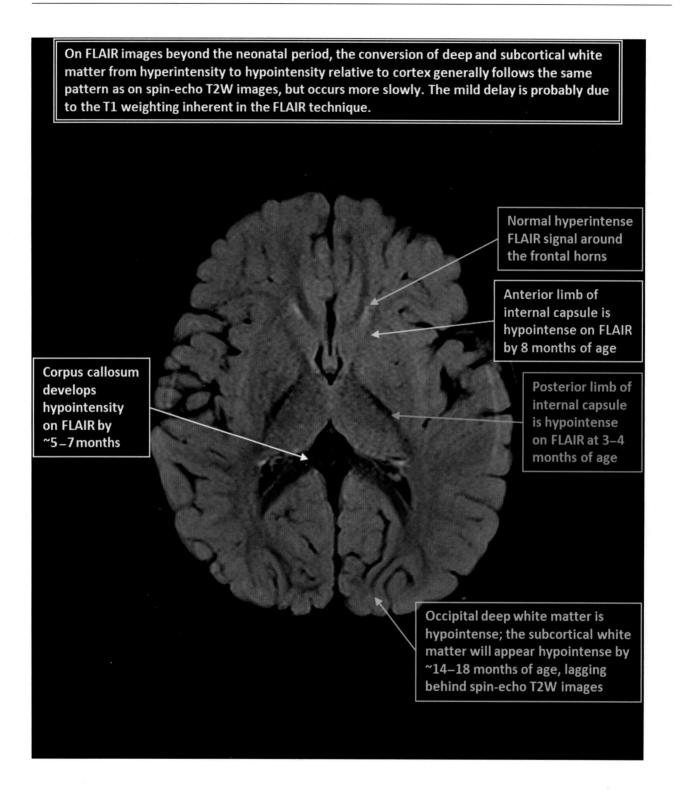

Normal hyperintense FLAIR signal around the frontal horns

Anterior limb of internal capsule is hypointense on FLAIR by 8 months of age

Corpus callosum develops hypointensity on FLAIR by ~5–7 months

Posterior limb of internal capsule is hypointense on FLAIR at 3–4 months of age

Occipital deep white matter is hypointense; the subcortical white matter will appear hypointense by ~14–18 months of age, lagging behind spin-echo T2W images

On FLAIR images beyond the neonatal period, the conversion of deep and subcortical white matter from hyperintensity to hypointensity relative to cortex generally follows the same pattern as on spin-echo T2W images, but occurs more slowly. The mild delay is probably due to the T1 weighting inherent in the FLAIR technique.

Occipital deep white matter is hypointense; the subcortical white matter will appear hypointense by ~14–18 months of age, lagging behind spin-echo T2W images

On FLAIR images beyond the neonatal period, the conversion of deep and subcortical white matter from hyperintensity to hypointensity relative to cortex generally follows the same pattern as on spin-echo T2W images, but occurs more slowly. The mild delay is probably due to the T1 weighting inherent in the FLAIR technique.

Anterior temporal white matter is starting to become hypointense on FLAIR

Normal hyperintense FLAIR signal around the occipital horns is more visible than on spin-echo T2W images

Occipital deep white matter is hypointense; the subcortical white matter will appear hypointense by ~14–18 months of age, lagging behind spin-echo T2W images

The dorsal pons is intermediate in signal compared to the hypointensity of the ventral pons; this contrast very gradually fades but may persist into adulthood

On FLAIR images beyond the neonatal period, the conversion of deep and subcortical white matter from hyperintensity to hypointensity relative to cortex generally follows the same pattern as on spin-echo T2W images, but occurs more slowly. The mild delay is probably due to the T1 weighting inherent in the FLAIR technique.

Anterior temporal white matter is starting to become hypointense on FLAIR

Normal hyperintense FLAIR signal around the occipital horns is more visible than on spin-echo T2W images

The dorsal pons is intermediate in signal compared to the hypointensity of the ventral pons; this contrast very gradually fades but may persist into adulthood

On FLAIR images beyond the neonatal period, the conversion of deep and subcortical white matter from hyperintensity to hypointensity relative to cortex generally follows the same pattern as on spin-echo T2W images, but occurs more slowly. The mild delay is probably due to the T1 weighting inherent in the FLAIR technique.

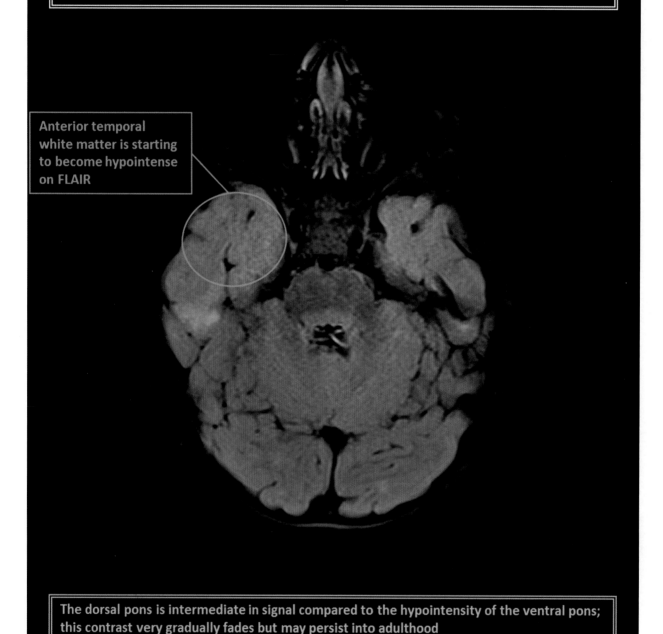

Anterior temporal white matter is starting to become hypointense on FLAIR

The dorsal pons is intermediate in signal compared to the hypointensity of the ventral pons; this contrast very gradually fades but may persist into adulthood

On FLAIR images beyond the neonatal period, the conversion of deep and subcortical white matter from hyperintensity to hypointensity relative to cortex generally follows the same pattern as on spin-echo T2W images, but occurs more slowly. The mild delay is probably due to the T1 weighting inherent in the FLAIR technique.

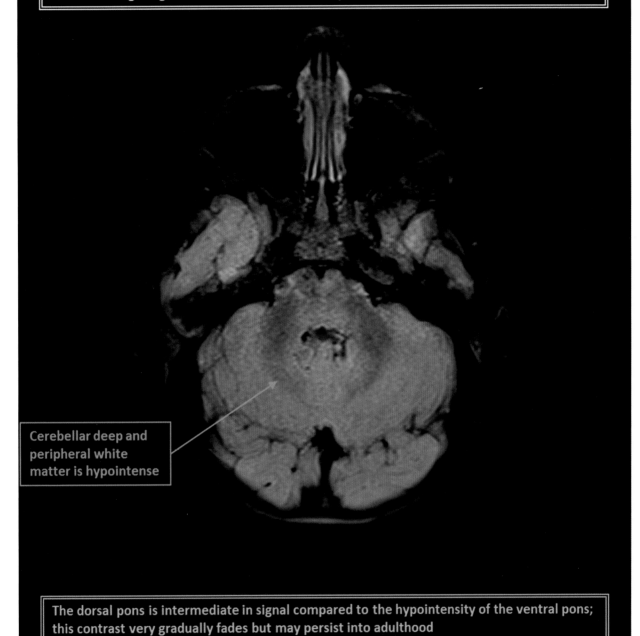

Cerebellar deep and peripheral white matter is hypointense

The dorsal pons is intermediate in signal compared to the hypointensity of the ventral pons; this contrast very gradually fades but may persist into adulthood

1 Year 6 Months, Coronal TSE T2

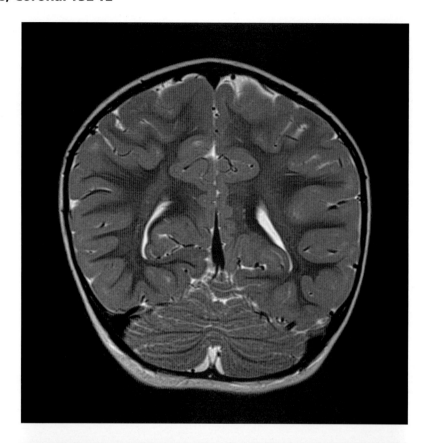

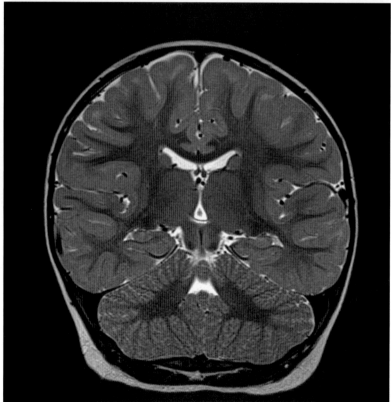

1 Year 6 Months, Coronal TSE T2 Images 1–4

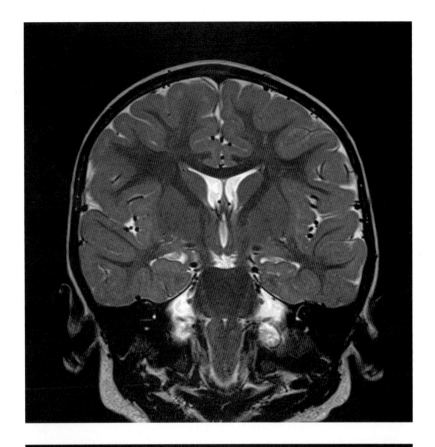

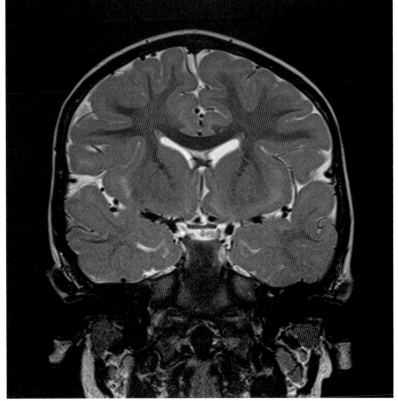

2 Years, Axial TSE T2

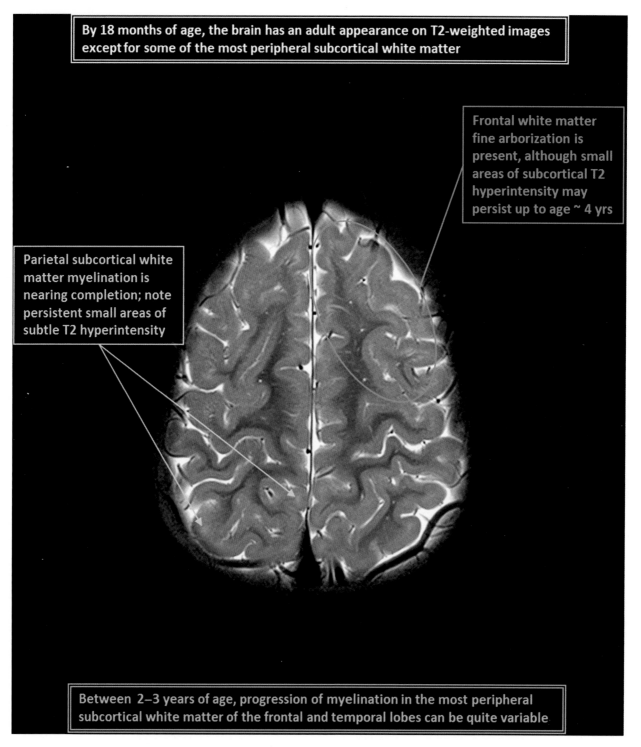

By 18 months of age, the brain has an adult appearance on T2-weighted images except for some of the most peripheral subcortical white matter

Frontal white matter fine arborization is present, although small areas of subcortical T2 hyperintensity may persist up to age ~ 4 yrs

Parietal subcortical white matter myelination is nearing completion; note persistent small areas of subtle T2 hyperintensity

Between 2–3 years of age, progression of myelination in the most peripheral subcortical white matter of the frontal and temporal lobes can be quite variable.

2 Years, Axial TSE T2 Images 1–10

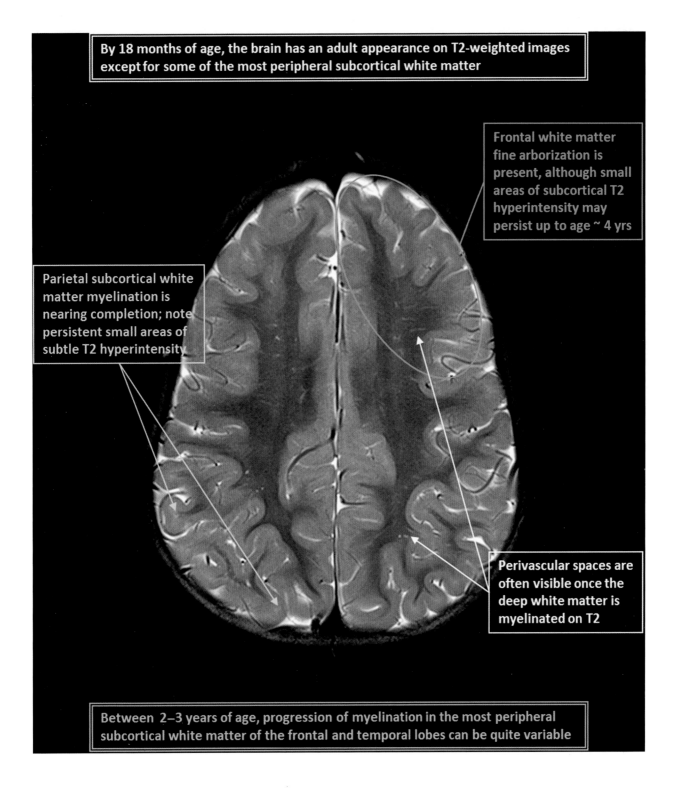

By 18 months of age, the brain has an adult appearance on T2-weighted images except for some of the most peripheral subcortical white matter

Frontal white matter fine arborization is present, although small areas of subcortical T2 hyperintensity may persist up to age ~ 4 yrs

Parietal subcortical white matter myelination is nearing completion; note persistent small areas of subtle T2 hyperintensity

Perivascular spaces are often visible once the deep white matter is myelinated on T2

Between 2–3 years of age, progression of myelination in the most peripheral subcortical white matter of the frontal and temporal lobes can be quite variable

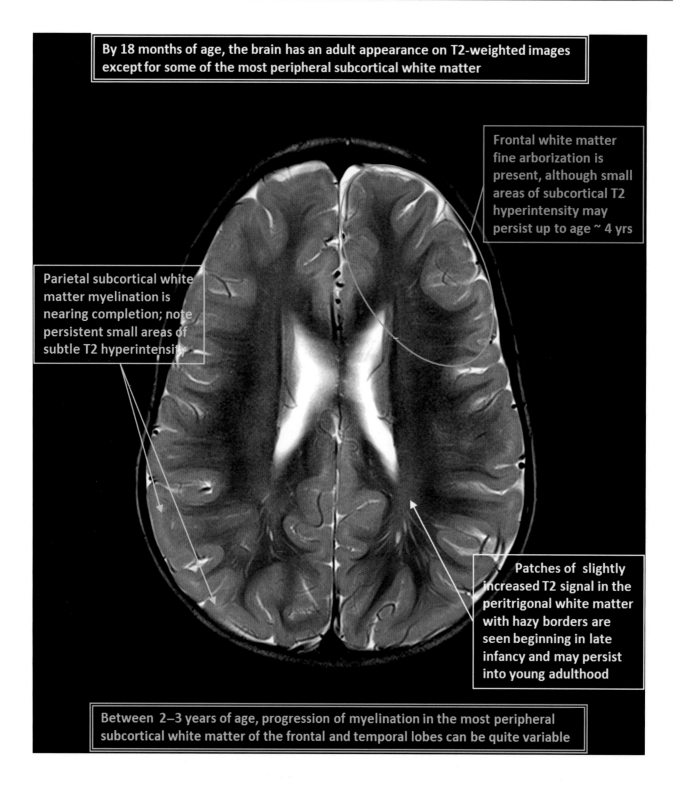

By 18 months of age, the brain has an adult appearance on T2-weighted images except for some of the most peripheral subcortical white matter

Frontal white matter fine arborization is present, although small areas of subcortical T2 hyperintensity may persist up to age ~ 4 yrs

Parietal subcortical white matter myelination is nearing completion; note persistent small areas of subtle T2 hyperintensity

Patches of slightly increased T2 signal in the peritrigonal white matter with hazy borders are seen beginning in late infancy and may persist into young adulthood

Between 2–3 years of age, progression of myelination in the most peripheral subcortical white matter of the frontal and temporal lobes can be quite variable

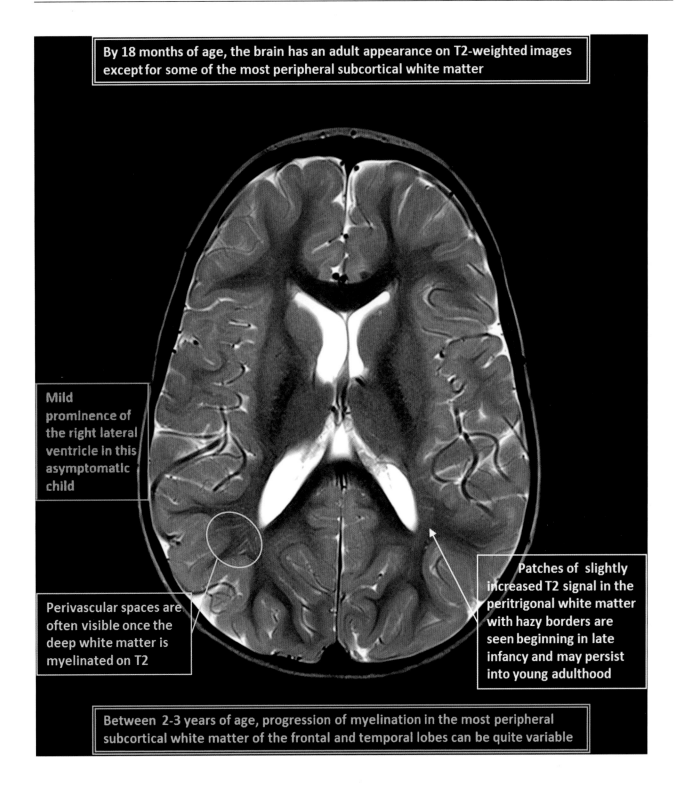

By 18 months of age, the brain has an adult appearance on T2-weighted images except for some of the most peripheral subcortical white matter

Mild prominence of the right lateral ventricle in this asymptomatic child

Perivascular spaces are often visible once the deep white matter is myelinated on T2

Patches of slightly increased T2 signal in the peritrigonal white matter with hazy borders are seen beginning in late infancy and may persist into young adulthood

Between 2-3 years of age, progression of myelination in the most peripheral subcortical white matter of the frontal and temporal lobes can be quite variable

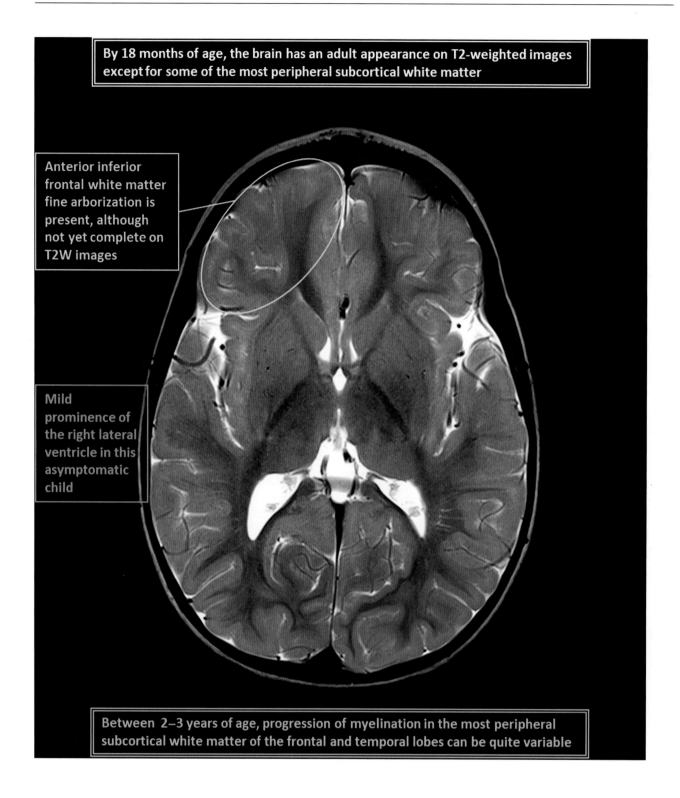

By 18 months of age, the brain has an adult appearance on T2-weighted images except for some of the most peripheral subcortical white matter

Anterior inferior frontal white matter fine arborization is present, although not yet complete on T2W images

Mild prominence of the right lateral ventricle in this asymptomatic child

Between 2–3 years of age, progression of myelination in the most peripheral subcortical white matter of the frontal and temporal lobes can be quite variable

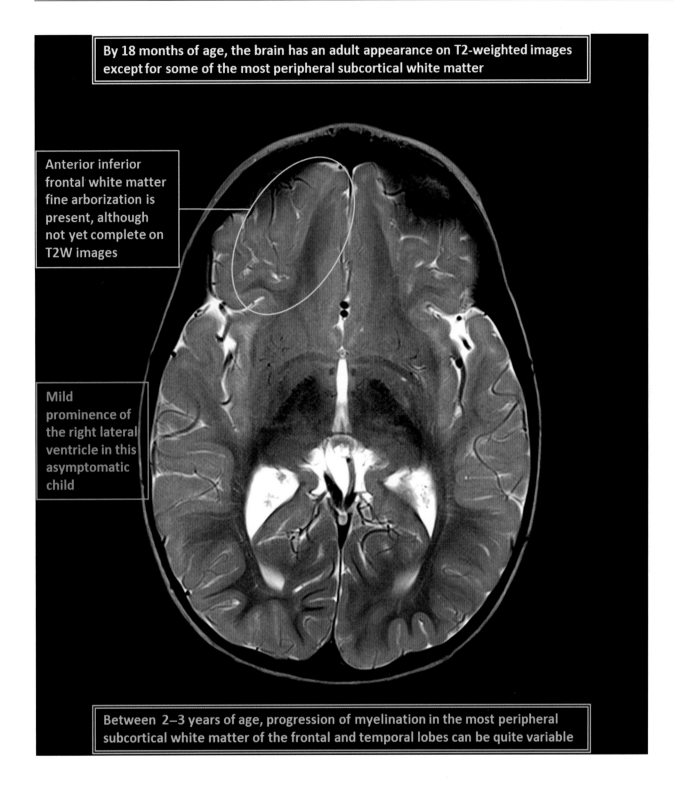

By 18 months of age, the brain has an adult appearance on T2-weighted images except for some of the most peripheral subcortical white matter

Anterior inferior frontal white matter fine arborization is present, although not yet complete on T2W images

Mild prominence of the right lateral ventricle in this asymptomatic child

Between 2–3 years of age, progression of myelination in the most peripheral subcortical white matter of the frontal and temporal lobes can be quite variable

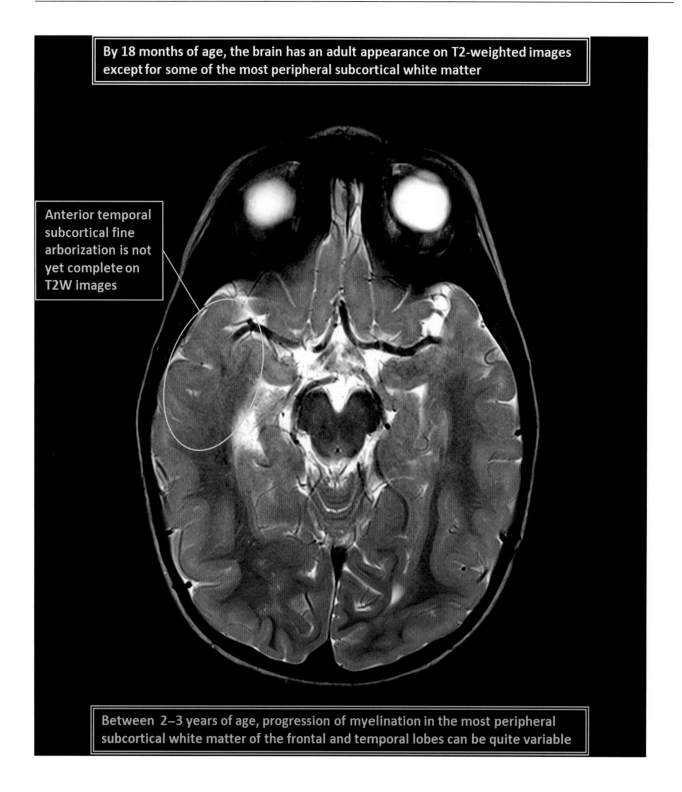

By 18 months of age, the brain has an adult appearance on T2-weighted images except for some of the most peripheral subcortical white matter

Anterior temporal subcortical fine arborization is not yet complete on T2W images

Between 2–3 years of age, progression of myelination in the most peripheral subcortical white matter of the frontal and temporal lobes can be quite variable

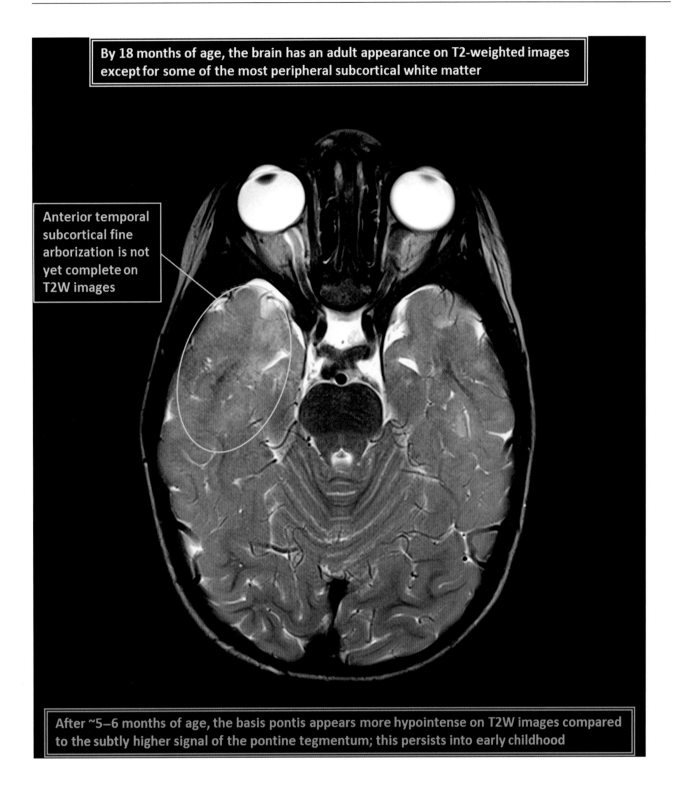

By 18 months of age, the brain has an adult appearance on T2-weighted images except for some of the most peripheral subcortical white matter

Anterior temporal subcortical fine arborization is not yet complete on T2W images

After ~5–6 months of age, the basis pontis appears more hypointense on T2W images compared to the subtly higher signal of the pontine tegmentum; this persists into early childhood

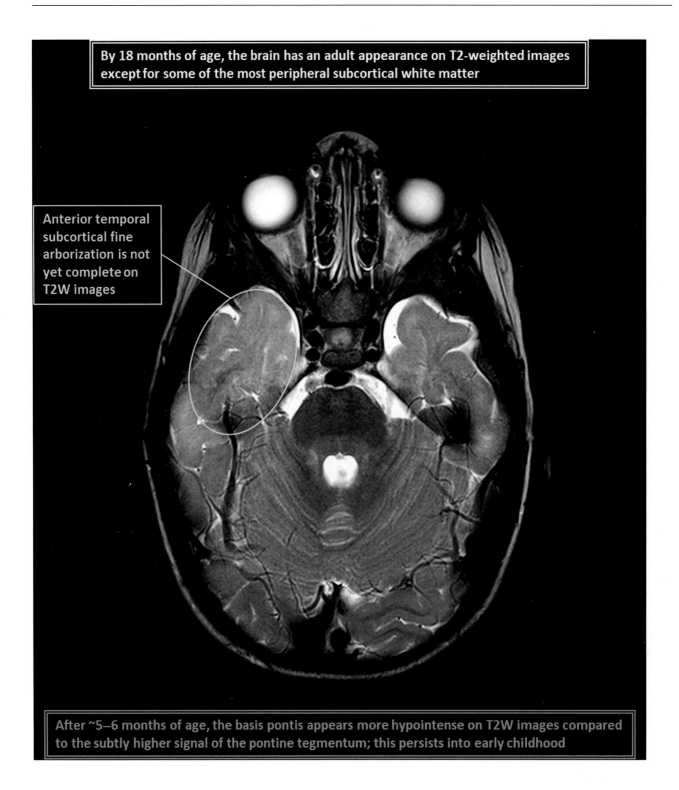

By 18 months of age, the brain has an adult appearance on T2-weighted images except for some of the most peripheral subcortical white matter

Anterior temporal subcortical fine arborization is not yet complete on T2W images

After ~5–6 months of age, the basis pontis appears more hypointense on T2W images compared to the subtly higher signal of the pontine tegmentum; this persists into early childhood

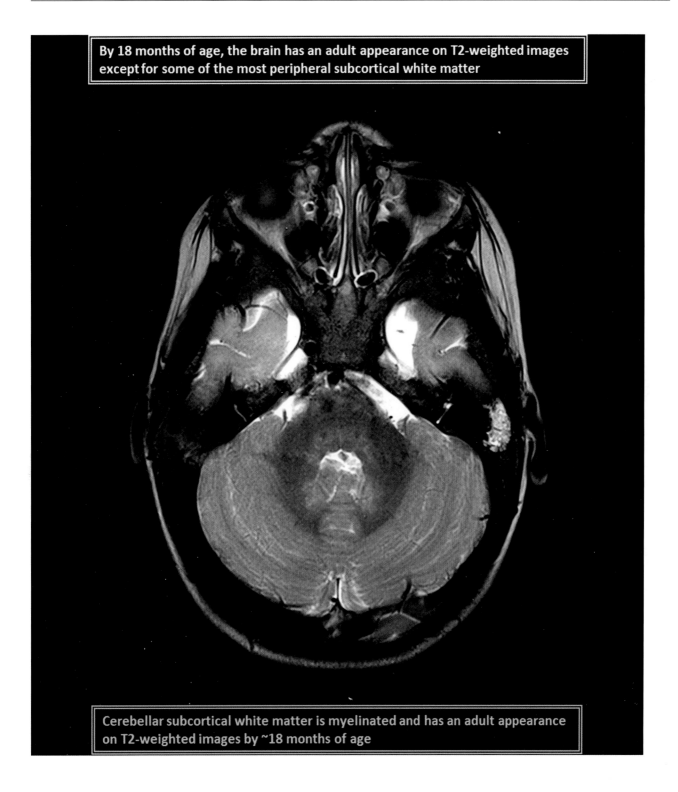

By 18 months of age, the brain has an adult appearance on T2-weighted images except for some of the most peripheral subcortical white matter

Cerebellar subcortical white matter is myelinated and has an adult appearance on T2-weighted images by ~18 months of age

2 Years, Axial FLAIR

> On FLAIR images beyond the neonatal period, the conversion of deep and subcortical white matter from hyperintensity to hypointensity relative to cortex generally follows the same pattern as on spin-echo T2W images, but occurs more slowly. The mild delay is probably due to the T1 weighting inherent in the FLAIR technique.

Frontal subcortical white matter hypointensity is evident by ~20–24 months of age, lagging slightly behind spin-echo T2W images

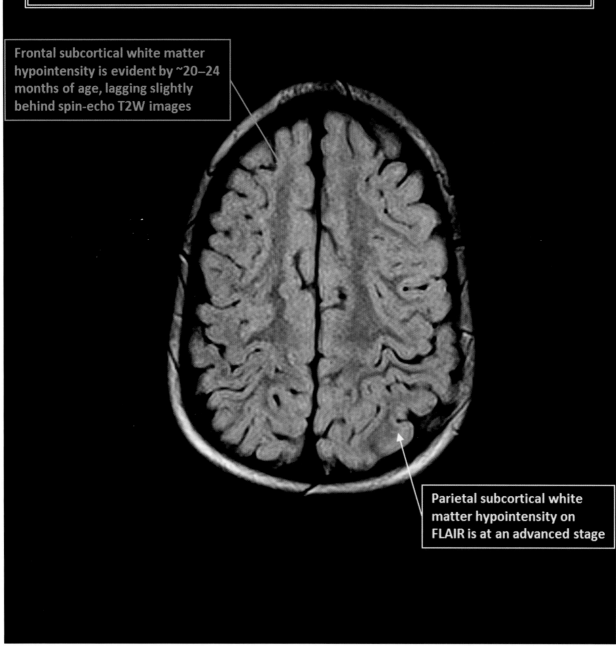

Parietal subcortical white matter hypointensity on FLAIR is at an advanced stage

2 Years, Axial FLAIR Images 1–10

On FLAIR images beyond the neonatal period, the conversion of deep and subcortical white matter from hyperintensity to hypointensity relative to cortex generally follows the same pattern as on spin-echo T2W images, but occurs more slowly. The mild delay is probably due to the T1 weighting inherent in the FLAIR technique.

Frontal subcortical white matter hypointensity is evident by ~20–24 months of age, lagging slightly behind spin-echo T2W images

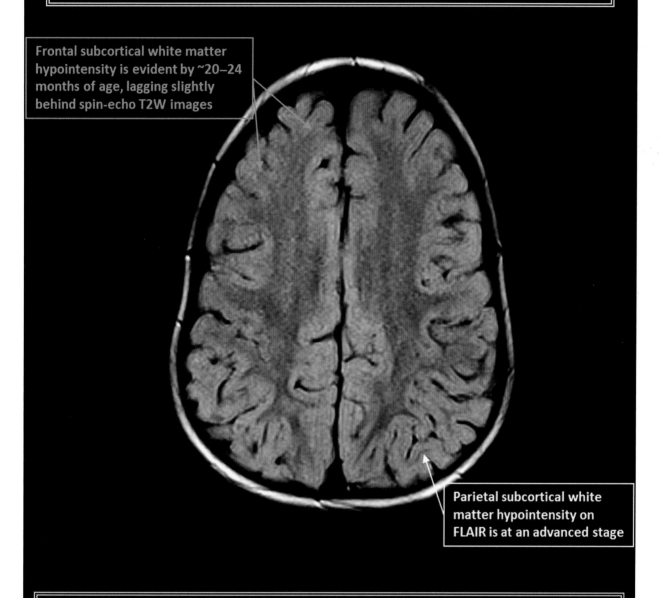

Parietal subcortical white matter hypointensity on FLAIR is at an advanced stage

Note the hazy, mildly increased FLAIR signal in the centrum semiovale and corona radiata. This is generally most apparent at 3T imaging, where it may persist to a lesser degree into adulthood.

On FLAIR images beyond the neonatal period, the conversion of deep and subcortical white matter from hyperintensity to hypointensity relative to cortex generally follows the same pattern as on spin-echo T2W images, but occurs more slowly. The mild delay is probably due to the T1 weighting inherent in the FLAIR technique.

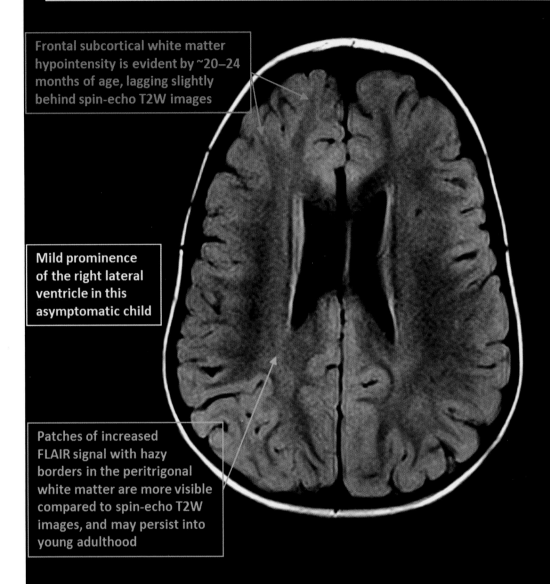

Frontal subcortical white matter hypointensity is evident by ~20–24 months of age, lagging slightly behind spin-echo T2W images

Mild prominence of the right lateral ventricle in this asymptomatic child

Patches of increased FLAIR signal with hazy borders in the peritrigonal white matter are more visible compared to spin-echo T2W images, and may persist into young adulthood

Note the hazy, mildly increased FLAIR signal in the centrum semiovale and corona radiata. This is generally most apparent at 3T imaging, where it may persist to a lesser degree into adulthood.

On FLAIR images beyond the neonatal period, the conversion of deep and subcortical white matter from hyperintensity to hypointensity relative to cortex generally follows the same pattern as on spin-echo T2W images, but occurs more slowly. The mild delay is probably due to the T1 weighting inherent in the FLAIR technique.

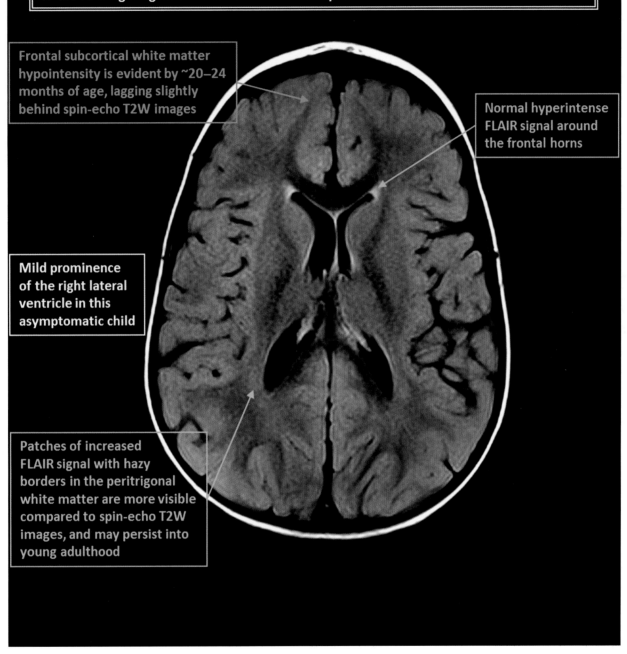

Frontal subcortical white matter hypointensity is evident by ~20–24 months of age, lagging slightly behind spin-echo T2W images

Normal hyperintense FLAIR signal around the frontal horns

Mild prominence of the right lateral ventricle in this asymptomatic child

Patches of increased FLAIR signal with hazy borders in the peritrigonal white matter are more visible compared to spin-echo T2W images, and may persist into young adulthood

On FLAIR images beyond the neonatal period, the conversion of deep and subcortical white matter from hyperintensity to hypointensity relative to cortex generally follows the same pattern as on spin-echo T2W images, but occurs more slowly. The mild delay is probably due to the T1 weighting inherent in the FLAIR technique.

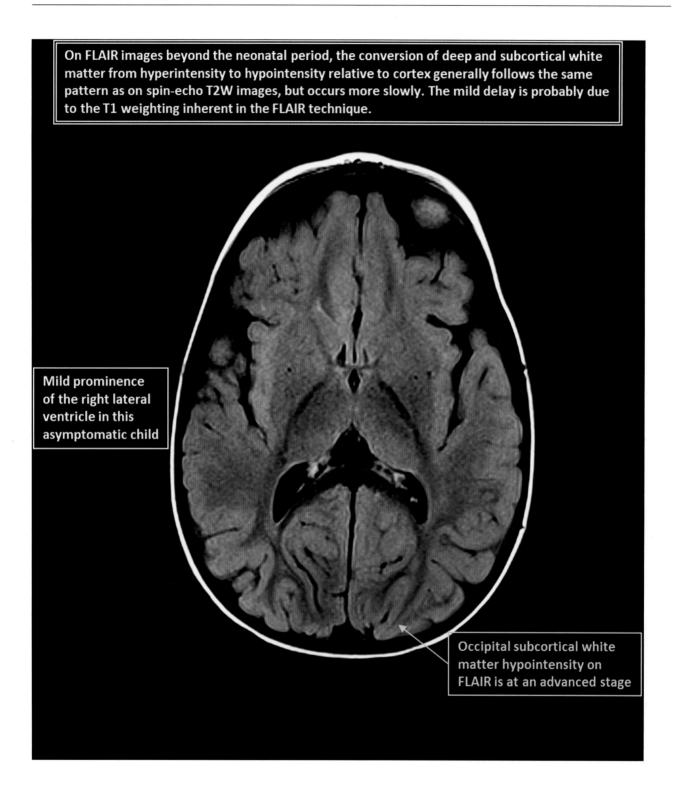

Mild prominence of the right lateral ventricle in this asymptomatic child

Occipital subcortical white matter hypointensity on FLAIR is at an advanced stage

On FLAIR images beyond the neonatal period, the conversion of deep and subcortical white matter from hyperintensity to hypointensity relative to cortex generally follows the same pattern as on spin-echo T2W images, but occurs more slowly. The mild delay is probably due to the T1 weighting inherent in the FLAIR technique.

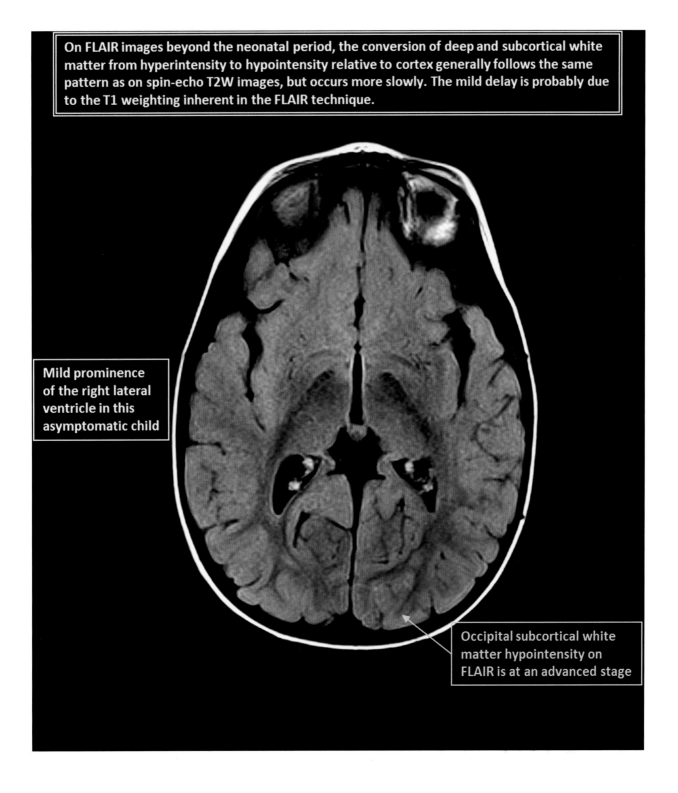

Mild prominence of the right lateral ventricle in this asymptomatic child

Occipital subcortical white matter hypointensity on FLAIR is at an advanced stage

On FLAIR images beyond the neonatal period, the conversion of deep and subcortical white matter from hyperintensity to hypointensity relative to cortex generally follows the same pattern as on spin-echo T2W images, but occurs more slowly. The mild delay is probably due to the T1 weighting inherent in the FLAIR technique.

Anterior temporal deep white matter appears hypointense at ~22–25 months of age, lagging behind spin-echo T2W images

Mild prominence of the right lateral ventricle in this asymptomatic child

Normal hyperintense FLAIR signal around the occipital horns is more visible than on spin-echo T2W images

Occipital subcortical white matter hypointensity on FLAIR is at an advanced stage

On FLAIR images beyond the neonatal period, the conversion of deep and subcortical white matter from hyperintensity to hypointensity relative to cortex generally follows the same pattern as on spin-echo T2W images, but occurs more slowly. The mild delay is probably due to the T1 weighting inherent in the FLAIR technique.

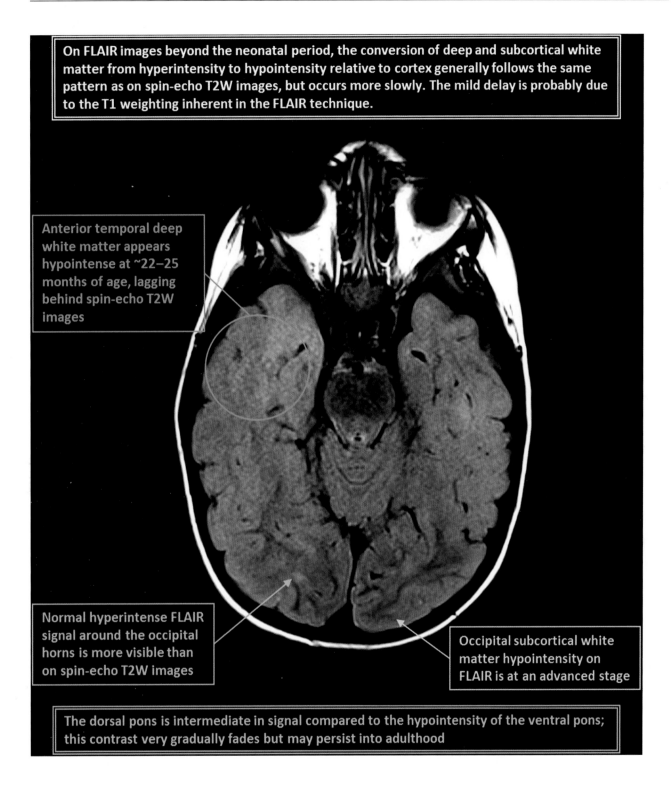

Anterior temporal deep white matter appears hypointense at ~22–25 months of age, lagging behind spin-echo T2W images

Normal hyperintense FLAIR signal around the occipital horns is more visible than on spin-echo T2W images

Occipital subcortical white matter hypointensity on FLAIR is at an advanced stage

The dorsal pons is intermediate in signal compared to the hypointensity of the ventral pons; this contrast very gradually fades but may persist into adulthood

On FLAIR images beyond the neonatal period, the conversion of deep and subcortical white matter from hyperintensity to hypointensity relative to cortex generally follows the same pattern as on spin-echo T2W images, but occurs more slowly. The mild delay is probably due to the T1 weighting inherent in the FLAIR technique.

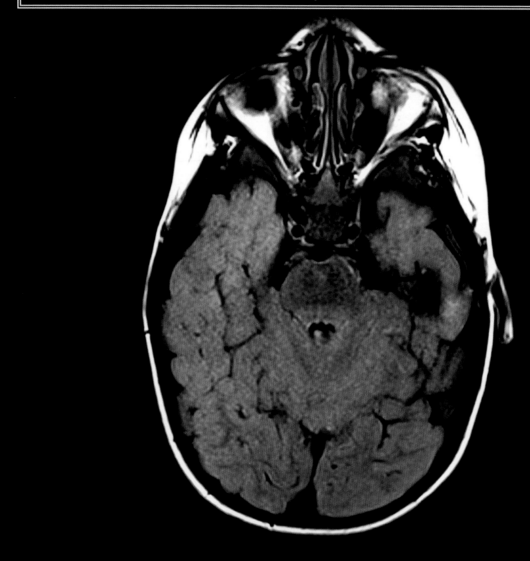

The dorsal pons is intermediate in signal compared to the hypointensity of the ventral pons; this contrast very gradually fades but may persist into adulthood

On FLAIR images beyond the neonatal period, the conversion of deep and subcortical white matter from hyperintensity to hypointensity relative to cortex generally follows the same pattern as on spin-echo T2W images, but occurs more slowly. The mild delay is probably due to the T1 weighting inherent in the FLAIR technique.

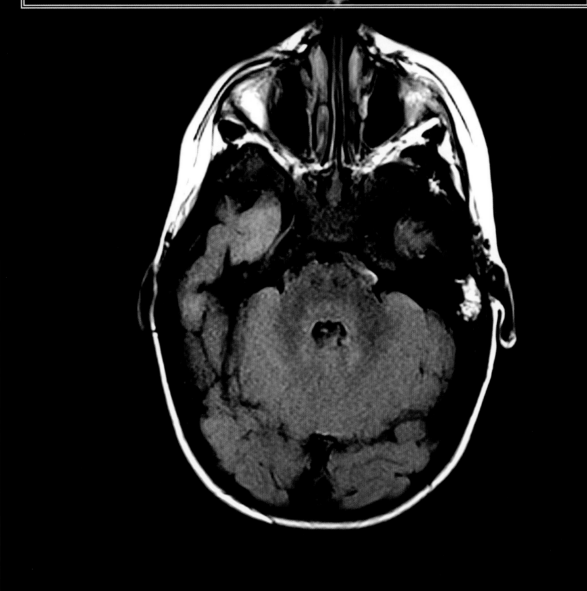

The dorsal pons is intermediate in signal compared to the hypointensity of the ventral pons; this contrast very gradually fades but may persist into adulthood

2 Years, Coronal TSE T2

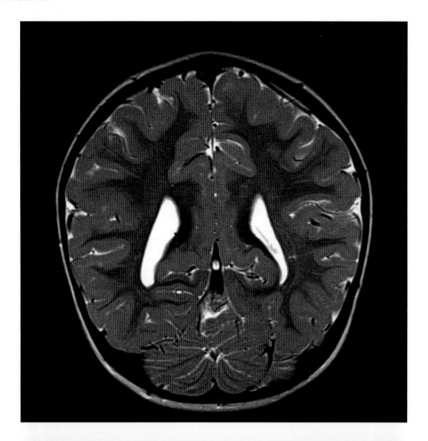

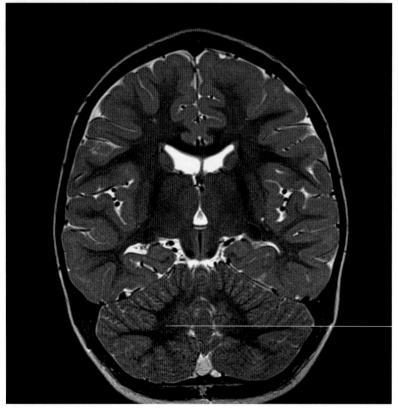

2 Years, Coronal TSE T2 Images 1–4

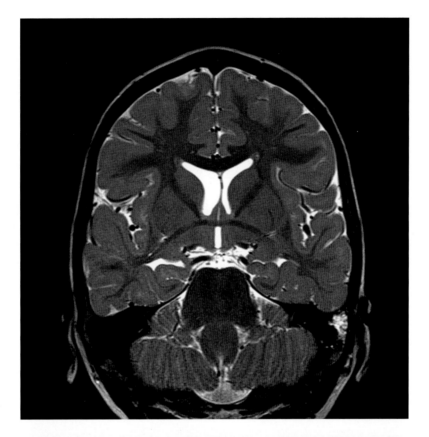

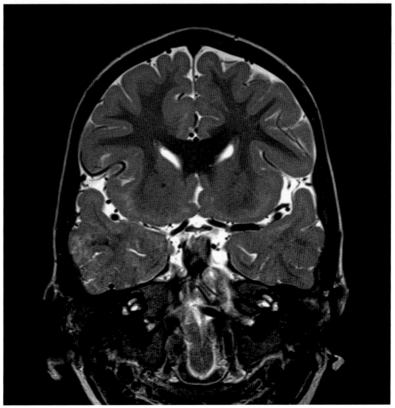

3 Years, Axial TSE T2

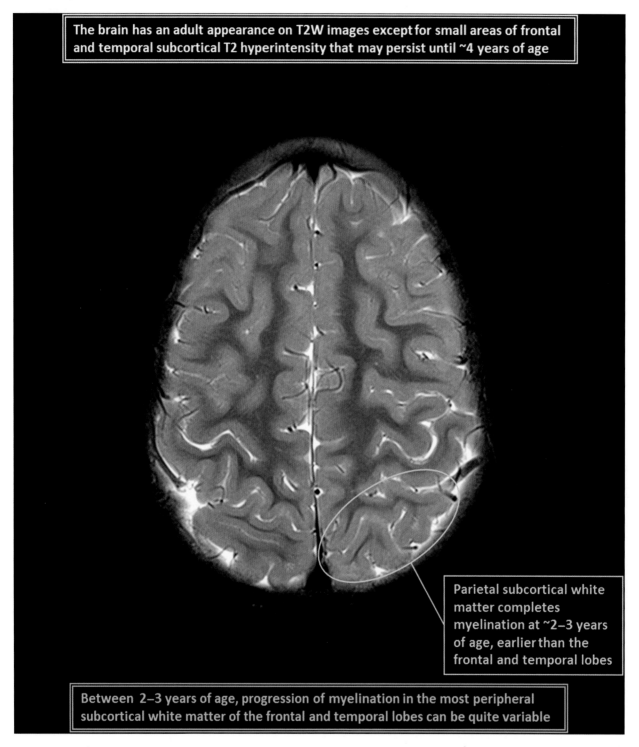

The brain has an adult appearance on T2W images except for small areas of frontal and temporal subcortical T2 hyperintensity that may persist until ~4 years of age

Parietal subcortical white matter completes myelination at ~2–3 years of age, earlier than the frontal and temporal lobes

Between 2–3 years of age, progression of myelination in the most peripheral subcortical white matter of the frontal and temporal lobes can be quite variable

3 Years, Axial TSE T2 Images 1–10

The brain has an adult appearance on T2W images except for small areas of frontal and temporal subcortical T2 hyperintensity that may persist until ~4 years of age

Parietal subcortical white matter completes myelination at ~2–3 years of age, earlier than the frontal and temporal lobes

Between 2–3 years of age, progression of myelination in the most peripheral subcortical white matter of the frontal and temporal lobes can be quite variable

The brain has an adult appearance on T2W images except for small areas of frontal and temporal subcortical T2 hyperintensity that may persist until ~4 years of age

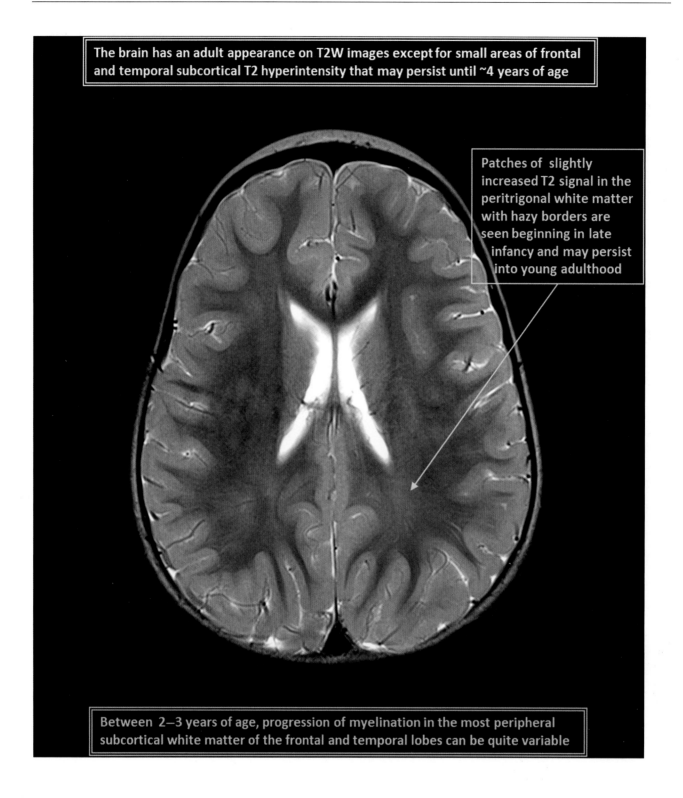

Patches of slightly increased T2 signal in the peritrigonal white matter with hazy borders are seen beginning in late infancy and may persist into young adulthood

Between 2–3 years of age, progression of myelination in the most peripheral subcortical white matter of the frontal and temporal lobes can be quite variable

The brain has an adult appearance on T2W images except for small areas of frontal and temporal subcortical T2 hyperintensity that may persist until ~4 years of age

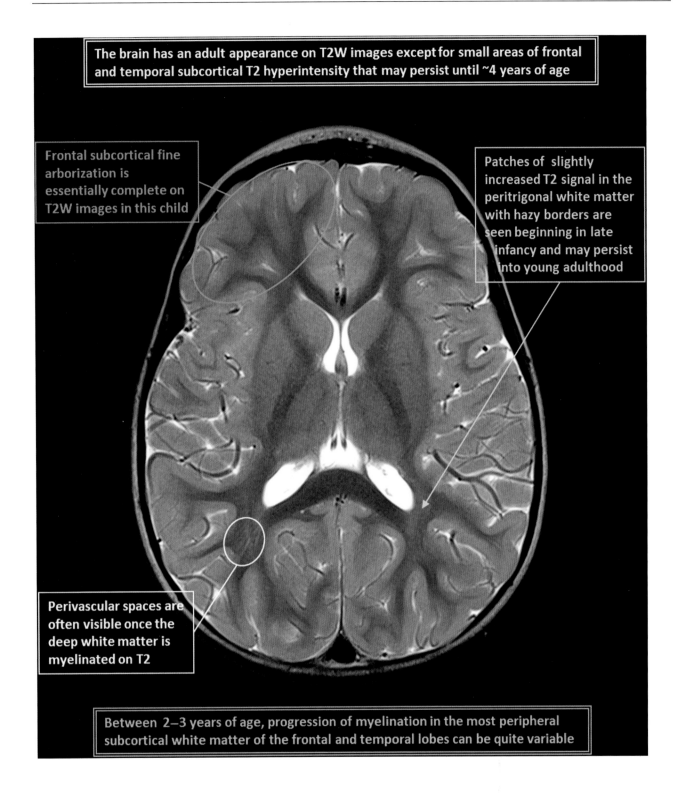

Frontal subcortical fine arborization is essentially complete on T2W images in this child

Patches of slightly increased T2 signal in the peritrigonal white matter with hazy borders are seen beginning in late infancy and may persist into young adulthood

Perivascular spaces are often visible once the deep white matter is myelinated on T2

Between 2–3 years of age, progression of myelination in the most peripheral subcortical white matter of the frontal and temporal lobes can be quite variable

The brain has an adult appearance on T2W images except for small areas of frontal and temporal subcortical T2 hyperintensity that may persist until ~4 years of age

Frontal subcortical fine arborization is essentially complete on T2W images in this child

Between 2–3 years of age, progression of myelination in the most peripheral subcortical white matter of the frontal and temporal lobes can be quite variable

The brain has an adult appearance on T2W images except for small areas of frontal and temporal subcortical T2 hyperintensity that may persist until ~4 years of age

Frontal subcortical fine arborization is essentially complete on T2W images in this child

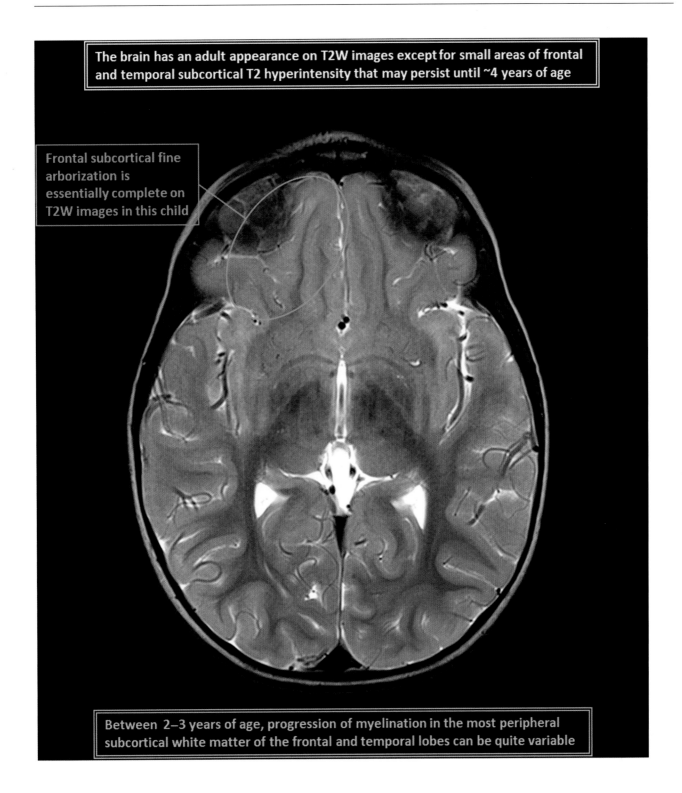

Between 2–3 years of age, progression of myelination in the most peripheral subcortical white matter of the frontal and temporal lobes can be quite variable

The brain has an adult appearance on T2W images except for small areas of frontal and temporal subcortical T2 hyperintensity that may persist until ~4 years of age

Anterior temporal subcortical fine arborization is one of the last areas to complete myelination on T2

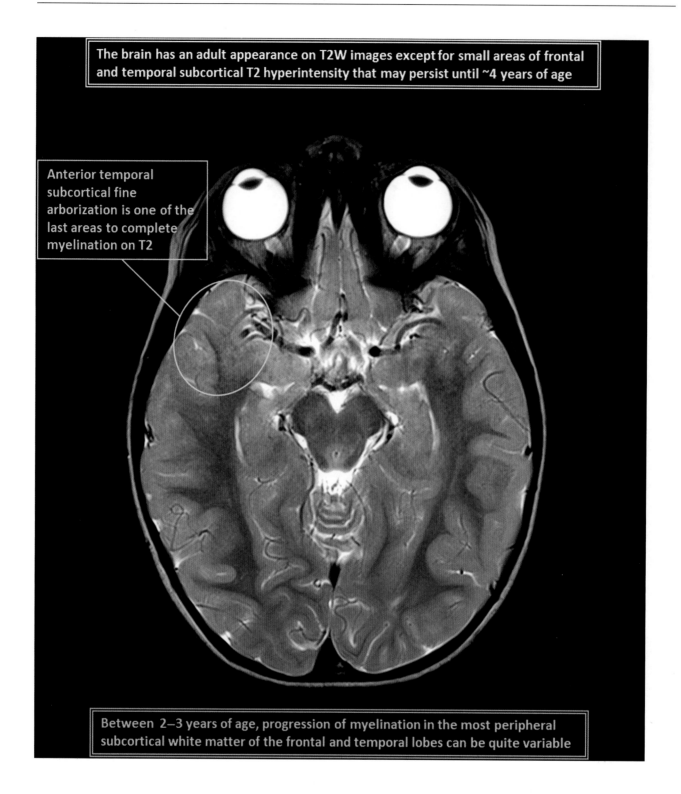

Between 2–3 years of age, progression of myelination in the most peripheral subcortical white matter of the frontal and temporal lobes can be quite variable

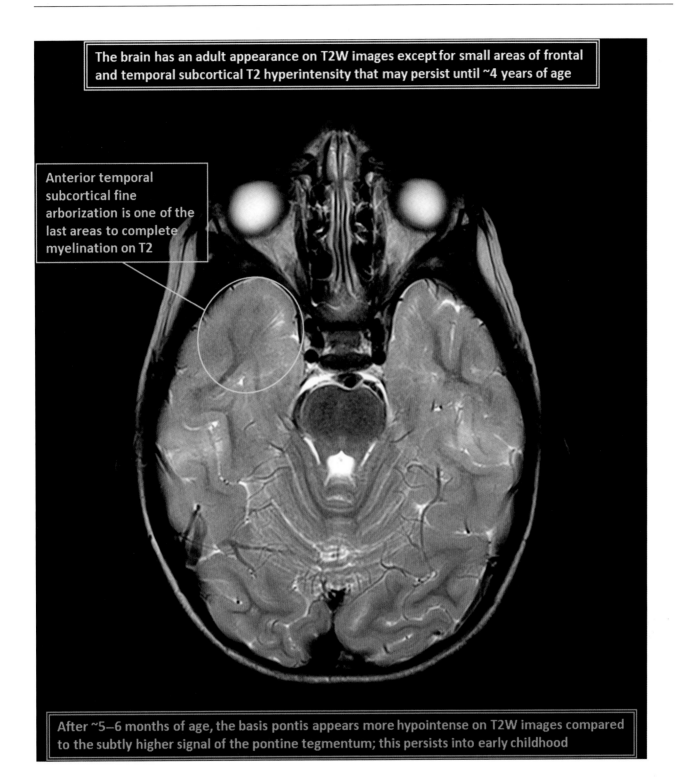

The brain has an adult appearance on T2W images except for small areas of frontal and temporal subcortical T2 hyperintensity that may persist until ~4 years of age

Anterior temporal subcortical fine arborization is one of the last areas to complete myelination on T2

After ~5–6 months of age, the basis pontis appears more hypointense on T2W images compared to the subtly higher signal of the pontine tegmentum; this persists into early childhood

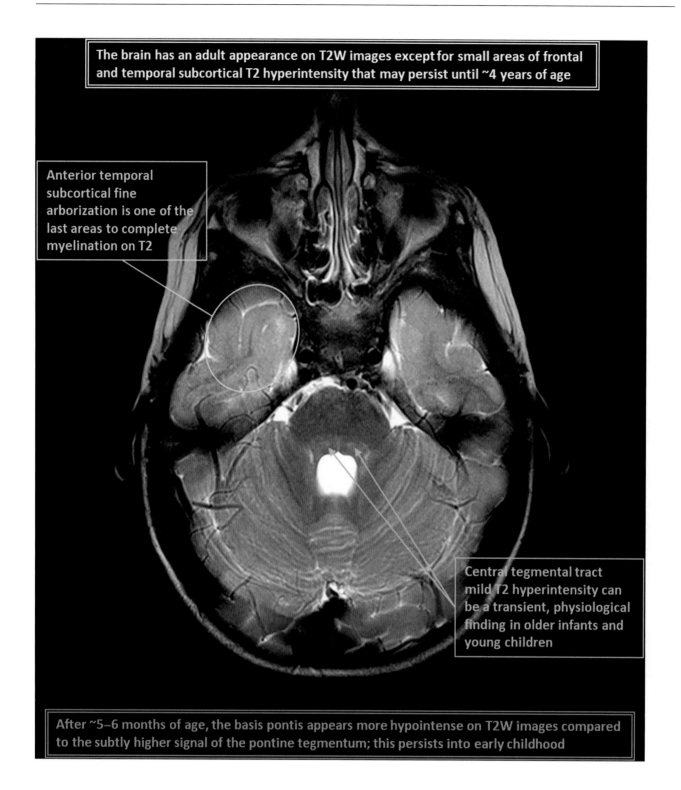

The brain has an adult appearance on T2W images except for small areas of frontal and temporal subcortical T2 hyperintensity that may persist until ~4 years of age

Anterior temporal subcortical fine arborization is one of the last areas to complete myelination on T2

Central tegmental tract mild T2 hyperintensity can be a transient, physiological finding in older infants and young children

After ~5–6 months of age, the basis pontis appears more hypointense on T2W images compared to the subtly higher signal of the pontine tegmentum; this persists into early childhood

The brain has an adult appearance on T2W images except for small areas of frontal and temporal subcortical T2 hyperintensity that may persist until ~4 years of age

After ~5–6 months of age, the basis pontis appears more hypointense on T2W images compared to the subtly higher signal of the pontine tegmentum; this persists into early childhood

3 Years, Axial FLAIR

On FLAIR images beyond the neonatal period, the conversion of deep and subcortical white matter from hyperintensity to hypointensity relative to cortex generally follows the same pattern as on spin-echo T2W images, but occurs more slowly. The mild delay is probably due to the T1 weighting inherent in the FLAIR technique.

Frontal subcortical white matter hypointensity is well developed but may continue to increase in contrast relative to cortex beyond the third year

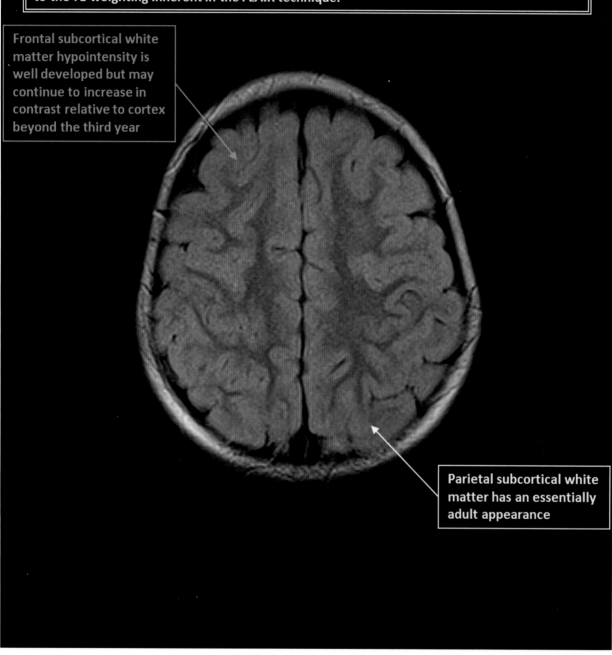

Parietal subcortical white matter has an essentially adult appearance

3 Years, Axial FLAIR Images 1–10

On FLAIR images beyond the neonatal period, the conversion of deep and subcortical white matter from hyperintensity to hypointensity relative to cortex generally follows the same pattern as on spin-echo T2W images, but occurs more slowly. The mild delay is probably due to the T1 weighting inherent in the FLAIR technique.

Frontal subcortical white matter hypointensity is well developed but may continue to increase in contrast relative to cortex beyond the third year

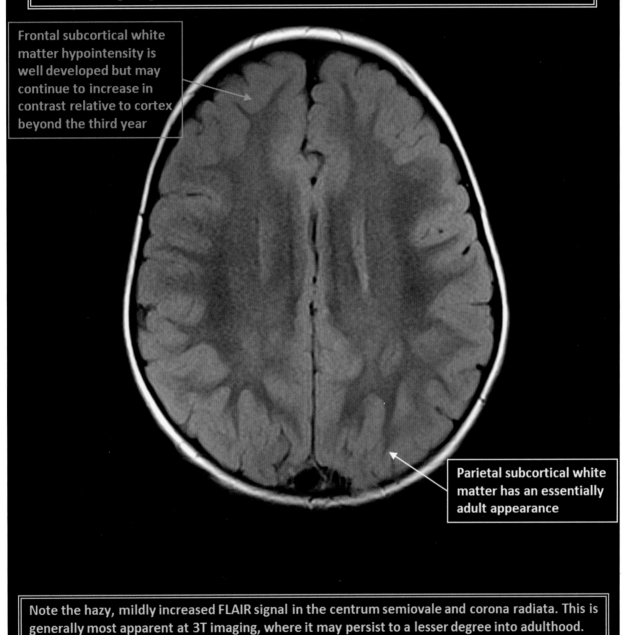

Parietal subcortical white matter has an essentially adult appearance

Note the hazy, mildly increased FLAIR signal in the centrum semiovale and corona radiata. This is generally most apparent at 3T imaging, where it may persist to a lesser degree into adulthood.

On FLAIR images beyond the neonatal period, the conversion of deep and subcortical white matter from hyperintensity to hypointensity relative to cortex generally follows the same pattern as on spin-echo T2W images, but occurs more slowly. The mild delay is probably due to the T1 weighting inherent in the FLAIR technique.

Frontal subcortical white matter hypointensity is well developed but may continue to increase in contrast relative to cortex beyond the third year

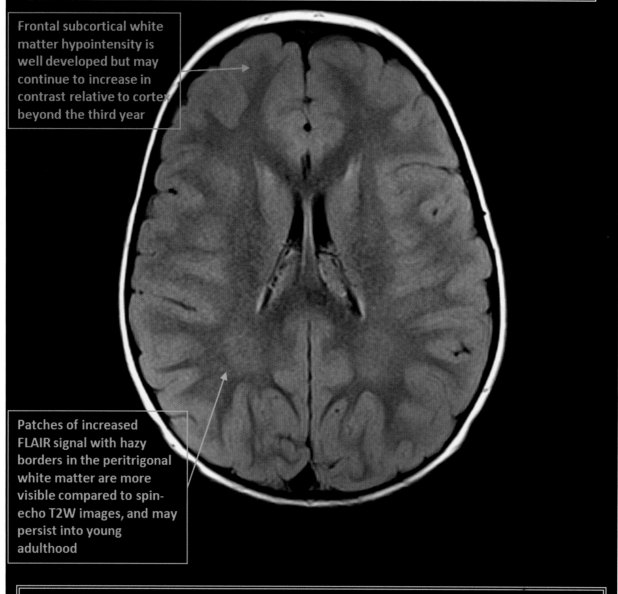

Patches of increased FLAIR signal with hazy borders in the peritrigonal white matter are more visible compared to spin-echo T2W images, and may persist into young adulthood

Note the hazy, mildly increased FLAIR signal in the centrum semiovale and corona radiata. This is generally most apparent at 3T imaging, where it may persist to a lesser degree into adulthood.

On FLAIR images beyond the neonatal period, the conversion of deep and subcortical white matter from hyperintensity to hypointensity relative to cortex generally follows the same pattern as on spin-echo T2W images, but occurs more slowly. The mild delay is probably due to the T1 weighting inherent in the FLAIR technique.

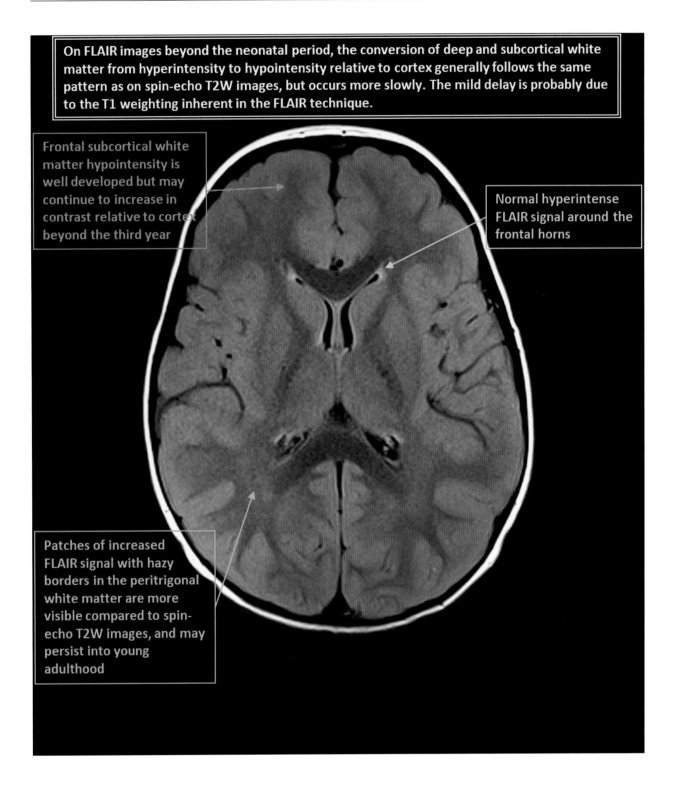

Frontal subcortical white matter hypointensity is well developed but may continue to increase in contrast relative to cortex beyond the third year

Normal hyperintense FLAIR signal around the frontal horns

Patches of increased FLAIR signal with hazy borders in the peritrigonal white matter are more visible compared to spin-echo T2W images, and may persist into young adulthood

On FLAIR images beyond the neonatal period, the conversion of deep and subcortical white matter from hyperintensity to hypointensity relative to cortex generally follows the same pattern as on spin-echo T2W images, but occurs more slowly. The mild delay is probably due to the T1 weighting inherent in the FLAIR technique.

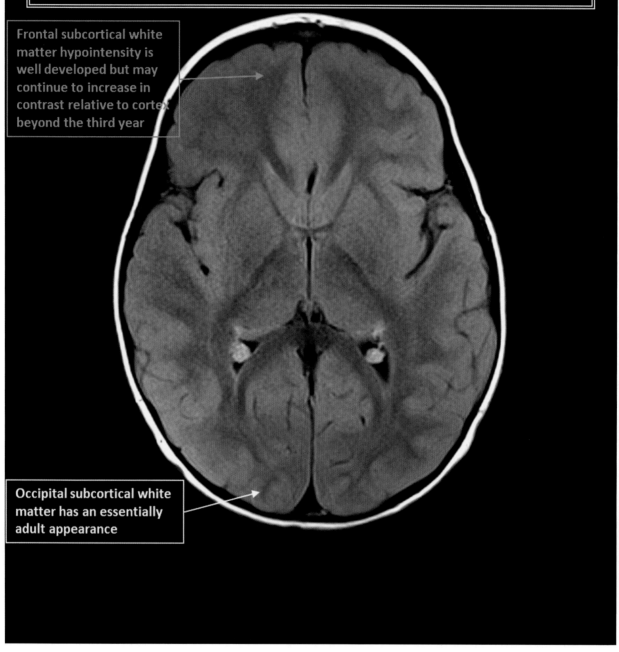

Frontal subcortical white matter hypointensity is well developed but may continue to increase in contrast relative to cortex beyond the third year

Occipital subcortical white matter has an essentially adult appearance

On FLAIR images beyond the neonatal period, the conversion of deep and subcortical white matter from hyperintensity to hypointensity relative to cortex generally follows the same pattern as on spin-echo T2W images, but occurs more slowly. The mild delay is probably due to the T1 weighting inherent in the FLAIR technique.

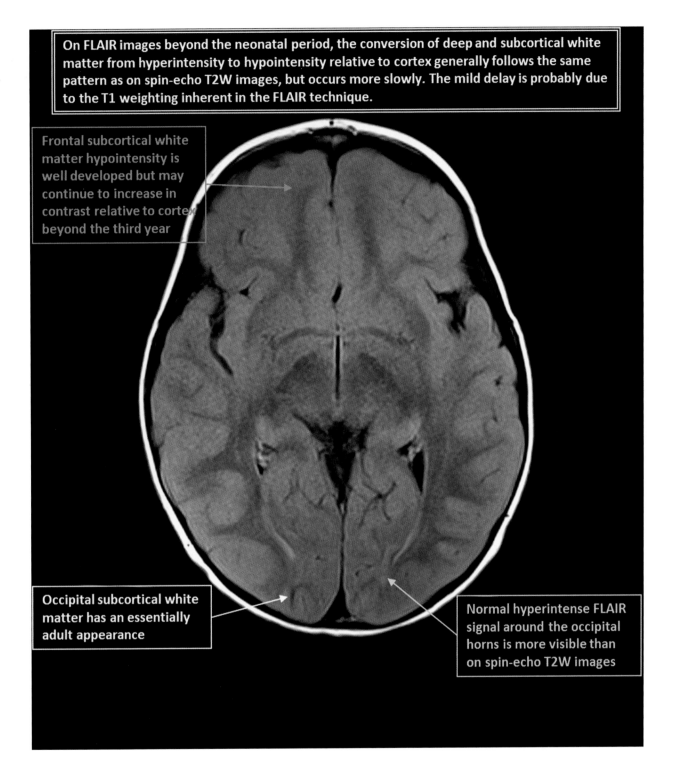

Frontal subcortical white matter hypointensity is well developed but may continue to increase in contrast relative to cortex beyond the third year

Occipital subcortical white matter has an essentially adult appearance

Normal hyperintense FLAIR signal around the occipital horns is more visible than on spin-echo T2W images

On FLAIR images beyond the neonatal period, the conversion of deep and subcortical white matter from hyperintensity to hypointensity relative to cortex generally follows the same pattern as on spin-echo T2W images, but occurs more slowly. The mild delay is probably due to the T1 weighting inherent in the FLAIR technique.

Anterior temporal deep white matter appears hypointense at ~22–25 months; the subcortical white matter may not become hypointense on FLAIR until after 2 years of age

Occipital subcortical white matter has an essentially adult appearance

On FLAIR images beyond the neonatal period, the conversion of deep and subcortical white matter from hyperintensity to hypointensity relative to cortex generally follows the same pattern as on spin-echo T2W images, but occurs more slowly. The mild delay is probably due to the T1 weighting inherent in the FLAIR technique.

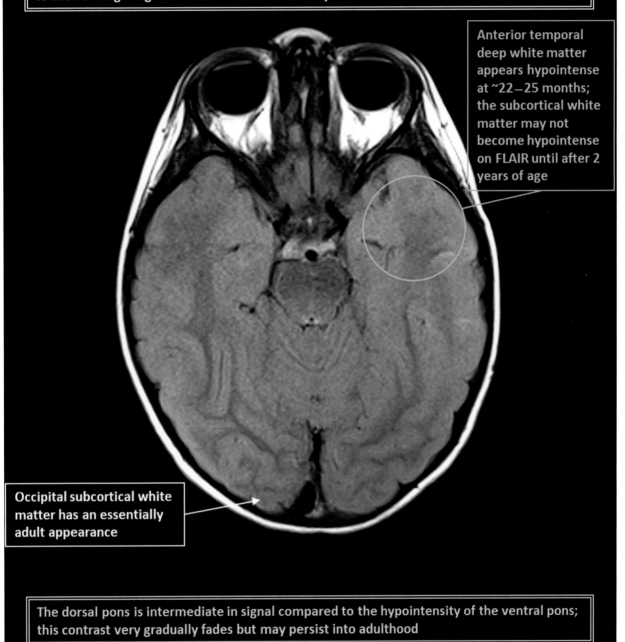

Anterior temporal deep white matter appears hypointense at ~22–25 months; the subcortical white matter may not become hypointense on FLAIR until after 2 years of age

Occipital subcortical white matter has an essentially adult appearance

The dorsal pons is intermediate in signal compared to the hypointensity of the ventral pons; this contrast very gradually fades but may persist into adulthood

On FLAIR images beyond the neonatal period, the conversion of deep and subcortical white matter from hyperintensity to hypointensity relative to cortex generally follows the same pattern as on spin-echo T2W images, but occurs more slowly. The mild delay is probably due to the T1 weighting inherent in the FLAIR technique.

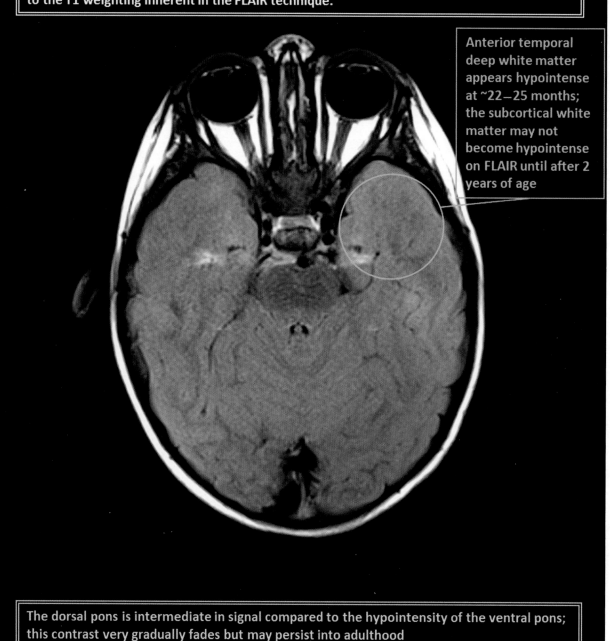

Anterior temporal deep white matter appears hypointense at ~22–25 months; the subcortical white matter may not become hypointense on FLAIR until after 2 years of age

The dorsal pons is intermediate in signal compared to the hypointensity of the ventral pons; this contrast very gradually fades but may persist into adulthood

On FLAIR images beyond the neonatal period, the conversion of deep and subcortical white matter from hyperintensity to hypointensity relative to cortex generally follows the same pattern as on spin-echo T2W images, but occurs more slowly. The mild delay is probably due to the T1 weighting inherent in the FLAIR technique.

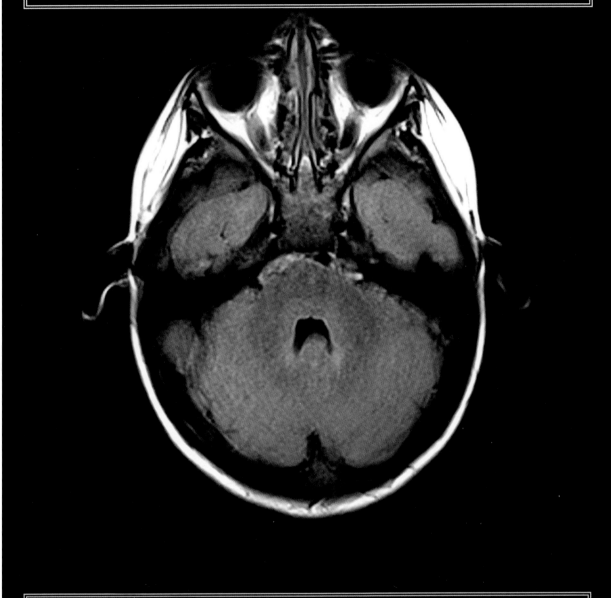

The dorsal pons is intermediate in signal compared to the hypointensity of the ventral pons; this contrast very gradually fades but may persist into adulthood

3 Years, Coronal TSE T2

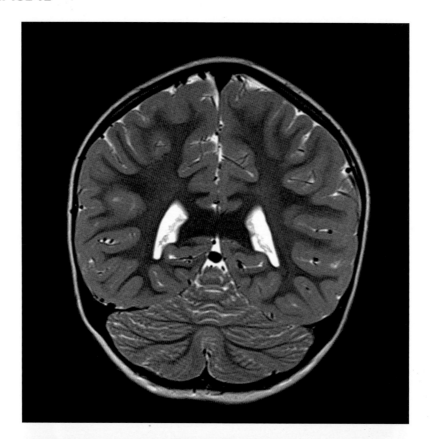

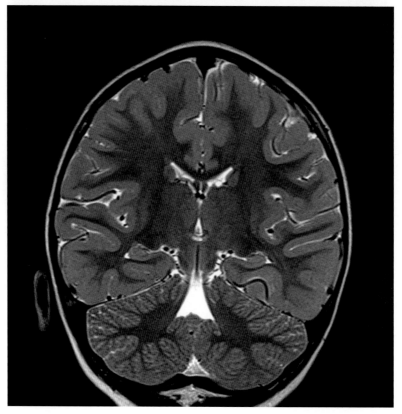

3 Years, Coronal TSE T2 Images 1–4

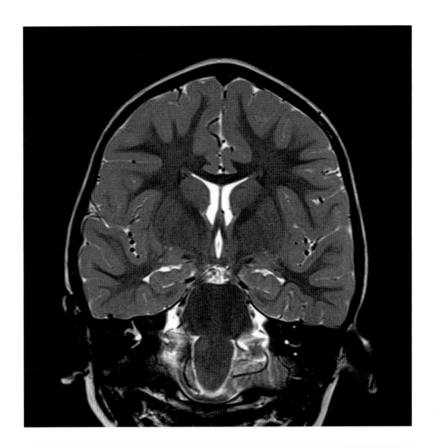

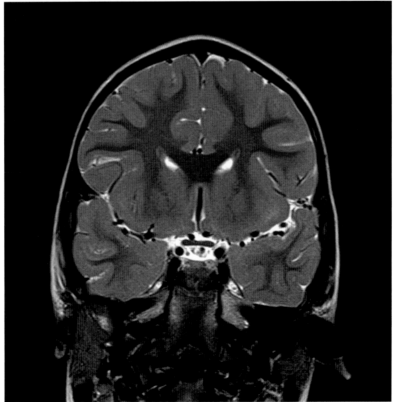

Anatomy Images, Age 3 Years

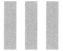

Axial T1 Images

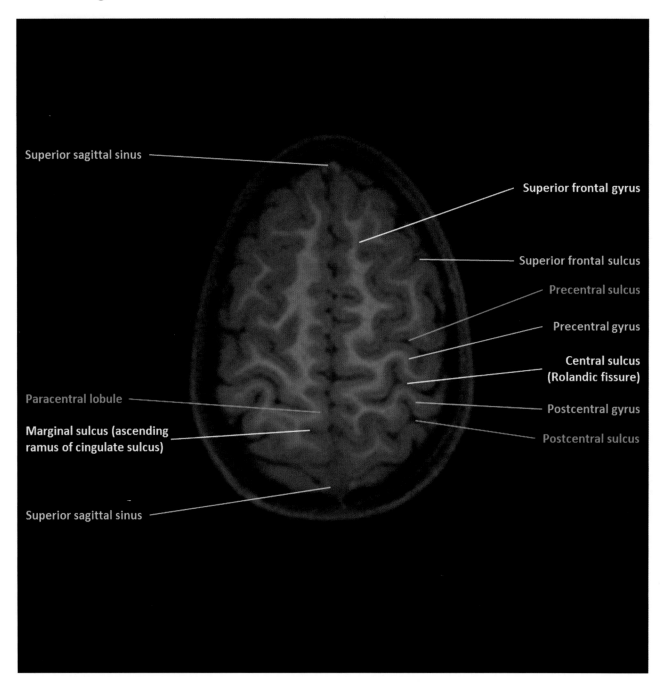

Superior sagittal sinus

Superior frontal gyrus

Superior frontal sulcus

Precentral sulcus

Precentral gyrus

Central sulcus (Rolandic fissure)

Postcentral gyrus

Paracentral lobule

Marginal sulcus (ascending ramus of cingulate sulcus)

Postcentral sulcus

Superior sagittal sinus

ANATOMY Axial T1 Images 1–30

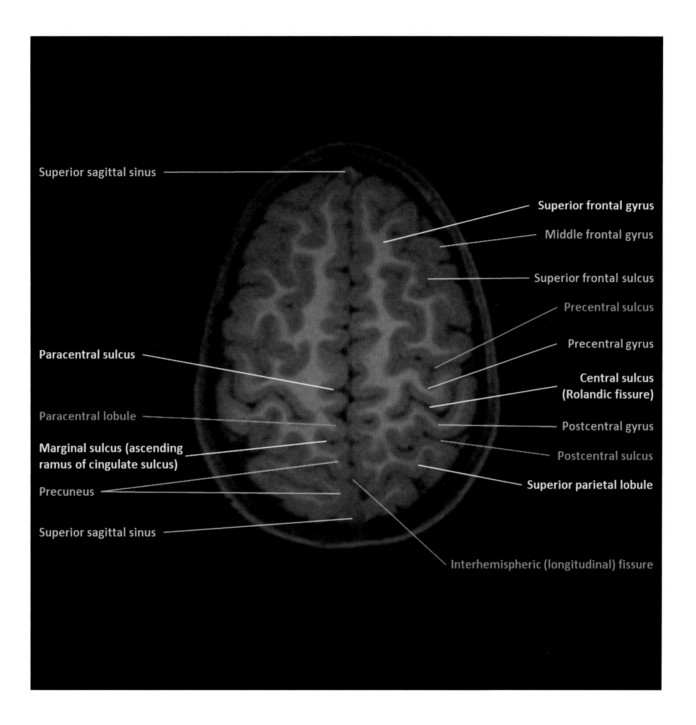

Superior sagittal sinus

Superior frontal gyrus

Middle frontal gyrus

Superior frontal sulcus

Precentral sulcus

Precentral gyrus

Paracentral sulcus

Central sulcus
(Rolandic fissure)

Paracentral lobule

Postcentral gyrus

Marginal sulcus (ascending
ramus of cingulate sulcus)

Postcentral sulcus

Precuneus

Superior parietal lobule

Superior sagittal sinus

Interhemispheric (longitudinal) fissure

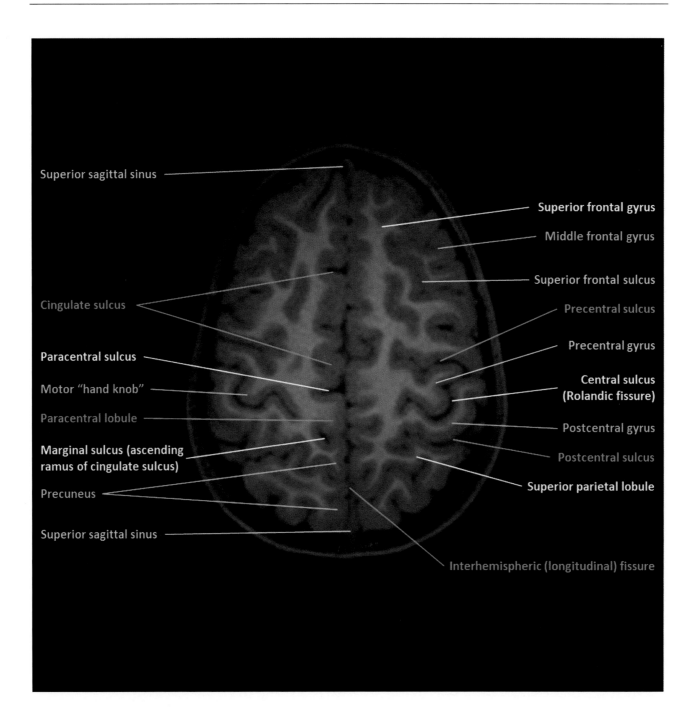

Superior sagittal sinus

Superior frontal gyrus

Middle frontal gyrus

Superior frontal sulcus

Precentral sulcus

Precentral gyrus

Cingulate sulcus

Paracentral sulcus

Motor "hand knob"

Central sulcus (Rolandic fissure)

Paracentral lobule

Postcentral gyrus

Marginal sulcus (ascending ramus of cingulate sulcus)

Postcentral sulcus

Superior parietal lobule

Precuneus

Superior sagittal sinus

Interhemispheric (longitudinal) fissure

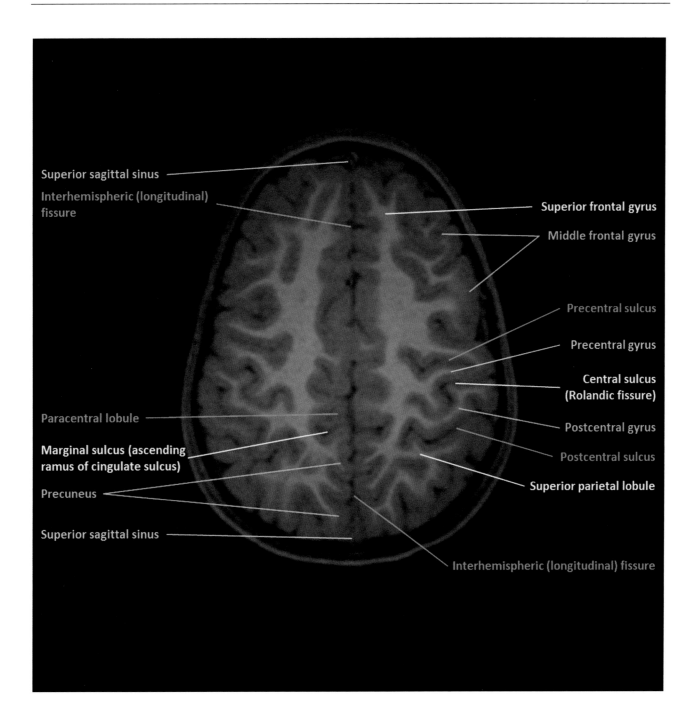

Superior sagittal sinus

Interhemispheric (longitudinal) fissure

Superior frontal gyrus

Middle frontal gyrus

Precentral sulcus

Precentral gyrus

Central sulcus (Rolandic fissure)

Postcentral gyrus

Postcentral sulcus

Superior parietal lobule

Paracentral lobule

Marginal sulcus (ascending ramus of cingulate sulcus)

Precuneus

Superior sagittal sinus

Interhemispheric (longitudinal) fissure

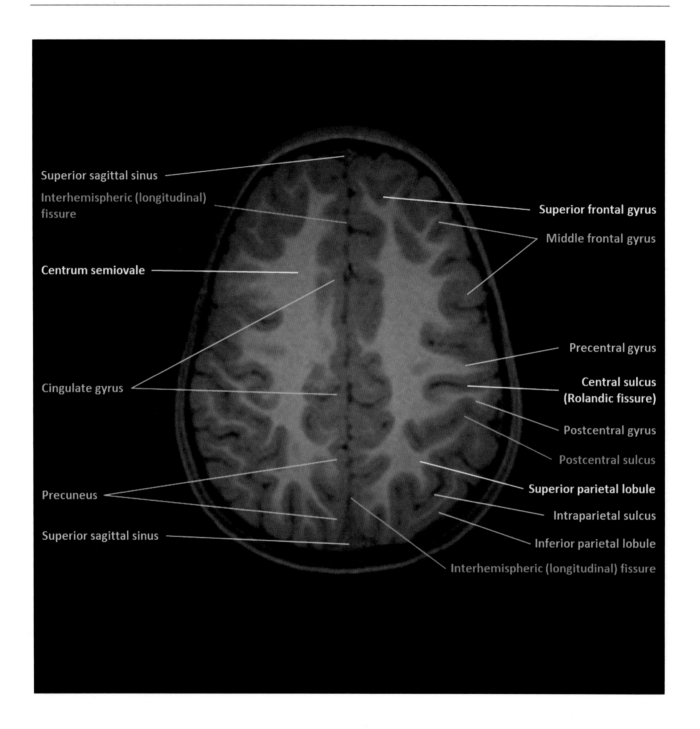

Superior sagittal sinus

Interhemispheric (longitudinal) fissure

Centrum semiovale

Cingulate gyrus

Precuneus

Superior sagittal sinus

Superior frontal gyrus

Middle frontal gyrus

Precentral gyrus

Central sulcus (Rolandic fissure)

Postcentral gyrus

Postcentral sulcus

Superior parietal lobule

Intraparietal sulcus

Inferior parietal lobule

Interhemispheric (longitudinal) fissure

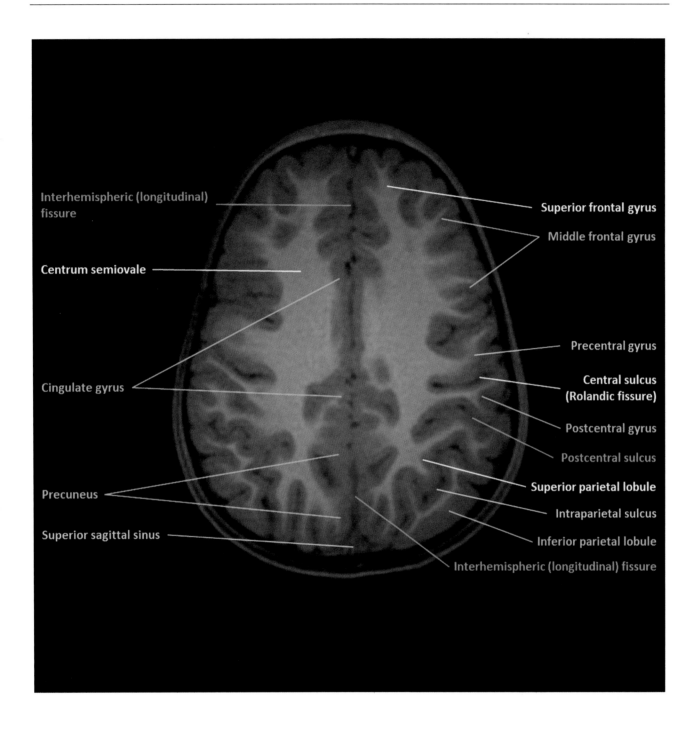

Interhemispheric (longitudinal) fissure

Centrum semiovale

Cingulate gyrus

Precuneus

Superior sagittal sinus

Superior frontal gyrus

Middle frontal gyrus

Precentral gyrus

Central sulcus (Rolandic fissure)

Postcentral gyrus

Postcentral sulcus

Superior parietal lobule

Intraparietal sulcus

Inferior parietal lobule

Interhemispheric (longitudinal) fissure

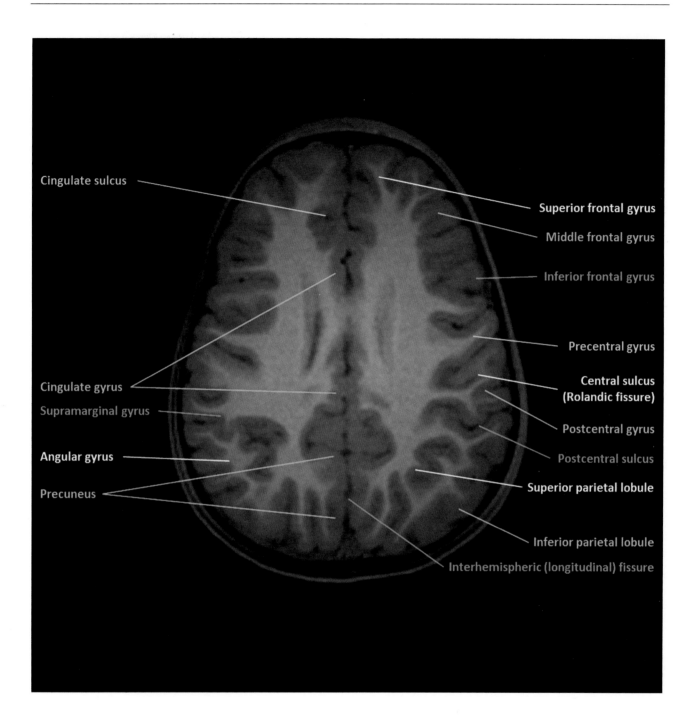

Cingulate sulcus

Superior frontal gyrus

Middle frontal gyrus

Inferior frontal gyrus

Precentral gyrus

Cingulate gyrus

**Central sulcus
(Rolandic fissure)**

Supramarginal gyrus

Postcentral gyrus

Postcentral sulcus

Angular gyrus

Superior parietal lobule

Precuneus

Inferior parietal lobule

Interhemispheric (longitudinal) fissure

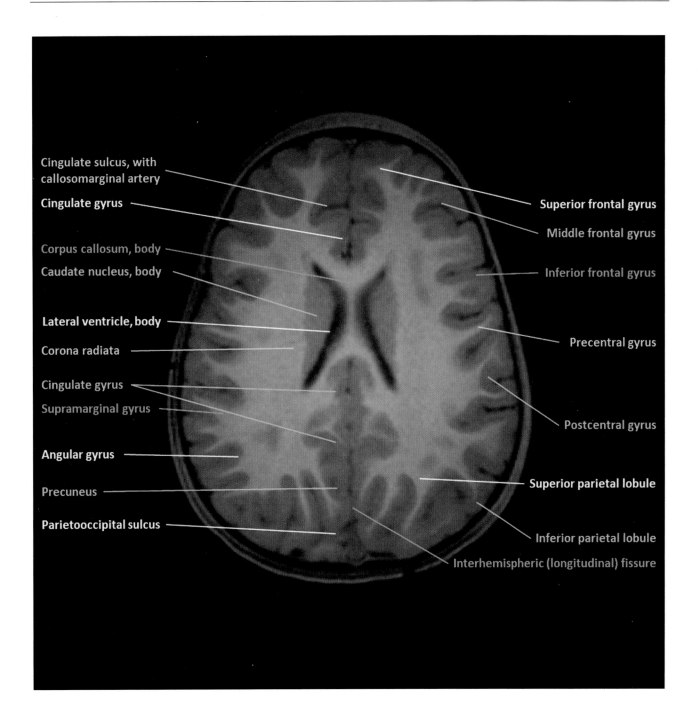

Cingulate sulcus, with callosomarginal artery

Cingulate gyrus

Corpus callosum, body

Caudate nucleus, body

Lateral ventricle, body

Corona radiata

Cingulate gyrus

Supramarginal gyrus

Angular gyrus

Precuneus

Parietooccipital sulcus

Superior frontal gyrus

Middle frontal gyrus

Inferior frontal gyrus

Precentral gyrus

Postcentral gyrus

Superior parietal lobule

Inferior parietal lobule

Interhemispheric (longitudinal) fissure

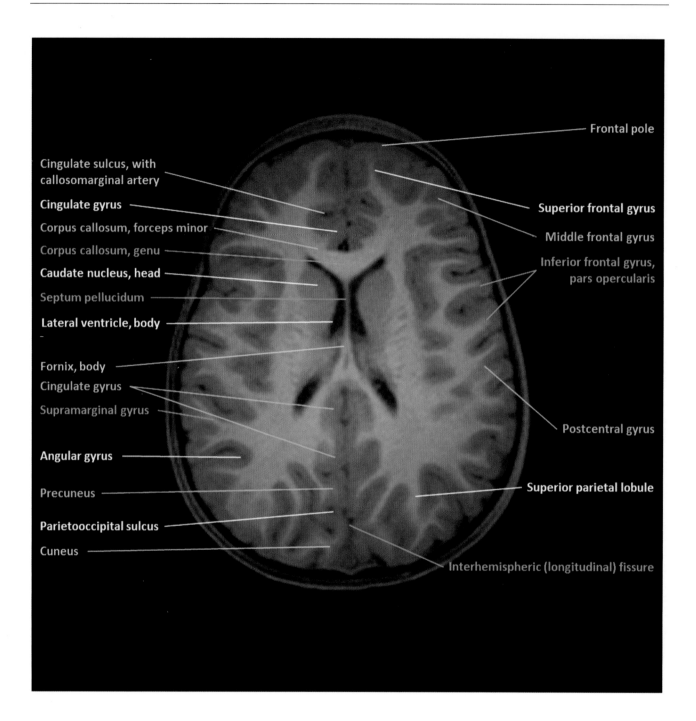

Frontal pole

Cingulate sulcus, with callosomarginal artery

Cingulate gyrus

Corpus callosum, forceps minor

Corpus callosum, genu

Caudate nucleus, head

Septum pellucidum

Lateral ventricle, body

Fornix, body

Cingulate gyrus

Supramarginal gyrus

Angular gyrus

Precuneus

Parietooccipital sulcus

Cuneus

Superior frontal gyrus

Middle frontal gyrus

Inferior frontal gyrus, pars opercularis

Postcentral gyrus

Superior parietal lobule

Interhemispheric (longitudinal) fissure

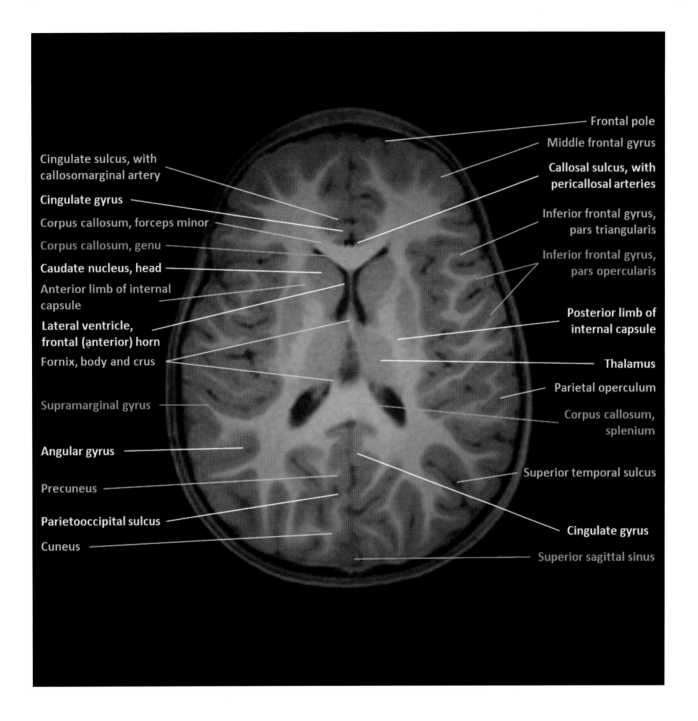

Cingulate sulcus, with
callosomarginal artery

Cingulate gyrus

Corpus callosum, forceps minor

Corpus callosum, genu

Caudate nucleus, head

Anterior limb of internal
capsule

**Lateral ventricle,
frontal (anterior) horn**

Fornix, body and crus

Supramarginal gyrus

Angular gyrus

Precuneus

Parietooccipital sulcus

Cuneus

Frontal pole

Middle frontal gyrus

**Callosal sulcus, with
pericallosal arteries**

Inferior frontal gyrus,
pars triangularis

Inferior frontal gyrus,
pars opercularis

**Posterior limb of
internal capsule**

Thalamus

Parietal operculum

Corpus callosum,
splenium

Superior temporal sulcus

Cingulate gyrus

Superior sagittal sinus

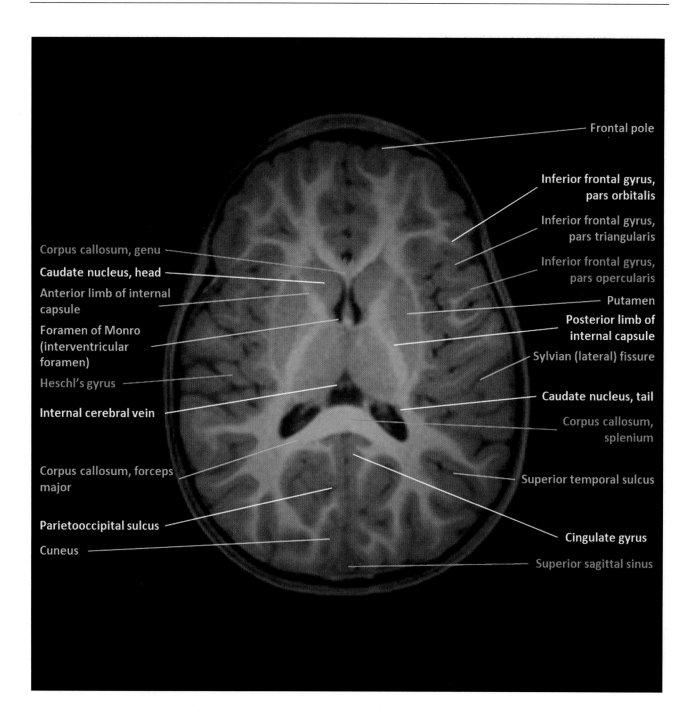

Frontal pole

**Inferior frontal gyrus,
pars orbitalis**

Inferior frontal gyrus,
pars triangularis

Inferior frontal gyrus,
pars opercularis

Putamen

**Posterior limb of
internal capsule**

Sylvian (lateral) fissure

Caudate nucleus, tail

Corpus callosum,
splenium

Superior temporal sulcus

Cingulate gyrus

Superior sagittal sinus

Corpus callosum, genu

Caudate nucleus, head

Anterior limb of internal
capsule

Foramen of Monro
(interventricular
foramen)

Heschl's gyrus

Internal cerebral vein

Corpus callosum, forceps
major

Parietooccipital sulcus

Cuneus

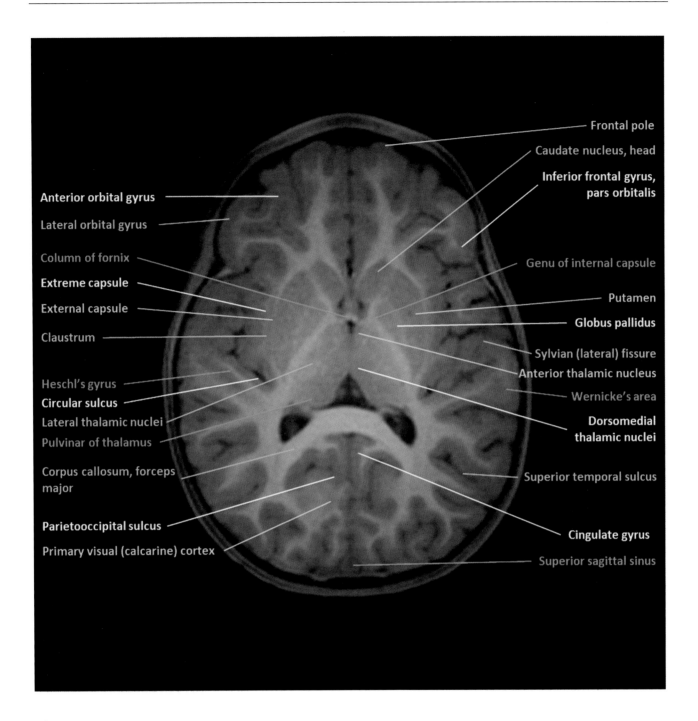

Frontal pole

Caudate nucleus, head

**Inferior frontal gyrus,
pars orbitalis**

Anterior orbital gyrus

Lateral orbital gyrus

Genu of internal capsule

Column of fornix

Extreme capsule

Putamen

External capsule

Globus pallidus

Claustrum

Sylvian (lateral) fissure

Anterior thalamic nucleus

Heschl's gyrus

Circular sulcus

Wernicke's area

Lateral thalamic nuclei

**Dorsomedial
thalamic nuclei**

Pulvinar of thalamus

Corpus callosum, forceps
major

Superior temporal sulcus

Parietooccipital sulcus

Cingulate gyrus

Primary visual (calcarine) cortex

Superior sagittal sinus

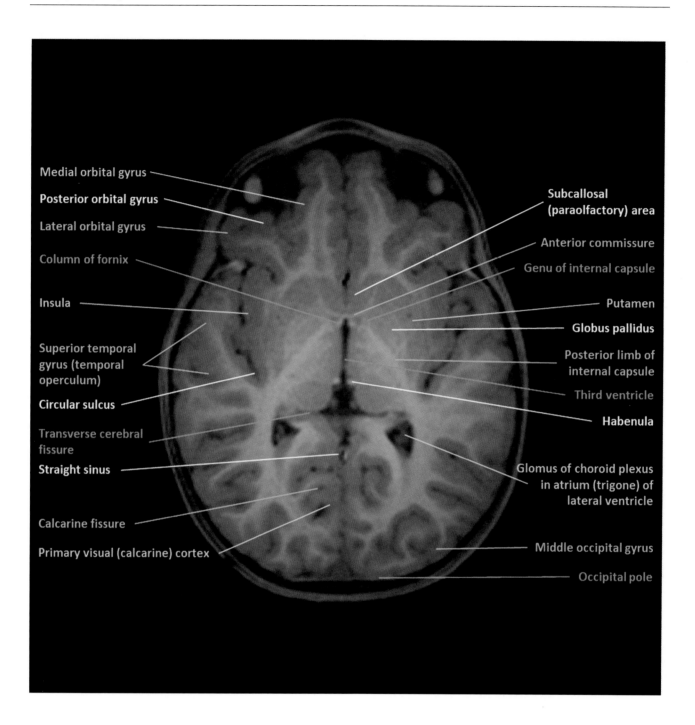

Medial orbital gyrus

Posterior orbital gyrus

Lateral orbital gyrus

Column of fornix

Insula

Superior temporal gyrus (temporal operculum)

Circular sulcus

Transverse cerebral fissure

Straight sinus

Calcarine fissure

Primary visual (calcarine) cortex

Subcallosal (paraolfactory) area

Anterior commissure

Genu of internal capsule

Putamen

Globus pallidus

Posterior limb of internal capsule

Third ventricle

Habenula

Glomus of choroid plexus in atrium (trigone) of lateral ventricle

Middle occipital gyrus

Occipital pole

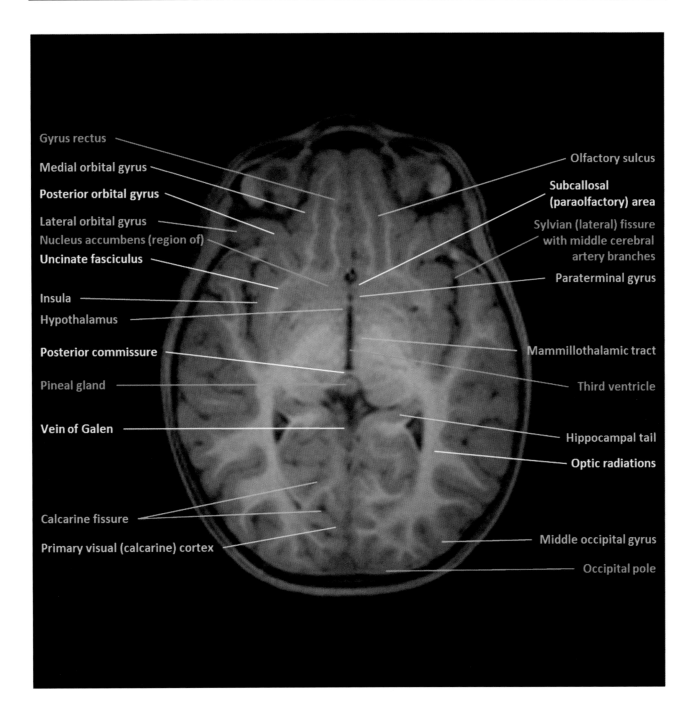

Gyrus rectus

Medial orbital gyrus

Posterior orbital gyrus

Lateral orbital gyrus

Nucleus accumbens (region of)

Uncinate fasciculus

Insula

Hypothalamus

Posterior commissure

Pineal gland

Vein of Galen

Calcarine fissure

Primary visual (calcarine) cortex

Olfactory sulcus

Subcallosal (paraolfactory) area

Sylvian (lateral) fissure with middle cerebral artery branches

Par50minal gyrus

Mammillothalamic tract

Third ventricle

Hippocampal tail

Optic radiations

Middle occipital gyrus

Occipital pole

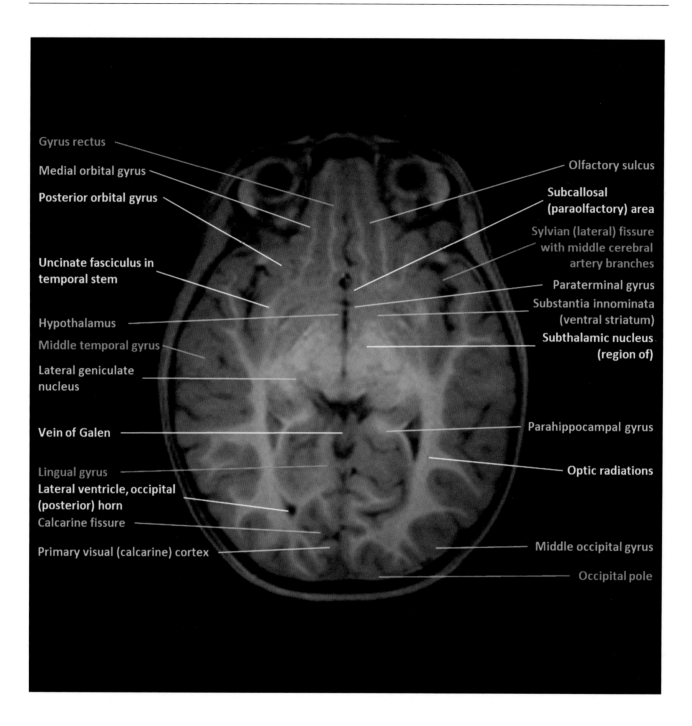

Gyrus rectus

Medial orbital gyrus

Posterior orbital gyrus

**Uncinate fasciculus in
temporal stem**

Hypothalamus

Middle temporal gyrus

Lateral geniculate
nucleus

Vein of Galen

Lingual gyrus

**Lateral ventricle, occipital
(posterior) horn**

Calcarine fissure

Primary visual (calcarine) cortex

Olfactory sulcus

**Subcallosal
(paraolfactory) area**

Sylvian (lateral) fissure
with middle cerebral
artery branches

Paraterminal gyrus

Substantia innominata
(ventral striatum)

**Subthalamic nucleus
(region of)**

Parahippocampal gyrus

Optic radiations

Middle occipital gyrus

Occipital pole

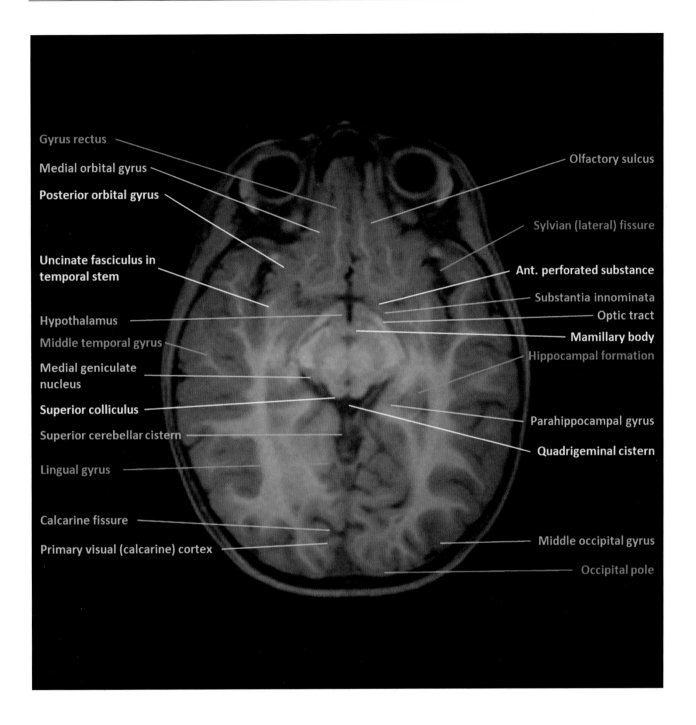

Gyrus rectus

Medial orbital gyrus

Posterior orbital gyrus

Uncinate fasciculus in temporal stem

Hypothalamus

Middle temporal gyrus

Medial geniculate nucleus

Superior colliculus

Superior cerebellar cistern

Lingual gyrus

Calcarine fissure

Primary visual (calcarine) cortex

Olfactory sulcus

Sylvian (lateral) fissure

Ant. perforated substance

Substantia innominata

Optic tract

Mamillary body

Hippocampal formation

Parahippocampal gyrus

Quadrigeminal cistern

Middle occipital gyrus

Occipital pole

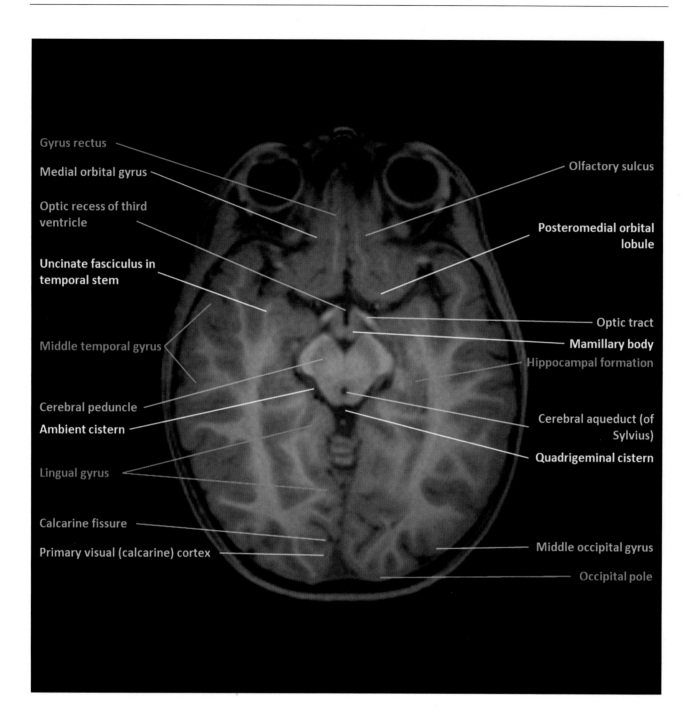

Gyrus rectus

Medial orbital gyrus

Optic recess of third ventricle

Uncinate fasciculus in temporal stem

Middle temporal gyrus

Cerebral peduncle

Ambient cistern

Lingual gyrus

Calcarine fissure

Primary visual (calcarine) cortex

Olfactory sulcus

Posteromedial orbital lobule

Optic tract

Mamillary body

Hippocampal formation

Cerebral aqueduct (of Sylvius)

Quadrigeminal cistern

Middle occipital gyrus

Occipital pole

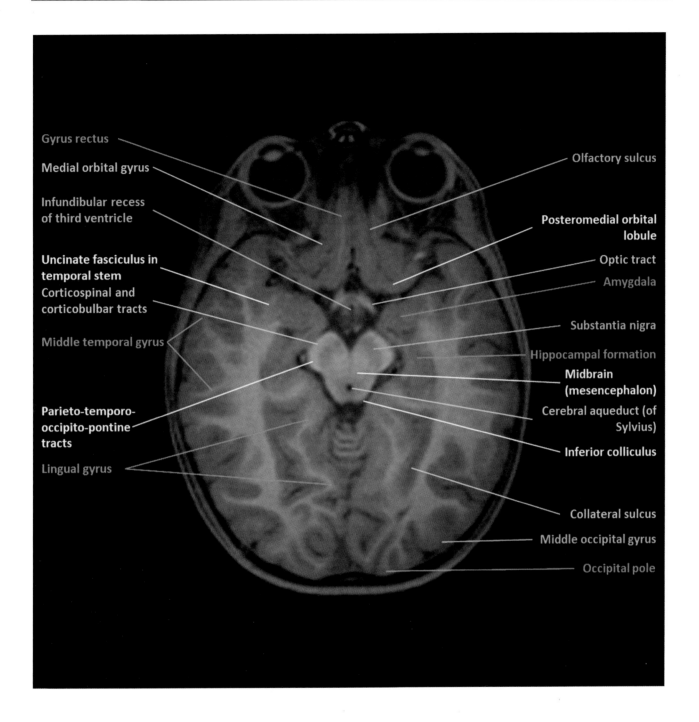

Gyrus rectus

Medial orbital gyrus

Infundibular recess
of third ventricle

**Uncinate fasciculus in
temporal stem**
Corticospinal and
corticobulbar tracts

Middle temporal gyrus

**Parieto-temporo-
occipito-pontine
tracts**

Lingual gyrus

Olfactory sulcus

**Posteromedial orbital
lobule**

Optic tract

Amygdala

Substantia nigra

Hippocampal formation

**Midbrain
(mesencephalon)**

Cerebral aqueduct (of
Sylvius)

Inferior colliculus

Collateral sulcus

Middle occipital gyrus

Occipital pole

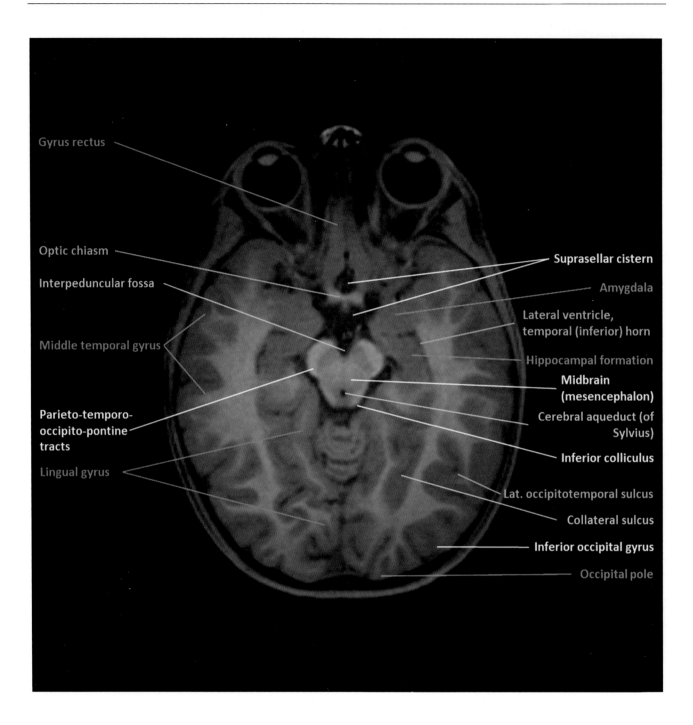

Gyrus rectus

Optic chiasm

Interpeduncular fossa

Middle temporal gyrus

**Parieto-temporo-
occipito-pontine
tracts**

Lingual gyrus

Suprasellar cistern

Amygdala

Lateral ventricle,
temporal (inferior) horn

Hippocampal formation

**Midbrain
(mesencephalon)**

Cerebral aqueduct (of
Sylvius)

Inferior colliculus

Lat. occipitotemporal sulcus

Collateral sulcus

Inferior occipital gyrus

Occipital pole

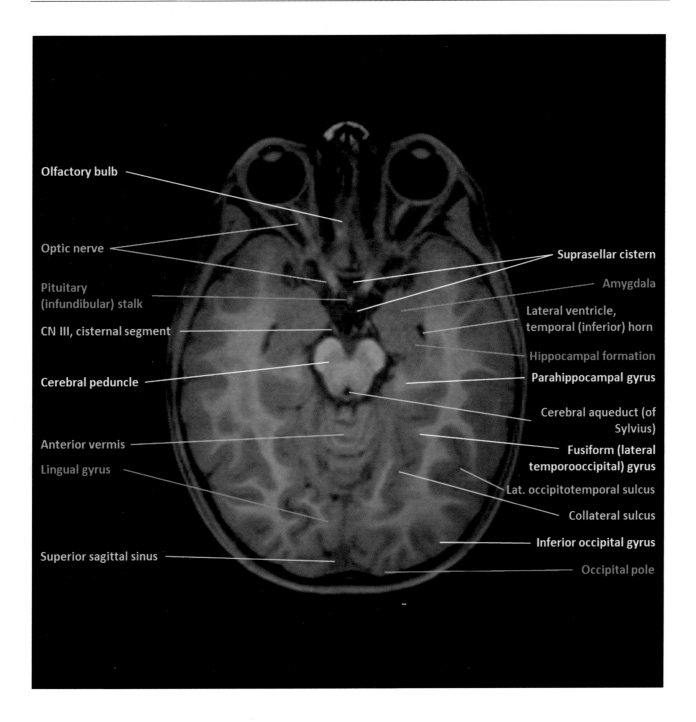

Olfactory bulb

Optic nerve

Pituitary (infundibular) stalk

CN III, cisternal segment

Cerebral peduncle

Anterior vermis

Lingual gyrus

Superior sagittal sinus

Suprasellar cistern

Amygdala

Lateral ventricle, temporal (inferior) horn

Hippocampal formation

Parahippocampal gyrus

Cerebral aqueduct (of Sylvius)

Fusiform (lateral temporooccipital) gyrus

Lat. occipitotemporal sulcus

Collateral sulcus

Inferior occipital gyrus

Occipital pole

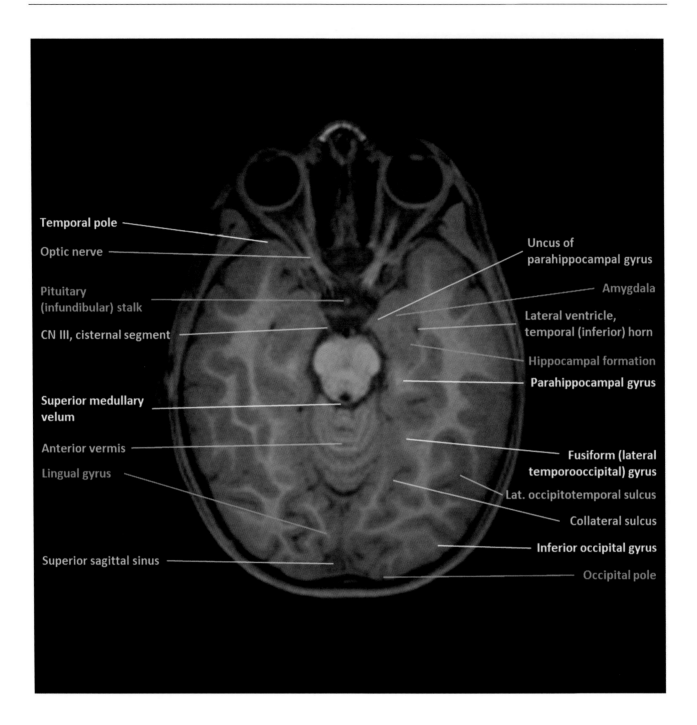

Temporal pole

Optic nerve

Pituitary (infundibular) stalk

CN III, cisternal segment

Superior medullary velum

Anterior vermis

Lingual gyrus

Superior sagittal sinus

Uncus of parahippocampal gyrus

Amygdala

Lateral ventricle, temporal (inferior) horn

Hippocampal formation

Parahippocampal gyrus

Fusiform (lateral temporooccipital) gyrus

Lat. occipitotemporal sulcus

Collateral sulcus

Inferior occipital gyrus

Occipital pole

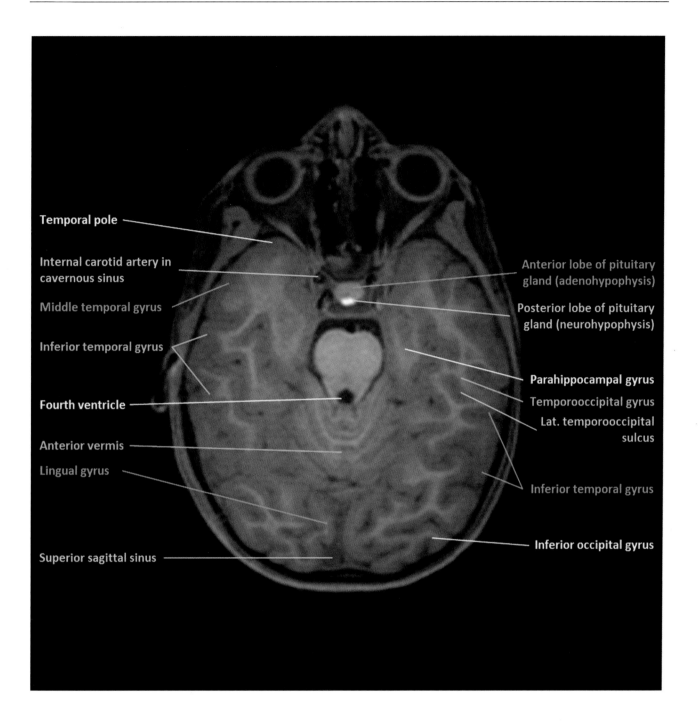

Temporal pole

Internal carotid artery in cavernous sinus

Middle temporal gyrus

Inferior temporal gyrus

Fourth ventricle

Anterior vermis

Lingual gyrus

Superior sagittal sinus

Anterior lobe of pituitary gland (adenohypophysis)

Posterior lobe of pituitary gland (neurohypophysis)

Parahippocampal gyrus

Temporooccipital gyrus

Lat. temporooccipital sulcus

Inferior temporal gyrus

Inferior occipital gyrus

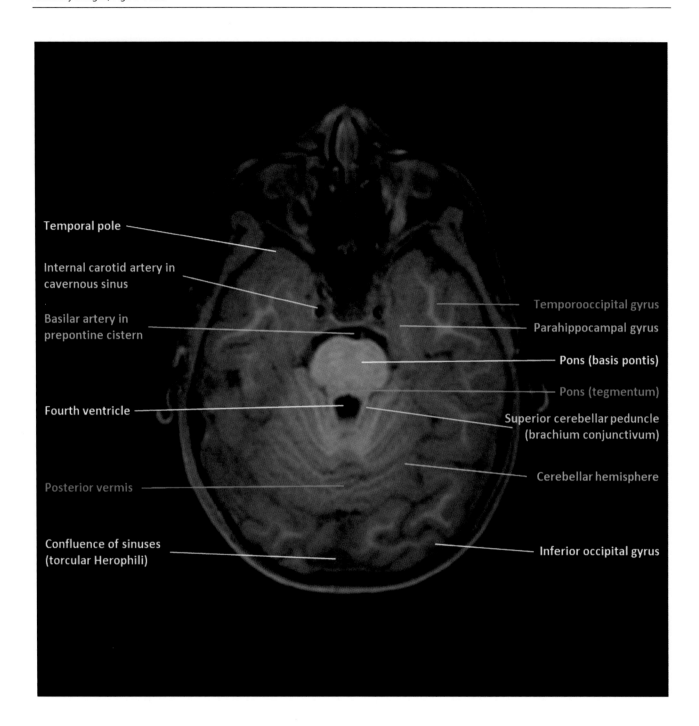

Temporal pole

Internal carotid artery in
cavernous sinus

Basilar artery in
prepontine cistern

Fourth ventricle

Posterior vermis

Confluence of sinuses
(torcular Herophili)

Temporooccipital gyrus

Parahippocampal gyrus

Pons (basis pontis)

Pons (tegmentum)

Superior cerebellar peduncle
(brachium conjunctivum)

Cerebellar hemisphere

Inferior occipital gyrus

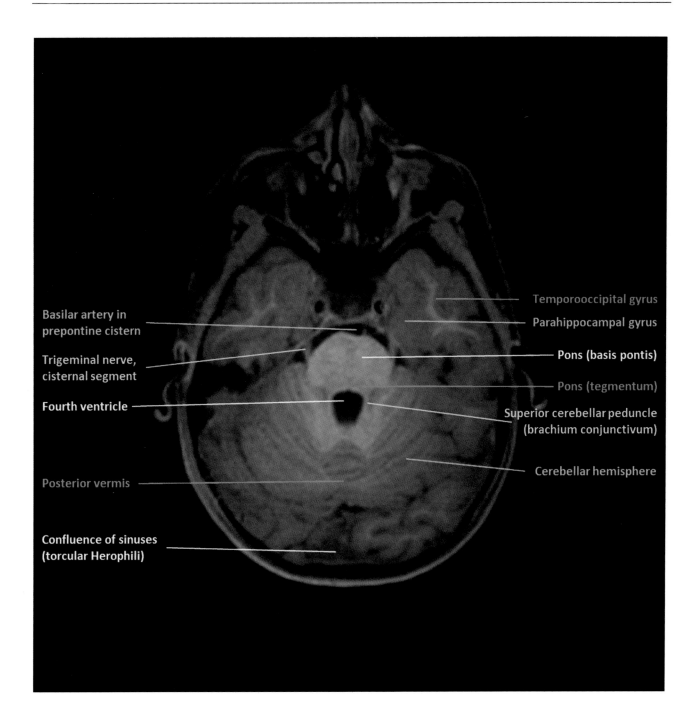

Basilar artery in
prepontine cistern

Trigeminal nerve,
cisternal segment

Fourth ventricle

Posterior vermis

Confluence of sinuses
(torcular Herophili)

Temporooccipital gyrus

Parahippocampal gyrus

Pons (basis pontis)

Pons (tegmentum)

Superior cerebellar peduncle
(brachium conjunctivum)

Cerebellar hemisphere

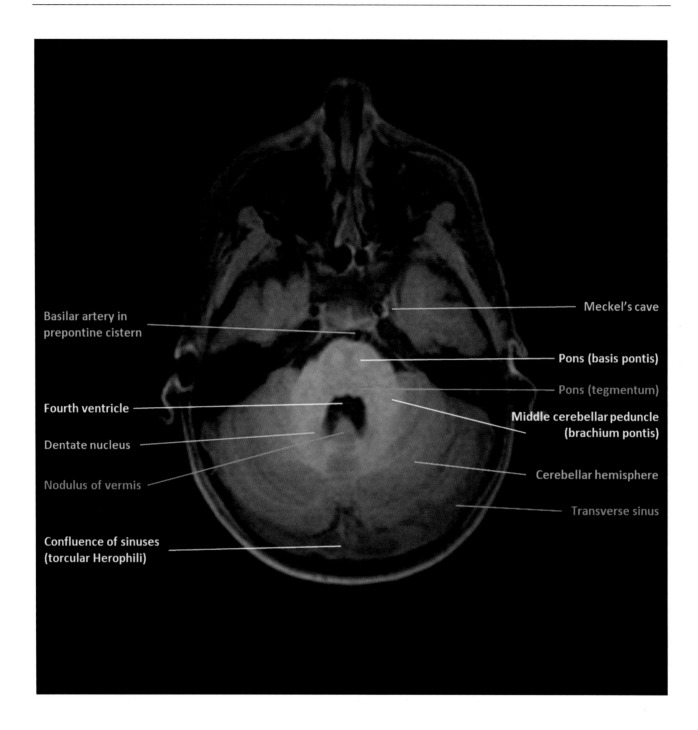

Basilar artery in
prepontine cistern

Meckel's cave

Pons (basis pontis)

Pons (tegmentum)

Fourth ventricle

**Middle cerebellar peduncle
(brachium pontis)**

Dentate nucleus

Cerebellar hemisphere

Nodulus of vermis

Transverse sinus

**Confluence of sinuses
(torcular Herophili)**

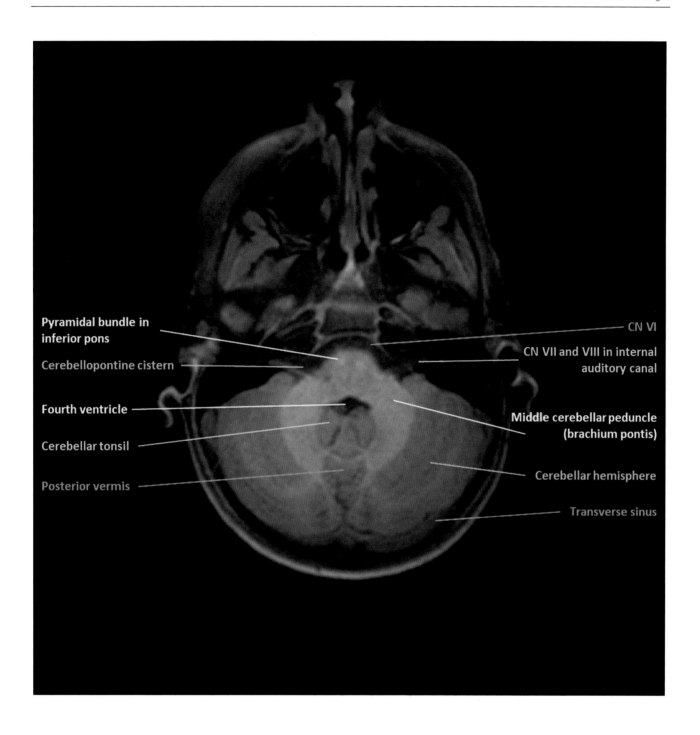

Pyramidal bundle in
inferior pons

Cerebellopontine cistern

Fourth ventricle

Cerebellar tonsil

Posterior vermis

CN VI

CN VII and VIII in internal
auditory canal

Middle cerebellar peduncle
(brachium pontis)

Cerebellar hemisphere

Transverse sinus

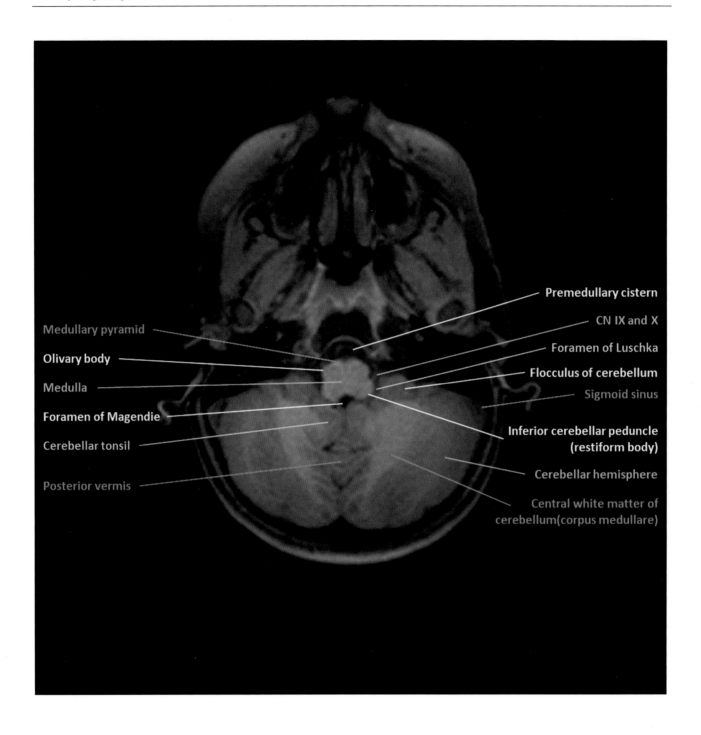

Medullary pyramid

Olivary body

Medulla

Foramen of Magendie

Cerebellar tonsil

Posterior vermis

Premedullary cistern

CN IX and X

Foramen of Luschka

Flocculus of cerebellum

Sigmoid sinus

Inferior cerebellar peduncle (restiform body)

Cerebellar hemisphere

Central white matter of cerebellum(corpus medullare)

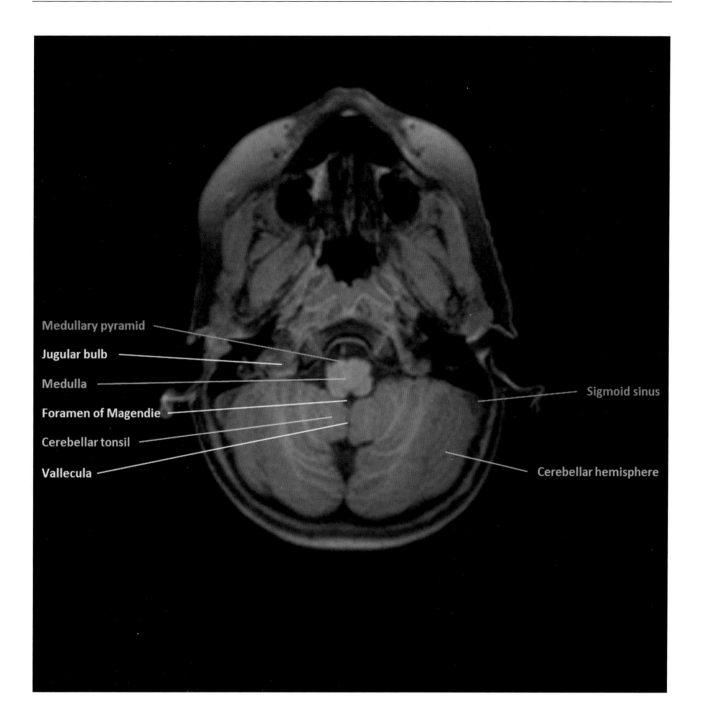

Medullary pyramid

Jugular bulb

Medulla

Foramen of Magendie

Cerebellar tonsil

Vallecula

Sigmoid sinus

Cerebellar hemisphere

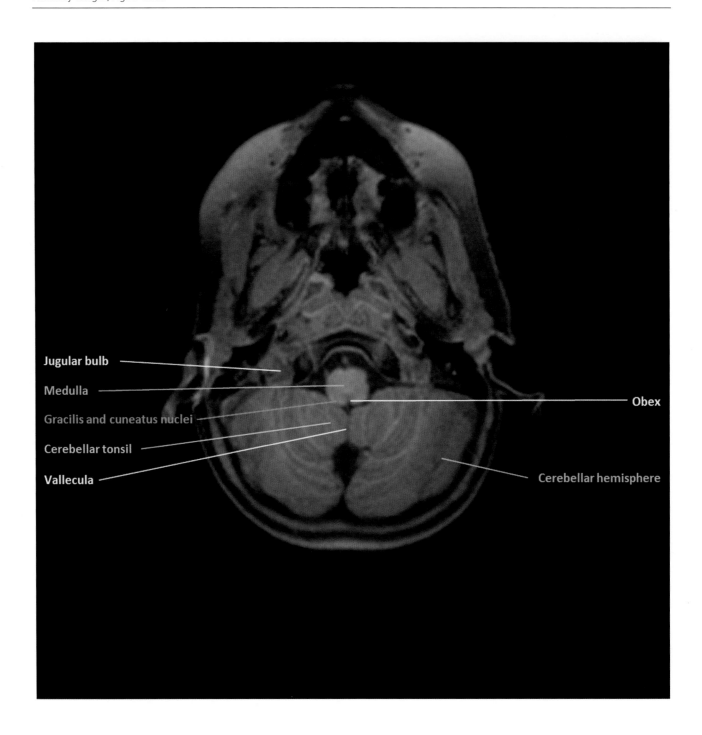

Jugular bulb

Medulla

Gracilis and cuneatus nuclei

Cerebellar tonsil

Vallecula

Obex

Cerebellar hemisphere

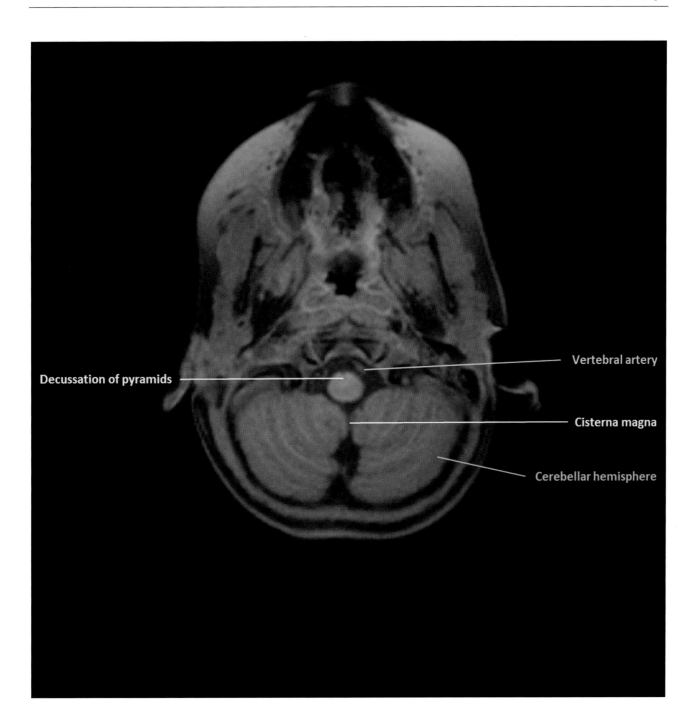

Decussation of pyramids

Vertebral artery

Cisterna magna

Cerebellar hemisphere

Coronal T1 Images

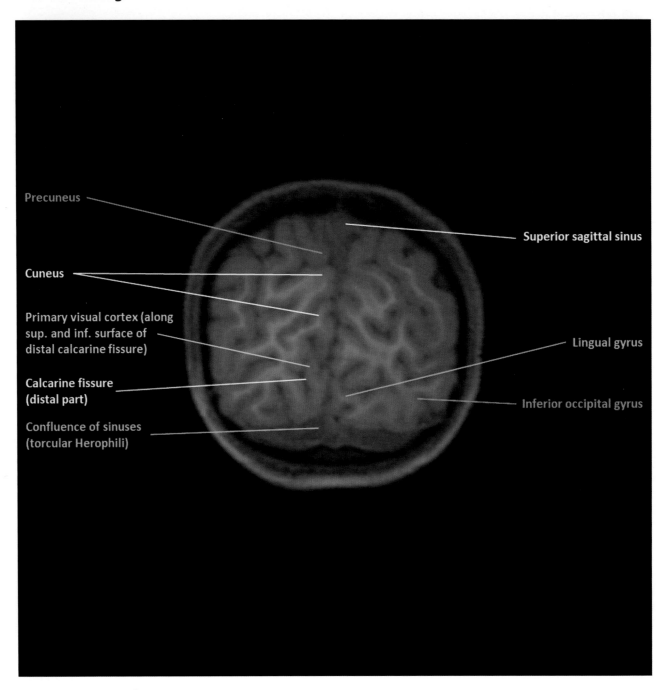

Precuneus

Superior sagittal sinus

Cuneus

Primary visual cortex (along sup. and inf. surface of distal calcarine fissure)

Lingual gyrus

Calcarine fissure (distal part)

Inferior occipital gyrus

Confluence of sinuses (torcular Herophili)

ANATOMY Coronal T1 Images 1–22

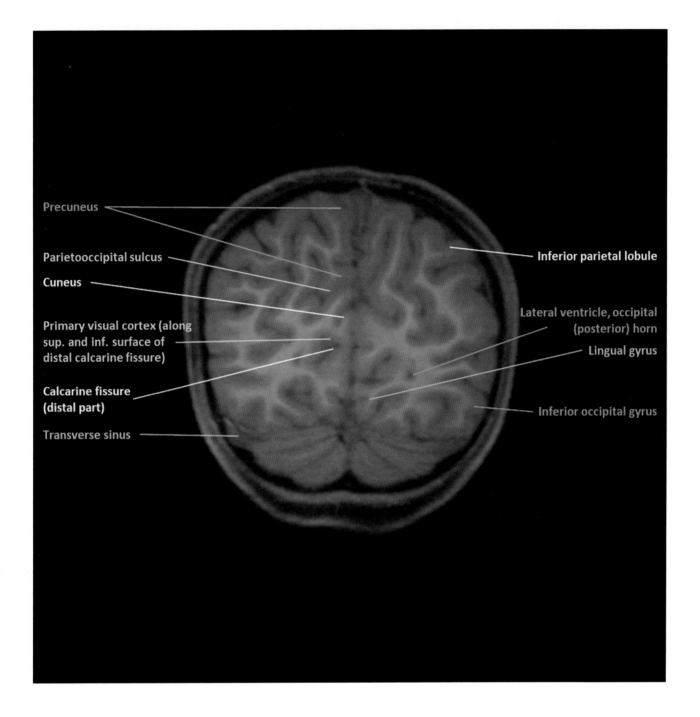

Precuneus

Parietooccipital sulcus

Cuneus

Primary visual cortex (along sup. and inf. surface of distal calcarine fissure)

Calcarine fissure (distal part)

Transverse sinus

Inferior parietal lobule

Lateral ventricle, occipital (posterior) horn

Lingual gyrus

Inferior occipital gyrus

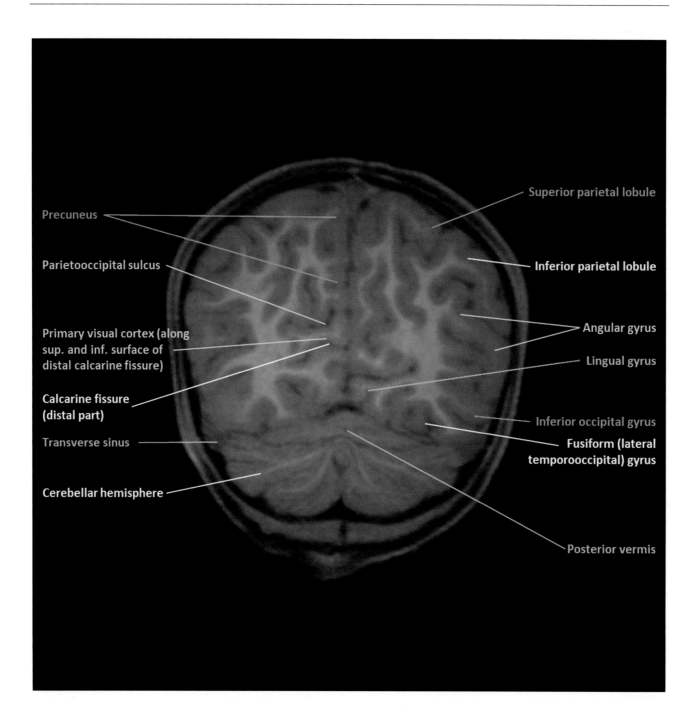

Precuneus

Parietooccipital sulcus

Primary visual cortex (along sup. and inf. surface of distal calcarine fissure)

Calcarine fissure (distal part)

Transverse sinus

Cerebellar hemisphere

Superior parietal lobule

Inferior parietal lobule

Angular gyrus

Lingual gyrus

Inferior occipital gyrus

Fusiform (lateral temporooccipital) gyrus

Posterior vermis

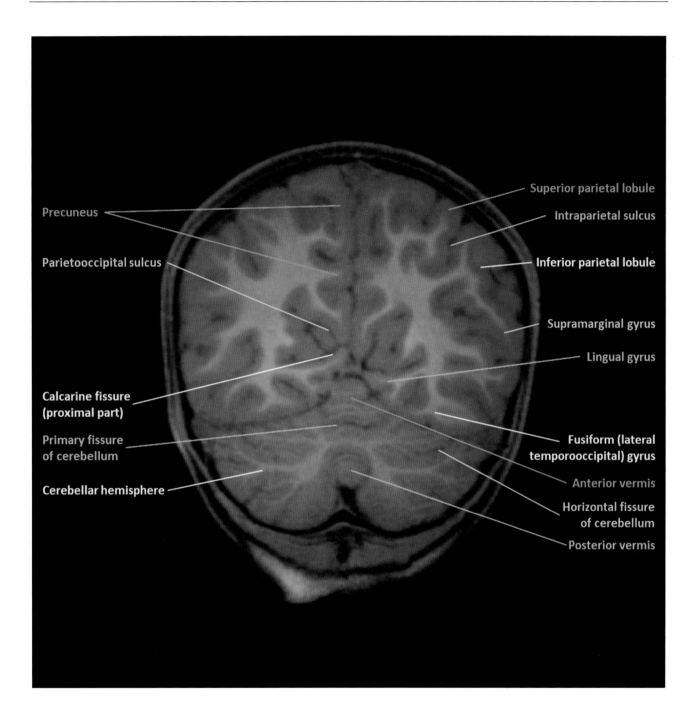

Precuneus

Parietooccipital sulcus

**Calcarine fissure
(proximal part)**

Primary fissure
of cerebellum

Cerebellar hemisphere

Superior parietal lobule

Intraparietal sulcus

Inferior parietal lobule

Supramarginal gyrus

Lingual gyrus

**Fusiform (lateral
temporooccipital) gyrus**

Anterior vermis

Horizontal fissure
of cerebellum

Posterior vermis

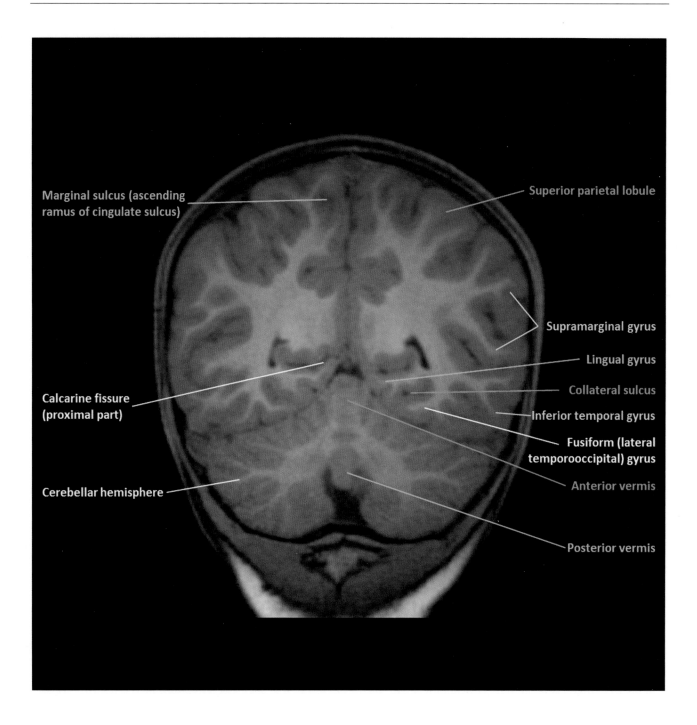

Marginal sulcus (ascending ramus of cingulate sulcus)

Superior parietal lobule

Supramarginal gyrus

Lingual gyrus

Collateral sulcus

Calcarine fissure (proximal part)

Inferior temporal gyrus

Fusiform (lateral temporooccipital) gyrus

Anterior vermis

Cerebellar hemisphere

Posterior vermis

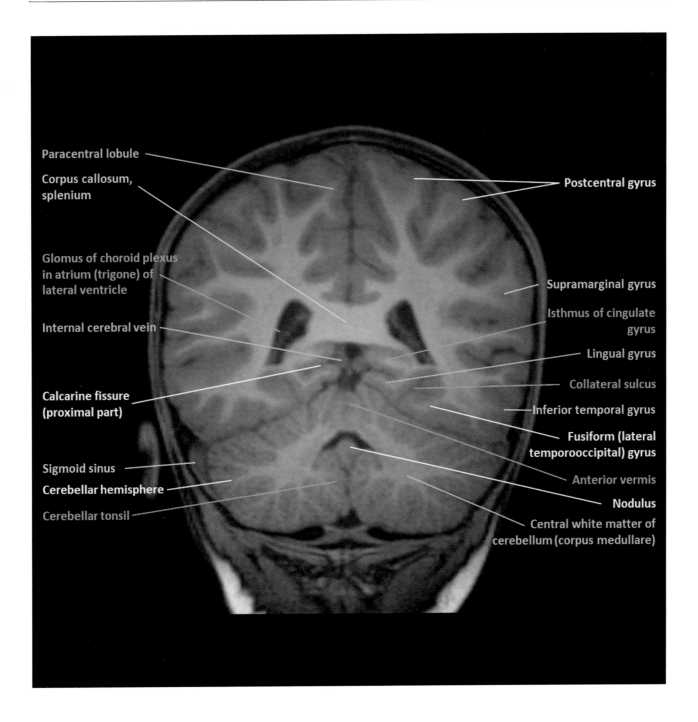

Paracentral lobule

Corpus callosum, splenium

Glomus of choroid plexus in atrium (trigone) of lateral ventricle

Internal cerebral vein

Calcarine fissure (proximal part)

Sigmoid sinus

Cerebellar hemisphere

Cerebellar tonsil

Postcentral gyrus

Supramarginal gyrus

Isthmus of cingulate gyrus

Lingual gyrus

Collateral sulcus

Inferior temporal gyrus

Fusiform (lateral temporooccipital) gyrus

Anterior vermis

Nodulus

Central white matter of cerebellum (corpus medullare)

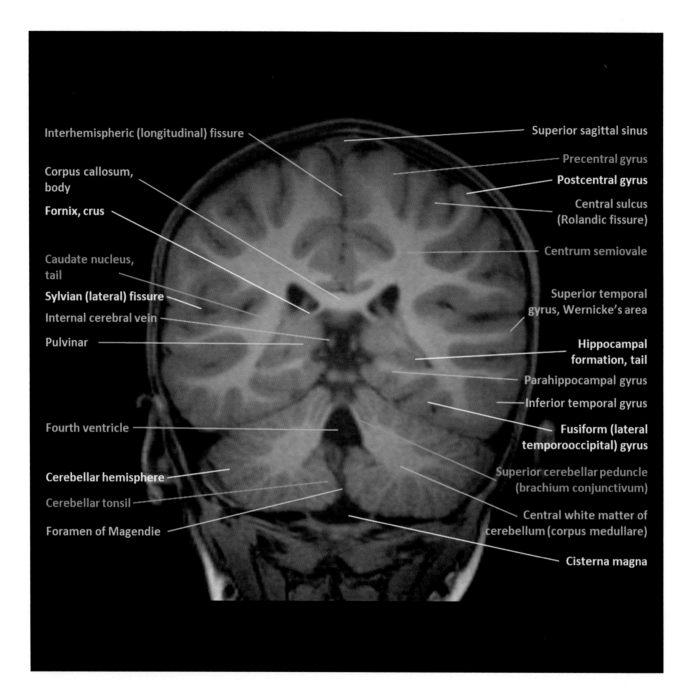

Interhemispheric (longitudinal) fissure

Corpus callosum, body

Fornix, crus

Caudate nucleus, tail

Sylvian (lateral) fissure

Internal cerebral vein

Pulvinar

Fourth ventricle

Cerebellar hemisphere

Cerebellar tonsil

Foramen of Magendie

Superior sagittal sinus

Precentral gyrus

Postcentral gyrus

Central sulcus (Rolandic fissure)

Centrum semiovale

Superior temporal gyrus, Wernicke's area

Hippocampal formation, tail

Parahippocampal gyrus

Inferior temporal gyrus

Fusiform (lateral temporooccipital) gyrus

Superior cerebellar peduncle (brachium conjunctivum)

Central white matter of cerebellum (corpus medullare)

Cisterna magna

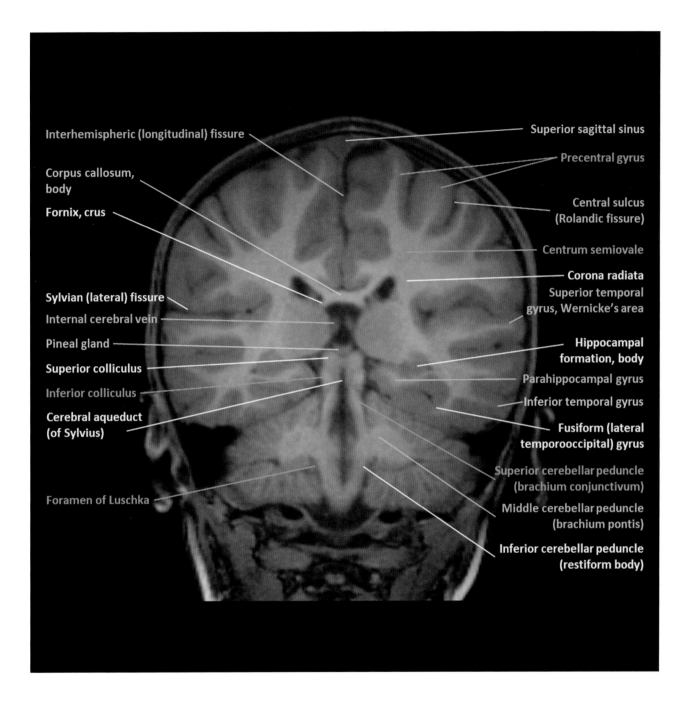

Interhemispheric (longitudinal) fissure

Corpus callosum, body

Fornix, crus

Sylvian (lateral) fissure

Internal cerebral vein

Pineal gland

Superior colliculus

Inferior colliculus

Cerebral aqueduct (of Sylvius)

Foramen of Luschka

Superior sagittal sinus

Precentral gyrus

Central sulcus (Rolandic fissure)

Centrum semiovale

Corona radiata

Superior temporal gyrus, Wernicke's area

Hippocampal formation, body

Parahippocampal gyrus

Inferior temporal gyrus

Fusiform (lateral temporooccipital) gyrus

Superior cerebellar peduncle (brachium conjunctivum)

Middle cerebellar peduncle (brachium pontis)

Inferior cerebellar peduncle (restiform body)

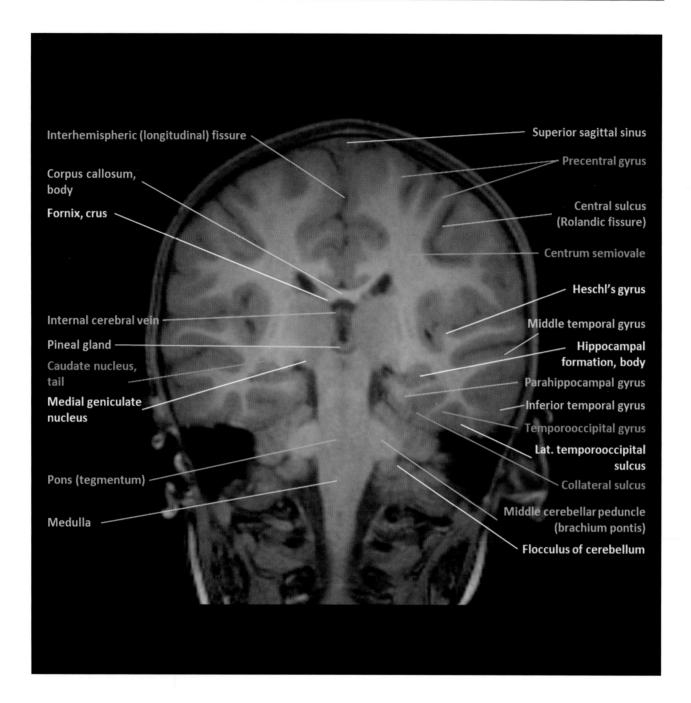

Interhemispheric (longitudinal) fissure

Corpus callosum, body

Fornix, crus

Internal cerebral vein

Pineal gland

Caudate nucleus, tail

Medial geniculate nucleus

Pons (tegmentum)

Medulla

Superior sagittal sinus

Precentral gyrus

Central sulcus (Rolandic fissure)

Centrum semiovale

Heschl's gyrus

Middle temporal gyrus

Hippocampal formation, body

Parahippocampal gyrus

Inferior temporal gyrus

Temporooccipital gyrus

Lat. temporooccipital sulcus

Collateral sulcus

Middle cerebellar peduncle (brachium pontis)

Flocculus of cerebellum

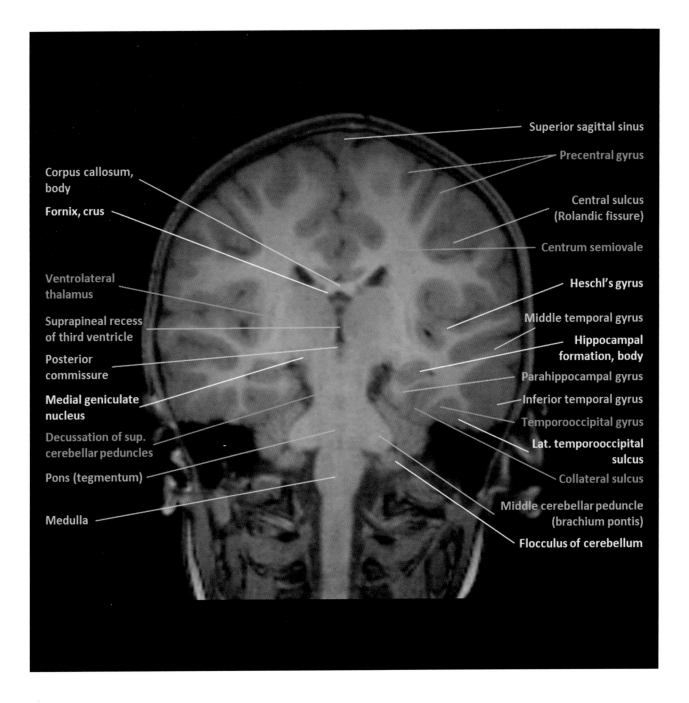

Superior sagittal sinus

Precentral gyrus

Central sulcus
(Rolandic fissure)

Centrum semiovale

Heschl's gyrus

Middle temporal gyrus

Hippocampal
formation, body

Parahippocampal gyrus

Inferior temporal gyrus

Temporooccipital gyrus

Lat. temporooccipital
sulcus

Collateral sulcus

Middle cerebellar peduncle
(brachium pontis)

Flocculus of cerebellum

Corpus callosum,
body

Fornix, crus

Ventrolateral
thalamus

Suprapineal recess
of third ventricle

Posterior
commissure

Medial geniculate
nucleus

Decussation of sup.
cerebellar peduncles

Pons (tegmentum)

Medulla

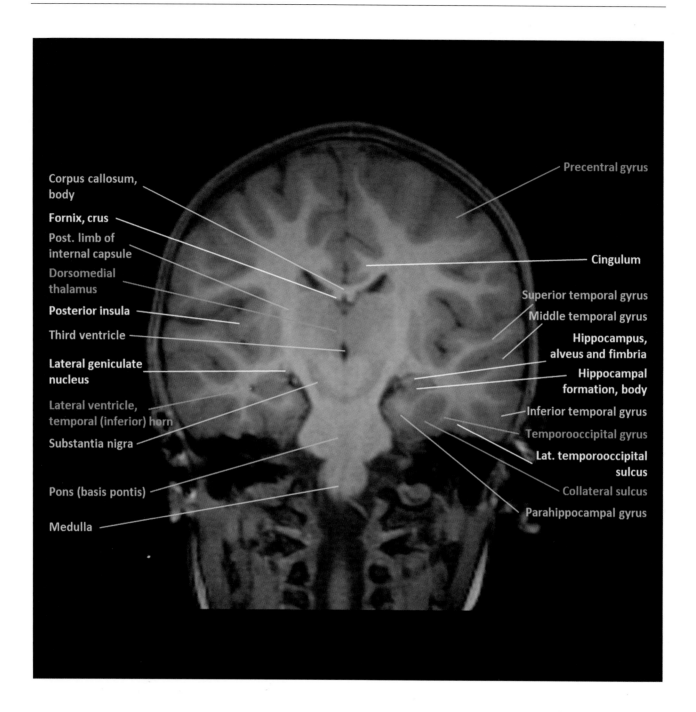

Corpus callosum, body

Fornix, crus

Post. limb of internal capsule

Dorsomedial thalamus

Posterior insula

Third ventricle

Lateral geniculate nucleus

Lateral ventricle, temporal (inferior) horn

Substantia nigra

Pons (basis pontis)

Medulla

Precentral gyrus

Cingulum

Superior temporal gyrus

Middle temporal gyrus

Hippocampus, alveus and fimbria

Hippocampal formation, body

Inferior temporal gyrus

Temporooccipital gyrus

Lat. temporooccipital sulcus

Collateral sulcus

Parahippocampal gyrus

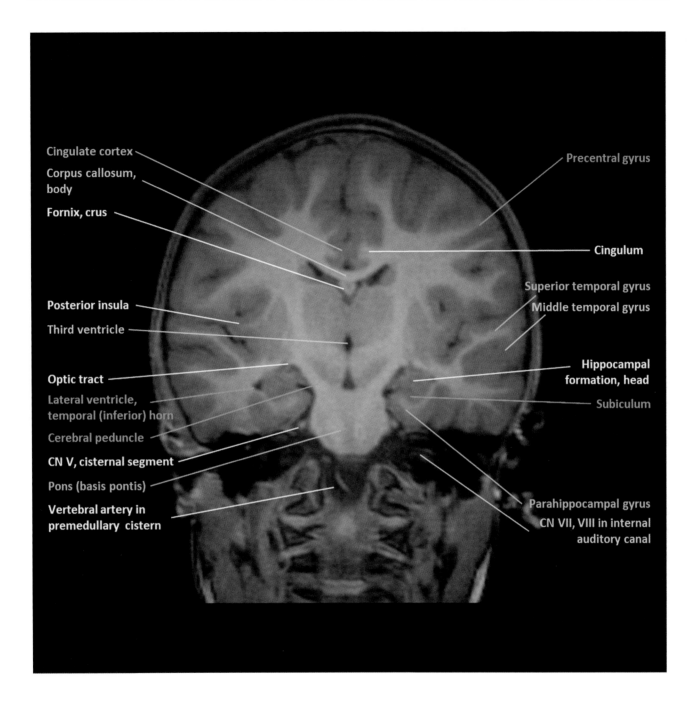

Cingulate cortex

Corpus callosum, body

Fornix, crus

Posterior insula

Third ventricle

Optic tract

Lateral ventricle, temporal (inferior) horn

Cerebral peduncle

CN V, cisternal segment

Pons (basis pontis)

Vertebral artery in premedullary cistern

Precentral gyrus

Cingulum

Superior temporal gyrus

Middle temporal gyrus

Hippocampal formation, head

Subiculum

Parahippocampal gyrus

CN VII, VIII in internal auditory canal

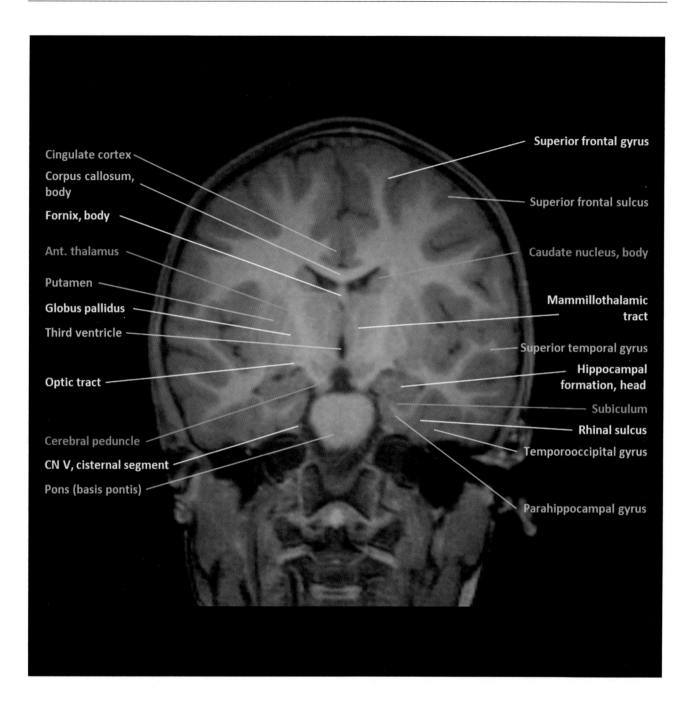

Cingulate cortex

Corpus callosum, body

Fornix, body

Ant. thalamus

Putamen

Globus pallidus

Third ventricle

Optic tract

Cerebral peduncle

CN V, cisternal segment

Pons (basis pontis)

Superior frontal gyrus

Superior frontal sulcus

Caudate nucleus, body

Mammillothalamic tract

Superior temporal gyrus

Hippocampal formation, head

Subiculum

Rhinal sulcus

Temporooccipital gyrus

Parahippocampal gyrus

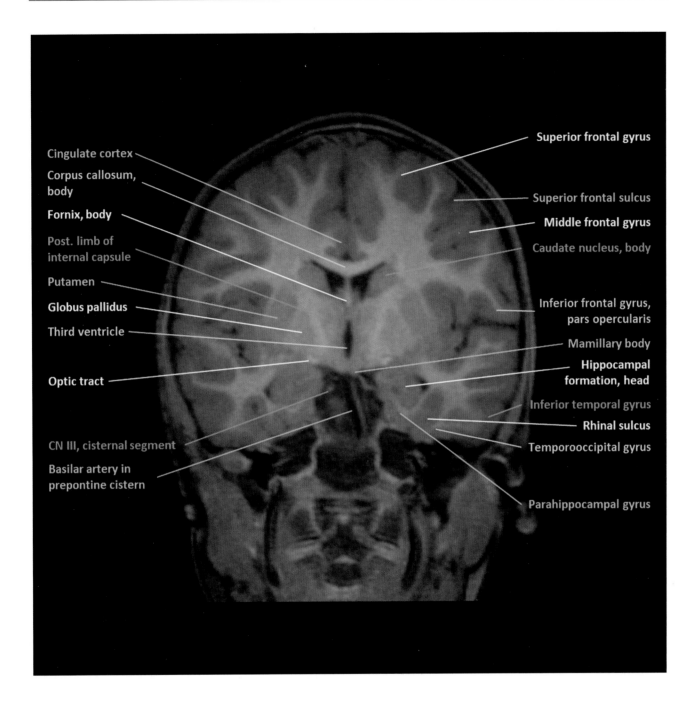

Cingulate cortex

Corpus callosum, body

Fornix, body

Post. limb of internal capsule

Putamen

Globus pallidus

Third ventricle

Optic tract

CN III, cisternal segment

Basilar artery in prepontine cistern

Superior frontal gyrus

Superior frontal sulcus

Middle frontal gyrus

Caudate nucleus, body

Inferior frontal gyrus, pars opercularis

Mamillary body

Hippocampal formation, head

Inferior temporal gyrus

Rhinal sulcus

Temporooccipital gyrus

Parahippocampal gyrus

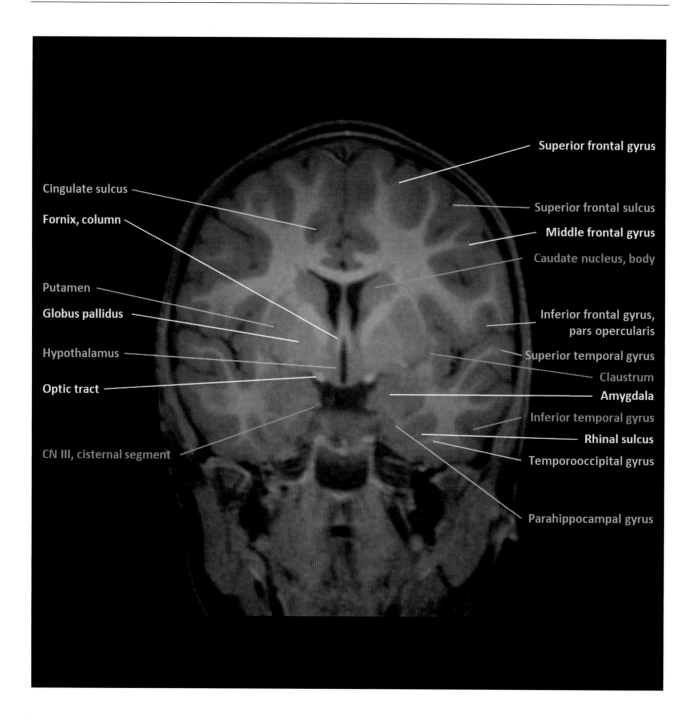

Cingulate sulcus

Fornix, column

Putamen

Globus pallidus

Hypothalamus

Optic tract

CN III, cisternal segment

Superior frontal gyrus

Superior frontal sulcus

Middle frontal gyrus

Caudate nucleus, body

Inferior frontal gyrus,
pars opercularis

Superior temporal gyrus

Claustrum

Amygdala

Inferior temporal gyrus

Rhinal sulcus

Temporooccipital gyrus

Parahippocampal gyrus

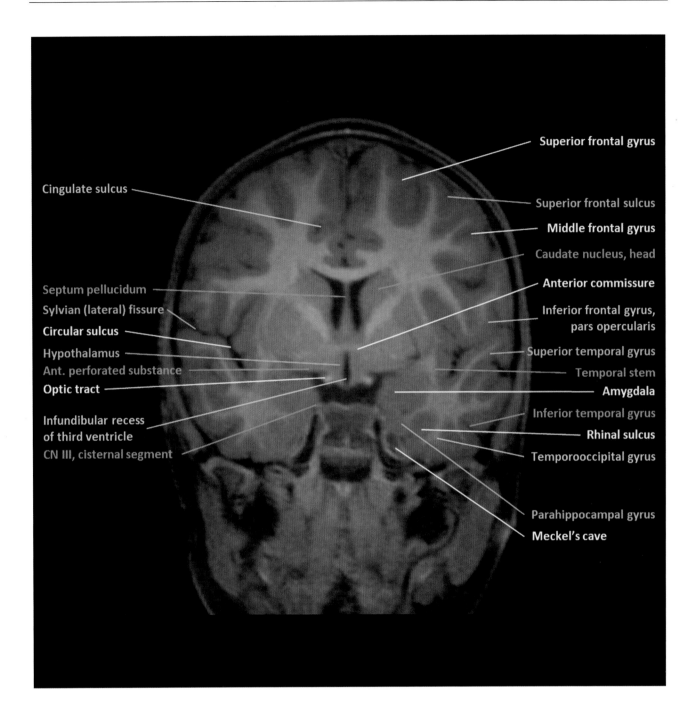

Cingulate sulcus

Septum pellucidum
Sylvian (lateral) fissure
Circular sulcus
Hypothalamus
Ant. perforated substance
Optic tract

Infundibular recess
of third ventricle
CN III, cisternal segment

Superior frontal gyrus

Superior frontal sulcus
Middle frontal gyrus
Caudate nucleus, head
Anterior commissure
Inferior frontal gyrus,
pars opercularis
Superior temporal gyrus
Temporal stem
Amygdala
Inferior temporal gyrus
Rhinal sulcus
Temporooccipital gyrus

Parahippocampal gyrus
Meckel's cave

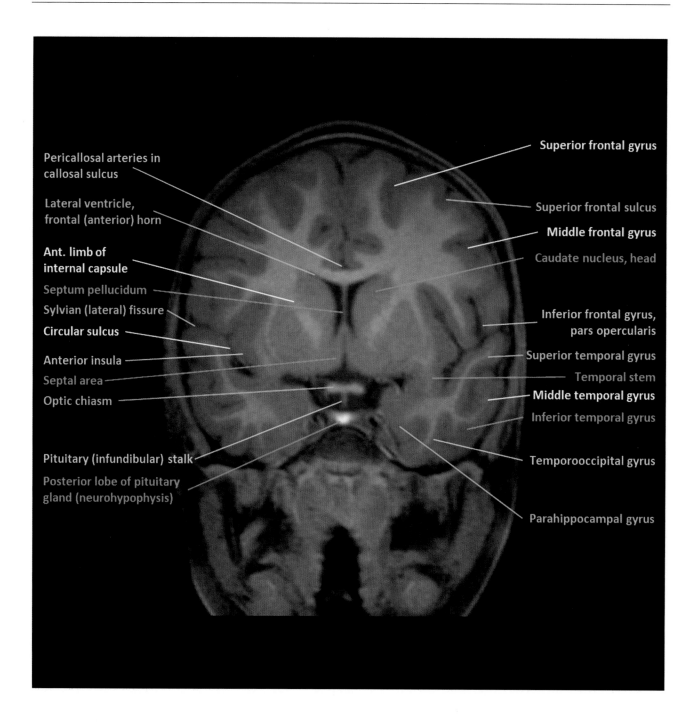

Pericallosal arteries in
callosal sulcus

Lateral ventricle,
frontal (anterior) horn

**Ant. limb of
internal capsule**

Septum pellucidum

Sylvian (lateral) fissure

Circular sulcus

Anterior insula

Septal area

Optic chiasm

Pituitary (infundibular) stalk

Posterior lobe of pituitary
gland (neurohypophysis)

Superior frontal gyrus

Superior frontal sulcus

Middle frontal gyrus

Caudate nucleus, head

Inferior frontal gyrus,
pars opercularis

Superior temporal gyrus

Temporal stem

Middle temporal gyrus

Inferior temporal gyrus

Temporooccipital gyrus

Parahippocampal gyrus

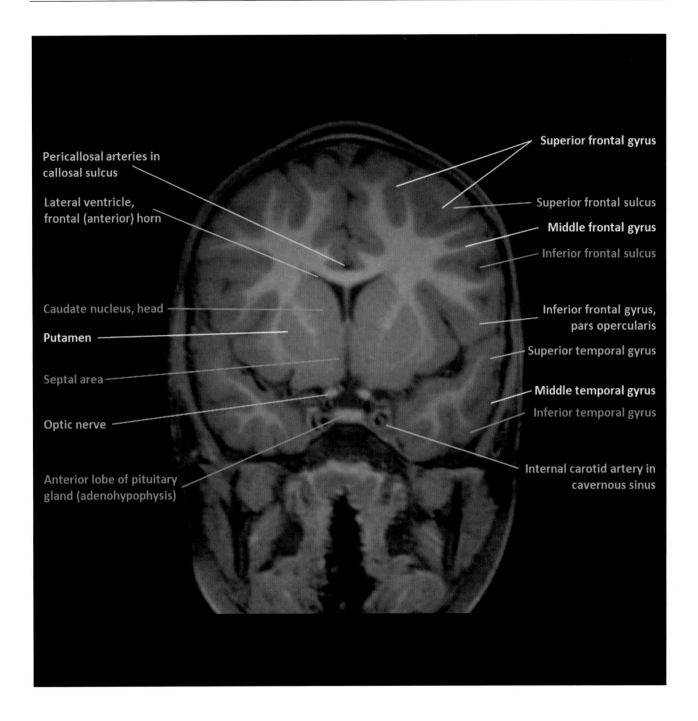

Pericallosal arteries in callosal sulcus

Lateral ventricle, frontal (anterior) horn

Caudate nucleus, head

Putamen

Septal area

Optic nerve

Anterior lobe of pituitary gland (adenohypophysis)

Superior frontal gyrus

Superior frontal sulcus

Middle frontal gyrus

Inferior frontal sulcus

Inferior frontal gyrus, pars opercularis

Superior temporal gyrus

Middle temporal gyrus

Inferior temporal gyrus

Internal carotid artery in cavernous sinus

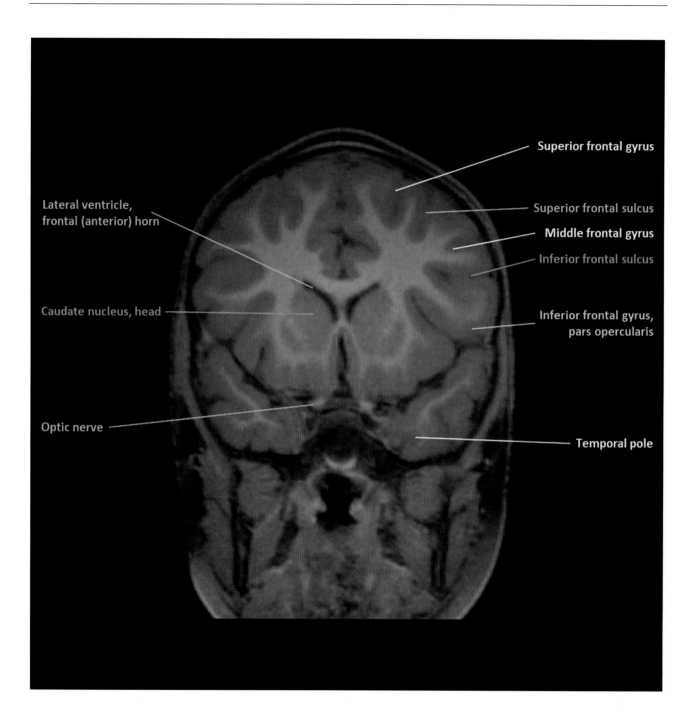

Superior frontal gyrus

Superior frontal sulcus

Middle frontal gyrus

Inferior frontal sulcus

Inferior frontal gyrus, pars opercularis

Temporal pole

Lateral ventricle, frontal (anterior) horn

Caudate nucleus, head

Optic nerve

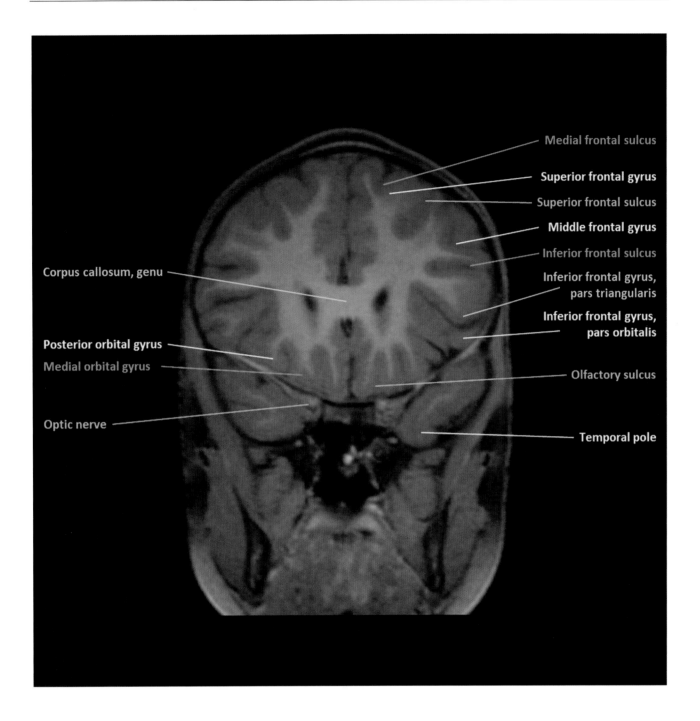

Medial frontal sulcus

Superior frontal gyrus

Superior frontal sulcus

Middle frontal gyrus

Inferior frontal sulcus

Inferior frontal gyrus, pars triangularis

Inferior frontal gyrus, pars orbitalis

Olfactory sulcus

Temporal pole

Corpus callosum, genu

Posterior orbital gyrus

Medial orbital gyrus

Optic nerve

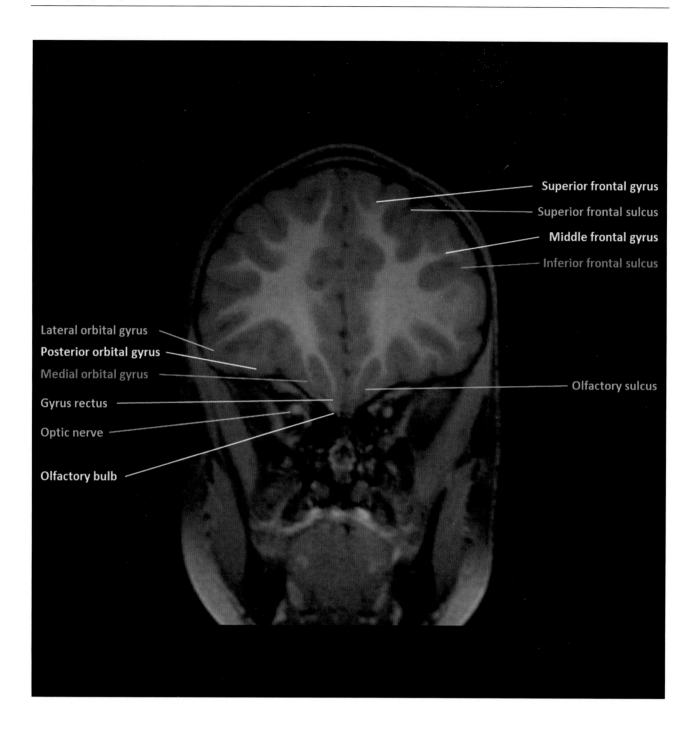

Superior frontal gyrus

Superior frontal sulcus

Middle frontal gyrus

Inferior frontal sulcus

Lateral orbital gyrus

Posterior orbital gyrus

Medial orbital gyrus

Olfactory sulcus

Gyrus rectus

Optic nerve

Olfactory bulb

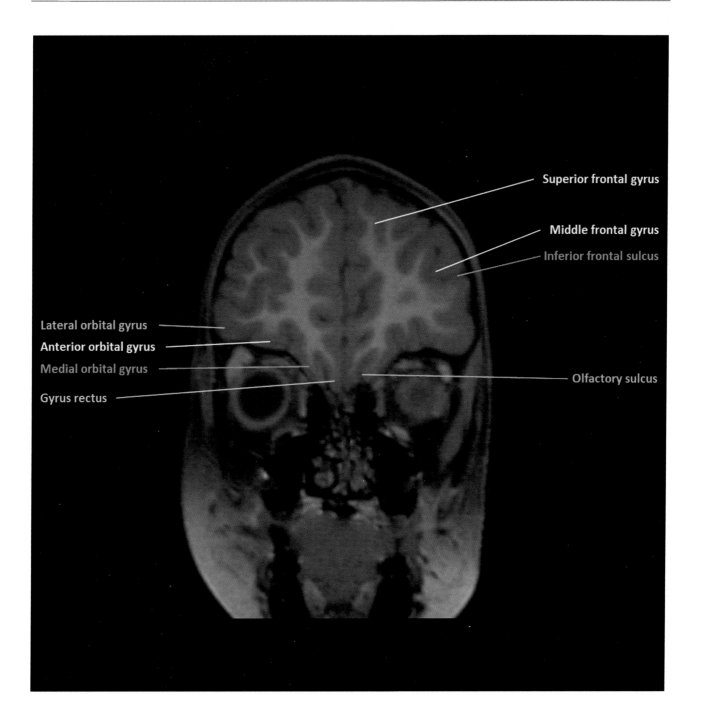

Superior frontal gyrus

Middle frontal gyrus

Inferior frontal sulcus

Lateral orbital gyrus

Anterior orbital gyrus

Medial orbital gyrus

Gyrus rectus

Olfactory sulcus

Sagittal T1 Images

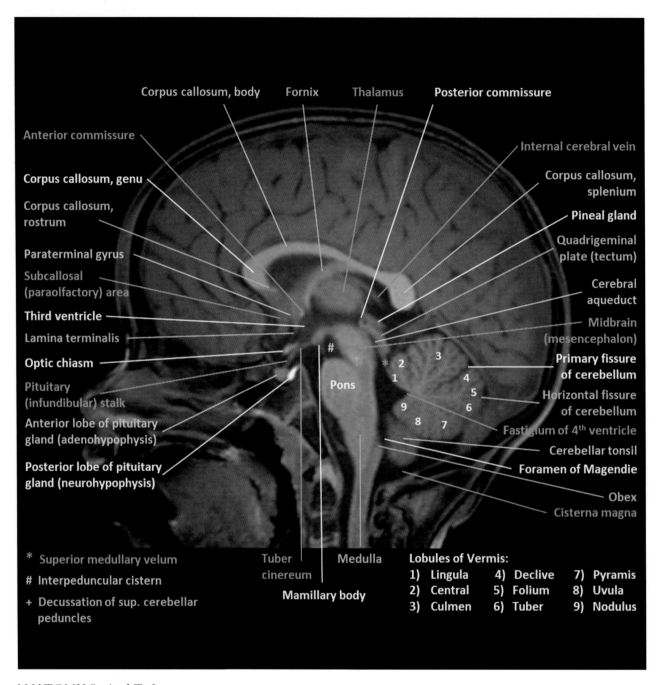

Corpus callosum, body Fornix Thalamus **Posterior commissure**

Anterior commissure

Corpus callosum, genu

Corpus callosum, rostrum

Paraterminal gyrus

Subcallosal (paraolfactory) area

Third ventricle

Lamina terminalis

Optic chiasm

Pituitary (infundibular) stalk

Anterior lobe of pituitary gland (adenohypophysis)

Posterior lobe of pituitary gland (neurohypophysis)

Internal cerebral vein

Corpus callosum, splenium

Pineal gland

Quadrigeminal plate (tectum)

Cerebral aqueduct

Midbrain (mesencephalon)

Primary fissure of cerebellum

Horizontal fissure of cerebellum

Fastigium of 4th ventricle

Cerebellar tonsil

Foramen of Magendie

Obex

Cisterna magna

Pons

Medulla

Tuber cinereum

Mamillary body

*   Superior medullary velum

\#   Interpeduncular cistern

\+   Decussation of sup. cerebellar peduncles

Lobules of Vermis:
1) Lingula	4) Declive	7) Pyramis
2) Central	5) Folium	8) Uvula
3) Culmen	6) Tuber	9) Nodulus

ANATOMY Sagittal T1 Images 1–11

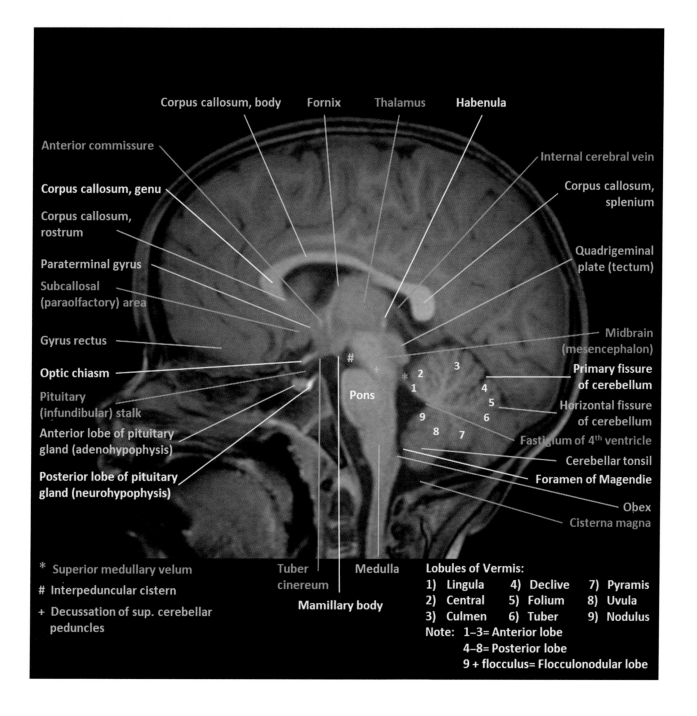

Corpus callosum, body   Fornix   Thalamus   **Habenula**

Anterior commissure

Corpus callosum, genu

Corpus callosum, rostrum

Parateminal gyrus

Subcallosal (paraolfactory) area

Gyrus rectus

Optic chiasm

Pituitary (infundibular) stalk

Anterior lobe of pituitary gland (adenohypophysis)

Posterior lobe of pituitary gland (neurohypophysis)

Internal cerebral vein

Corpus callosum, splenium

Quadrigeminal plate (tectum)

Midbrain (mesencephalon)

Primary fissure of cerebellum

Horizontal fissure of cerebellum

Fastigium of 4th ventricle

Cerebellar tonsil

Foramen of Magendie

Obex

Cisterna magna

Pons

Tuber cinereum   Medulla

Mamillary body

* Superior medullary velum

\# Interpeduncular cistern

\+ Decussation of sup. cerebellar peduncles

Lobules of Vermis:

1) Lingula   4) Declive   7) Pyramis
2) Central   5) Folium   8) Uvula
3) Culmen   6) Tuber   9) Nodulus

Note: 1–3= Anterior lobe
       4–8= Posterior lobe
       9 + flocculus= Flocculonodular lobe

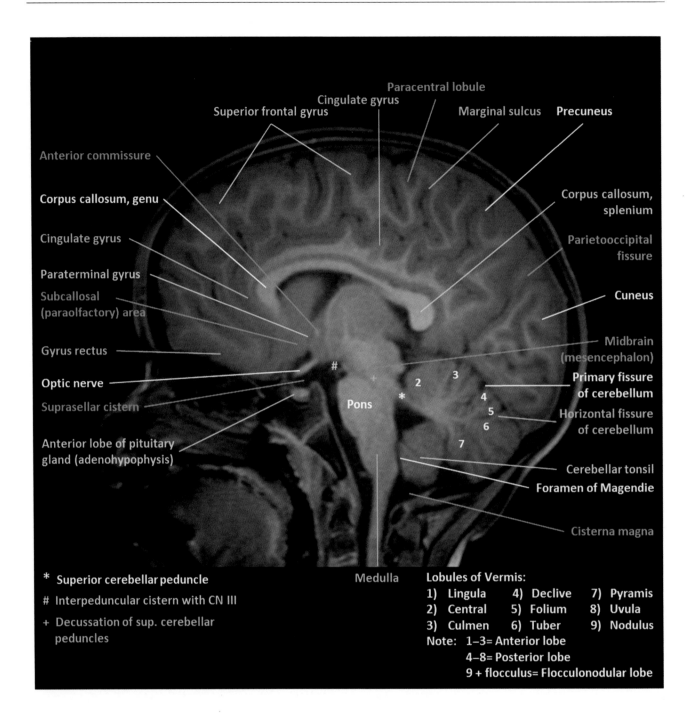

Paracentral lobule

Cingulate gyrus

Superior frontal gyrus

Marginal sulcus   **Precuneus**

Anterior commissure

Corpus callosum, genu

Corpus callosum, splenium

Cingulate gyrus

Parietooccipital fissure

Paraterminal gyrus

Subcallosal (paraolfactory) area

Cuneus

Gyrus rectus

Midbrain (mesencephalon)

Optic nerve

Primary fissure of cerebellum

Suprasellar cistern

Horizontal fissure of cerebellum

Anterior lobe of pituitary gland (adenohypophysis)

Cerebellar tonsil

Foramen of Magendie

Cisterna magna

Pons

Medulla

\#

\+

*

2

3

4

5

6

7

* Superior cerebellar peduncle

\# Interpeduncular cistern with CN III

\+ Decussation of sup. cerebellar peduncles

Lobules of Vermis:
1) Lingula   4) Declive   7) Pyramis
2) Central   5) Folium   8) Uvula
3) Culmen   6) Tuber   9) Nodulus

Note: 1–3= Anterior lobe
       4–8= Posterior lobe
       9 + flocculus= Flocculonodular lobe

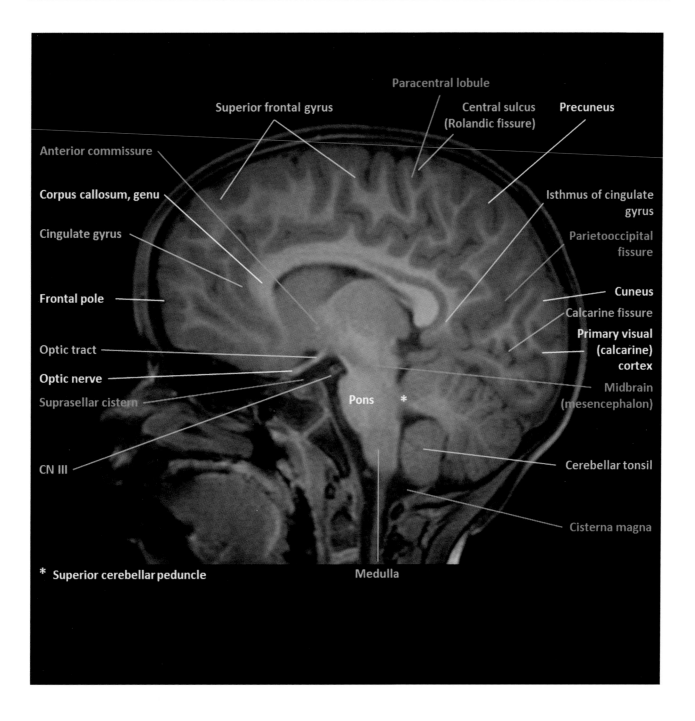

Paracentral lobule

Superior frontal gyrus

Central sulcus
(Rolandic fissure)

Precuneus

Anterior commissure

Corpus callosum, genu

Isthmus of cingulate
gyrus

Cingulate gyrus

Parietooccipital
fissure

Frontal pole

Cuneus

Calcarine fissure

Optic tract

**Primary visual
(calcarine)
cortex**

Optic nerve

Suprasellar cistern

Pons   *

Midbrain
(mesencephalon)

CN III

Cerebellar tonsil

Cisterna magna

* **Superior cerebellar peduncle**

Medulla

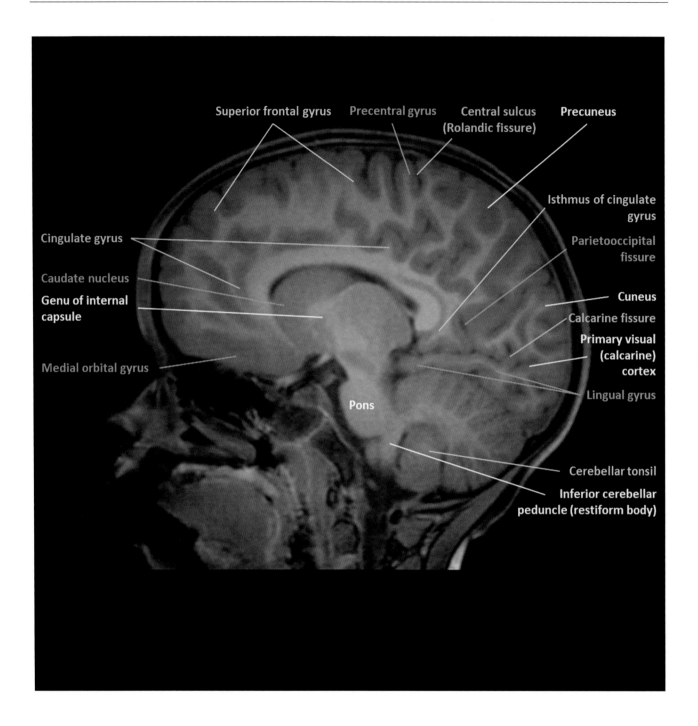

Superior frontal gyrus   Precentral gyrus   Central sulcus   Precuneus
                                              (Rolandic fissure)

Isthmus of cingulate
gyrus

Cingulate gyrus

Parietooccipital
fissure

Caudate nucleus

Cuneus

Genu of internal
capsule

Calcarine fissure

Primary visual
(calcarine)
cortex

Medial orbital gyrus

Lingual gyrus

Pons

Cerebellar tonsil

Inferior cerebellar
peduncle (restiform body)

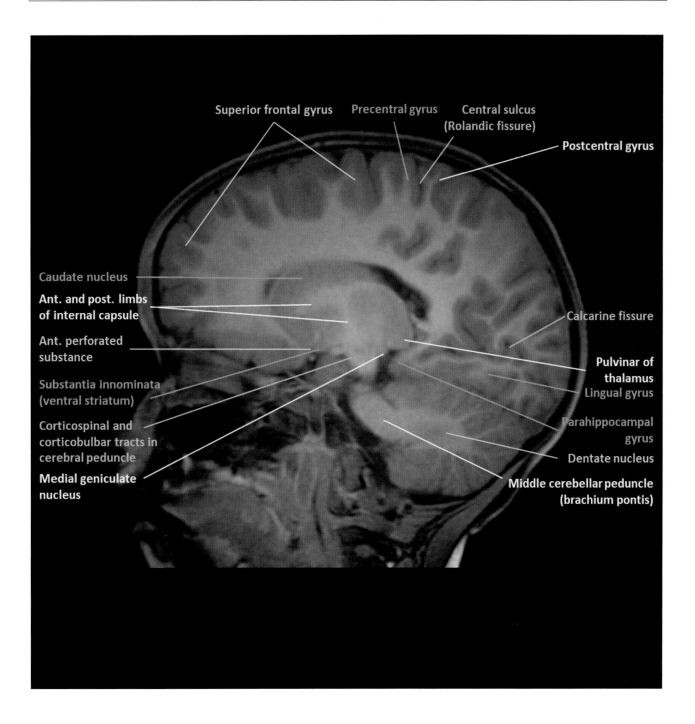

Superior frontal gyrus

Precentral gyrus

Central sulcus
(Rolandic fissure)

Postcentral gyrus

Caudate nucleus

**Ant. and post. limbs
of internal capsule**

Ant. perforated
substance

Substantia innominata
(ventral striatum)

Corticospinal and
corticobulbar tracts in
cerebral peduncle

**Medial geniculate
nucleus**

Calcarine fissure

**Pulvinar of
thalamus**
Lingual gyrus

Parahippocampal
gyrus

Dentate nucleus

**Middle cerebellar peduncle
(brachium pontis)**

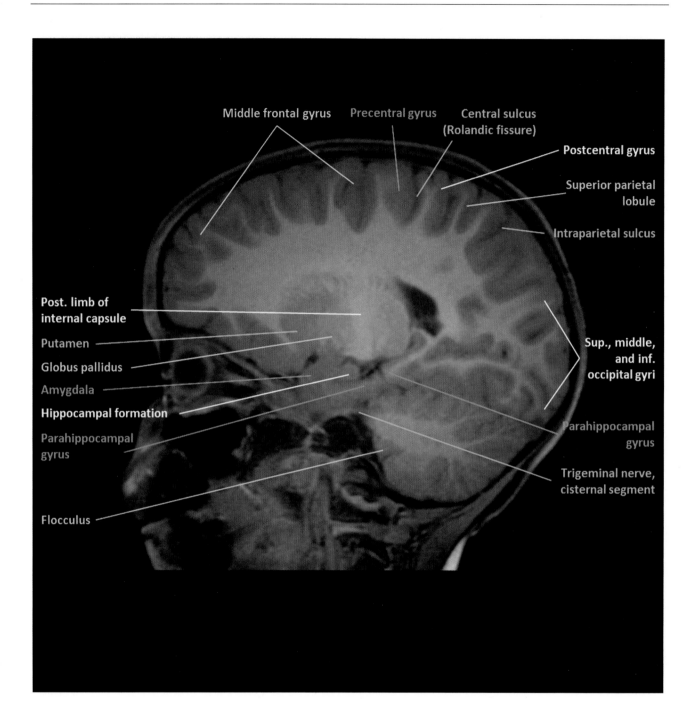

Middle frontal gyrus   Precentral gyrus   Central sulcus
(Rolandic fissure)

Postcentral gyrus

Superior parietal
lobule

Intraparietal sulcus

Post. limb of
internal capsule

Putamen

Globus pallidus

Amygdala

Hippocampal formation

Parahippocampal
gyrus

Flocculus

Sup., middle,
and inf.
occipital gyri

Parahippocampal
gyrus

Trigeminal nerve,
cisternal segment

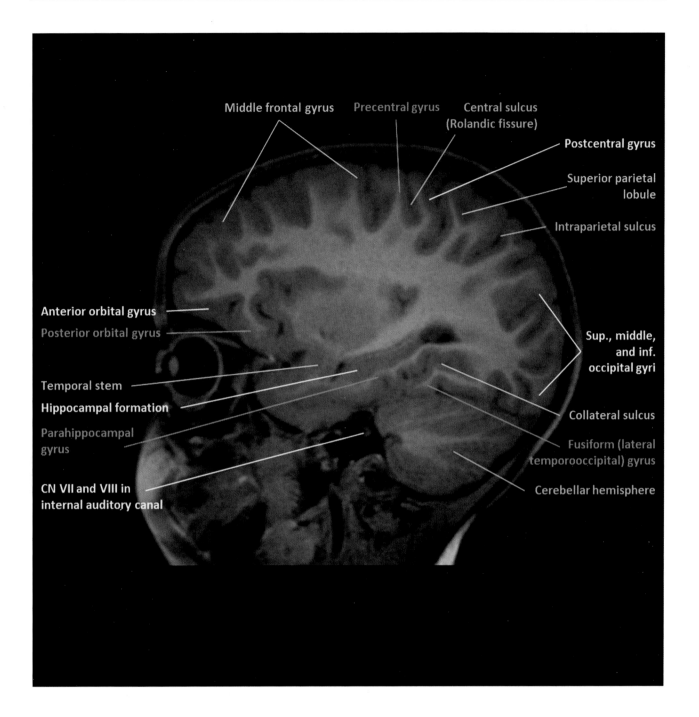

Middle frontal gyrus   Precentral gyrus   Central sulcus (Rolandic fissure)

Postcentral gyrus

Superior parietal lobule

Intraparietal sulcus

Anterior orbital gyrus

Posterior orbital gyrus

Sup., middle, and inf. occipital gyri

Temporal stem

Hippocampal formation

Parahippocampal gyrus

Collateral sulcus

Fusiform (lateral temporooccipital) gyrus

CN VII and VIII in internal auditory canal

Cerebellar hemisphere

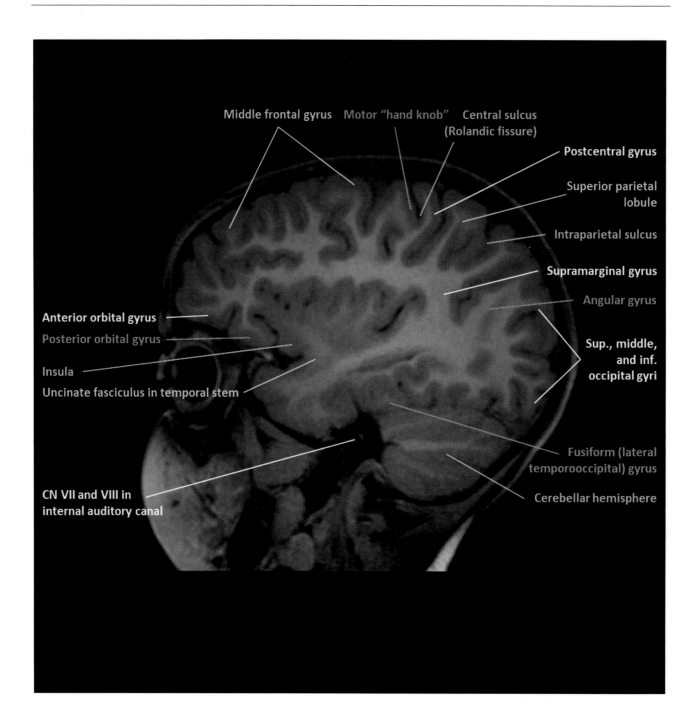

Middle frontal gyrus   Motor "hand knob"   Central sulcus (Rolandic fissure)

Postcentral gyrus

Superior parietal lobule

Intraparietal sulcus

Supramarginal gyrus

Angular gyrus

Sup., middle, and inf. occipital gyri

Anterior orbital gyrus

Posterior orbital gyrus

Insula

Uncinate fasciculus in temporal stem

CN VII and VIII in internal auditory canal

Fusiform (lateral temporooccipital) gyrus

Cerebellar hemisphere

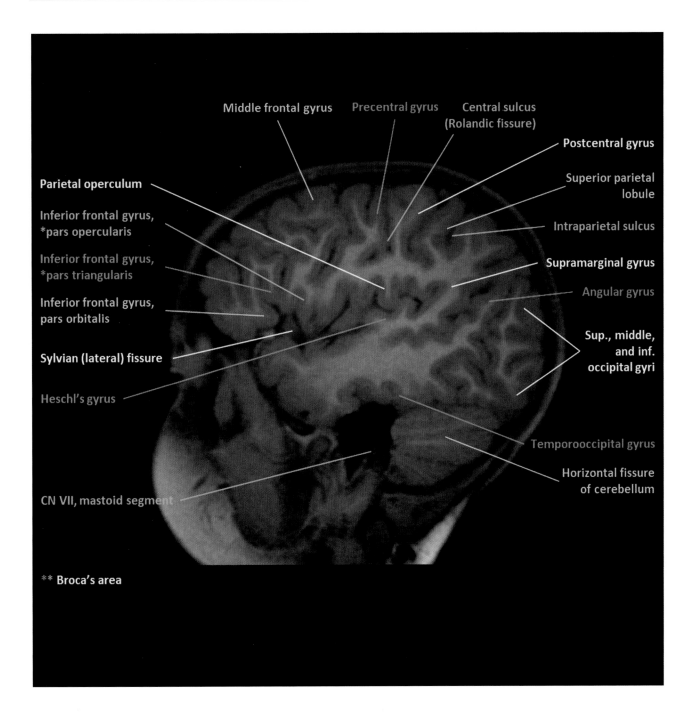

Middle frontal gyrus

Precentral gyrus

Central sulcus
(Rolandic fissure)

Postcentral gyrus

Superior parietal
lobule

Intraparietal sulcus

Supramarginal gyrus

Angular gyrus

Sup., middle,
and inf.
occipital gyri

Parietal operculum

Inferior frontal gyrus,
*pars opercularis

Inferior frontal gyrus,
*pars triangularis

Inferior frontal gyrus,
pars orbitalis

Sylvian (lateral) fissure

Heschl's gyrus

Temporooccipital gyrus

Horizontal fissure
of cerebellum

CN VII, mastoid segment

** Broca's area

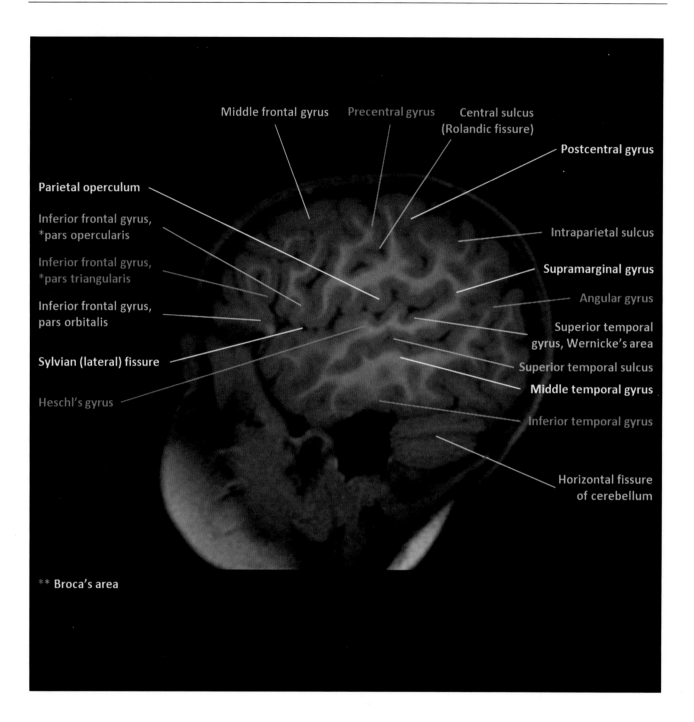

Middle frontal gyrus

Precentral gyrus

Central sulcus
(Rolandic fissure)

Postcentral gyrus

Parietal operculum

Inferior frontal gyrus,
*pars opercularis

Inferior frontal gyrus,
*pars triangularis

Inferior frontal gyrus,
pars orbitalis

Sylvian (lateral) fissure

Heschl's gyrus

Intraparietal sulcus

Supramarginal gyrus

Angular gyrus

Superior temporal
gyrus, Wernicke's area

Superior temporal sulcus

Middle temporal gyrus

Inferior temporal gyrus

Horizontal fissure
of cerebellum

** Broca's area

Glossary

An array of confusing and often imprecise terms exists to describe abnormalities of cerebral white matter. For the sake of accuracy, reference may be made to the following definitions when reporting on deviations from the normal pattern of myelination.

Delayed myelination: less myelination than normal for chronologic age corrected for prematurity, but progression of myelination is shown on follow-up MRI. Note that at least two MRIs separated in time must be obtained in order to determine if a true delay exists. Delayed myelination is nonspecific and has many possible etiologies, including hypoxic-ischemic insult, malnutrition, chromosomal abnormality, inborn errors of metabolism, infection, periventricular leukomalacia, congenital malformation, hydrocephalus, heart failure, endocrine abnormality, irradiation, and toxin exposure. Note that idiopathic developmental delay has not been found to be correlated with isolated delays in myelination on T2W imaging (68) but that volumetric assessment of white matter in developmentally delayed children beyond early childhood may reveal a reduction in brain myelination (75).

Demyelination: destruction, removal, or loss of myelin after it has been normally formed, with or without preservation of axons. Examples of acquired demyelinating diseases with an inflammatory component are multiple sclerosis, acute disseminated encephalomyelitis, and neuromyelitis optica. Additionally, many inborn errors of metabolism result in demyelination, as do some viruses and toxins.

Dysmyelination: an ambiguous term for disorders in which myelin is not formed or maintained properly, or myelination formation is delayed or arrested.

Hypomyelination: a significant, permanent deficit in myelin. This is diagnosed when there is an unchanged pattern of deficient myelination on two MRIs at least 6 months apart in a child older than 1 year. Hypomyelination is rare and has a specific differential diagnosis (76).

Leukodystrophy: a genetic disorder causing abnormal production or metabolism of myelin leading to a failure in myelination, hypomyelination, and/or progressive loss of myelin.

Myelination: the development of myelin lipid bilayer sheaths around axons.

Myelin disorder: a general term that includes delayed myelination, hypomyelination, demyelination, and dysmyelination.

Premyelination: normal diffusion anisotropy in maturing but still unmyelinated white matter that precedes the visible myelination-related changes on T1W and T2W images. Premyelination manifests on conventional DWI as subtly restricted diffusion.

Index

Page numbers followed by *f* or *t* indicate figures or tables, respectively. Numbers in *italics* indicate images.